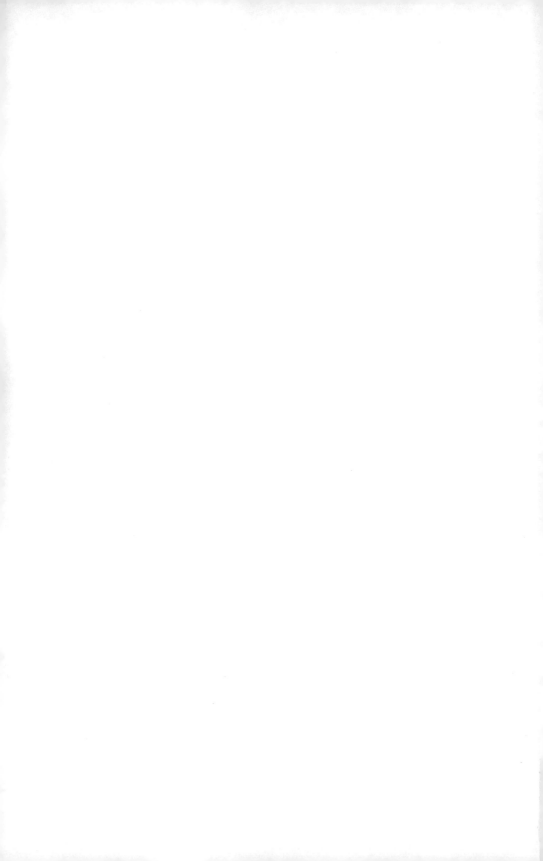

The Gene Therapy Plan

The Gene Therapy Plan

Taking Control of
Your Genetic Destiny
with Diet and Lifestyle

Mitchell L. Gaynor, M.D.

VIKING

VIKING
Published by the Penguin Group
Penguin Group (USA) LLC
375 Hudson Street
New York, New York 10014

USA | Canada | UK | Ireland | Australia | New Zealand | India | South Africa | China
penguin.com
A Penguin Random House Company

First published by Viking Penguin, a member of Penguin Group (USA) LLC, 2015

LIBRARY OF CONGRESS CATALOGING-IN-PUBLICATION DATA
Gaynor, Mitchell L., 1956–
The gene therapy plan : taking control of your genetic destiny with diet and lifestyle / Mitchell L. Gaynor, MD ; foreword by Mehmet C. Oz.
pages cm
Includes bibliographical references and index.
ISBN 978-0-670-01526-9 (hardback)
1. Genetic disorders—Diet therapy.   2. Nutrition—Genetic aspects.   3. Cooking for the sick.
4. Diet therapy.   I. Title.
QP144.G45G39 2015
616'.042—dc23

2014038544

Printed in the United States of America

10 9 8 7 6 5 4 3 2 1

Set in Minion Pro
Designed by Katy Riegel

To my mother

Contents

INTEGRATIVE MEDICINE IS progressively sweeping across the nation's medical schools, hospitals, and clinics. Academic and residency programs are helping to prepare young physicians to challenge the status quo by thinking beyond the borders of how we've been treating patients in Western society for seventy-five years. Integrative medicine is really about treating the entire patient.

During my time as a medical student, the education was very traditional in the sense that students were taught to view the mind and the body separately. And a lot of this educational approach is reflected in the way medicine is practiced today, especially as we are faced with growing specialties and diminishing primary care practices. By the time I completed my training, the dogma of medical practice focused on treating the body and its organs as separate entities. I was primed to pursue a career doing the same. But life whispers to us periodically, and the wisdom of forward-thinking physicians—including my father-in-law, the pioneering heart surgeon Gerald Lemole—shook me out of this rut and opened my mind to unconventional healing approaches. I began to push against the grain of conventional medicine in order to uncover ways of treating patients that weren't taught to me in medical school. Now don't get me wrong—I wholeheartedly believe in the power of science. But I've been in practice long enough and have come across many patients from all walks of life with different healing beliefs to appreciate the treasure of integrative medicine.

Fundamentally, I have been taught the importance of including the latest in cutting-edge ideas to help my patients, no matter what the source. As head of the Heart Institute at New York–Presbyterian Hospital, this includes developing the most innovative heart valve replacement approaches. As the director of the hospital's Complementary Medicine Program, I supported the integration of Eastern medical practices such as yoga and meditation. Stretching the spectrum of potential tools also demands that we obtain a complete clinical picture so we are able to prescribe medicines or procedures as well as relaxation techniques, exercises, and even foods that can help prevent and treat health problems.

The Gene Therapy Plan educates both patients and healers to accomplish this comprehensive goal. Dr. Mitchell Gaynor focuses on how we can use food to promote health. But more than just being about eating foods that are healthy for us, this book is about harnessing the power hidden in foods to change our genetic predisposition for disease, drawing from a branch of genetic study called ecogenetics. Ecogenetics is a growing field that applies the philosophy of personalized medicine by using specific substances to target a patient's genetic profile for developing diseases such as cancer, diabetes, and heart disease. By focusing on bioactive nutrients such as apigenin in pomegranates, EGCG in green tea, and curcumin in curry, physicians will be able to prescribe foods that operate at the level of your DNA to promote health. What's interesting is that once you put into practice consuming foods that target your gene *expression,* you progressively begin to lose those cravings for foods that are bad for you—such as highly refined carbohydrates.

I met Dr. Gaynor years ago, when a patient of his approached me about a heart operation. I was confused by the request since the chart clearly outlined metastatic cancer that would kill him within months. The patient smiled and asked me to check the date in the chart again. The cancer diagnosis was over five years old! I found out that my patient had been cured by Dr. Gaynor, and I have been sending him challenging cases ever since, including friends and family. Mitch is the founder and president of Gaynor Integrative Oncology, and he serves as a clinical assistant professor of medicine at Weill Cornell Medical College. As a renowned specialist in the field of oncology and integrative medicine, he has dedicated his career to combining medicinal practices with proven complementary therapies to treat his cancer patients, which makes him well positioned to write this book on the nutritional aspects of disease prevention.

Part of Dr. Gaynor's success as a well-respected cancer specialist is his ability to treat the entire person through a combination of allopathic approaches and alternative therapies. *The Gene Therapy Plan* offers practical advice as well as supplemental and juicing recipes that are easy to incorporate into your life. This book provides insight into the evolution of medicine by showing how eco-genetic food changes your genetic blueprint. The book provides scientific data to support age-old practices and alternative therapies, which is an important component to bridging the divide between Eastern and Western medicine. This is a key stepping point toward the globalization of medicine using conventional Western and unconventional alternative treatments with proven results together to treat the whole patient.

Mehmet C. Oz, M.D.
Vice Chair and Professor of Surgery, NYP–Columbia University
Coauthor, You: The Owner's Manual *health book series*

Introduction

"YOU ARE WHAT YOU EAT," my mother always told me. But it wasn't until after I'd finished my medical training and become a cancer specialist that I learned just how profoundly right she was.

My mother started teaching me about food and health when I was six. She had just been diagnosed with breast cancer, and she wanted me to be able to look after myself. Like most parents, she was concerned that I not load up on Cheetos and potato chips, but, more than that, her diagnosis had brought her into the movement toward unprocessed foods and vitamin supplements launched by Adelle Davis. So she taught me how to make nutritious snacks, and how to blend fruit and vegetable juices to achieve the most healthful effects with a taste I'd like. She also taught me how to prepare nutritious meals, and when she had to be in the hospital for long periods I'd be the one to make dinner for my father and older brother.

Unfortunately, our lessons in nutrition were cut short by my mother's death when I was nine. Her conversion to wholesome foods and supplements may have been too little, too late, but the odds were stacked heavily against her: during her pregnancy with my brother twelve years earlier, she had been treated with DES, a synthetic form of estrogen that we now know is associated with a much greater risk of breast cancer.

The loss was devastating, of course, but it also gave me a clear purpose in life. When my mother died, I made up my mind that I was going to find out why people's cells turned against them, as hers had, to cause debilitating, even fatal diseases. I also determined that I was going to do something about it.

I went to medical school, then took specialized training in hematology, the study of blood, and in oncology, the study of cancer, which included doing research at Rockefeller University to study molecular biology. This is a relatively new field that explores the fundamental building blocks of life at the physical and chemical level, especially the processes of genetic control. What I learned from Rockefeller's cutting-edge researchers gave me an entirely new perspective on the role of genes in determining health outcomes across the life span. And this new view of how genes function showed me that my mother's emphasis on the role of nutrition in health was absolutely on target.

Genes, the microscopic bundles of DNA that reside in the nucleus of each cell, control all cellular processes, including cell division. (Cancer, perhaps the most feared disease of all, develops when normal cell division—the process that allows children to grow bigger and healthy tissues to renew themselves—goes haywire.)

We inherit our genes from our parents and—according to what I'd learned in medical school—each person's genetic endowment was pretty much determined at the moment of conception and then remained stable throughout life. If the DNA you inherited from your parents made you robust and healthy, then—according to this theory—you were all set. If your genes made you susceptible to cancer, or obesity, or arthritis . . . well, that was just your fate. In this old way of thinking, health was largely the result of a genetic lottery, and there was nothing you could do to change the odds.

By the time I got to Rockefeller, though, advances in molecular biology had turned this static and predetermined view of health on its head. The new research showed that illness or health was not solely a matter of a "genetic destiny" coming from "good genes" or "bad genes" passed along from Mom or Dad. The picture that emerged was actually much more subtle and complex, and it gave each of us a much more active role to play in directing our own health outcomes through our nutritional and lifestyle choices.

Molecular biology teaches us that the individual's entire complement of more than twenty thousand genes—called his or her "genome"—contains myriad bits of information that instruct the cells to carry out essential functions. But not all of these genes are active all the time. Many are dormant, and the question of whether or not they become active and begin to influence our biology—either by making us more robust or by making us ill—is called "gene expression." The primary influence on gene expression is the environment in which we live, which is where our opportunity to exert a positive influence through nutrition enters in.

In the twenty-first century, our environment bombards us every day with an onslaught of pesticide residues, carcinogenic chemicals, large quantities of foodlike substances, which include refined sugar and dangerous fats. These substances in our food, in our air, and in our water interact with the genes in our cells, turning some on and some off. The worst of these chemicals can transform healthy cells into tumors, which is in large part why one in three Americans will develop cancer. In fact, 90 to 95 percent of cancers are linked to environmental toxicants.[1] But it is not just cancer that is caused by this chemical stew in which we live. Today we have an epidemic of thyroid disease, especially among middle-aged women, which almost always originates as an autoimmune condition triggered by environmental toxins. Nearly 20 percent of our children have a learning, emotional, or developmental disability, and the incidences of diabetes and asthma are skyrocketing. The environment's effect on our genes is implicated in all of these conditions as well.

But this dark cloud also contains a silver lining. We may have limited control over the level of toxins in our external environment, but each of us can exercise enormous control over what we introduce into our internal environment—which is to say, what we eat. By being more thoughtful and deliberate about our nutritional choices, we can not only reduce or eliminate many of the toxic influences interacting with our genes to cause disease, we can influence our genetic expression to activate the enzymes that can neutralize or remove toxic substances from our tissues, to stimulate cellular processes to boost our immune system, and to reverse the progression of disease, including cancer.

Using nutrients in this strategic way to combat disease and promote good health is called "nutrigenetics," and it is the core principle of the Gene Therapy Plan. *Nutrigenetics* is actually a subset of a broader approach called "*ecogenetics*," which is focused more broadly on how we live in our environment and how the environment as a whole interacts with the individual's genome to produce either health or disease. Our level of physical activity, for instance, may encourage (or discourage) the production of more inflammation-suppressing enzymes. Meanwhile, whether we are fat or lean affects whether we send out weaker (if we are lean) or stronger (if we are obese) signals to suppress cancer-killing substances.

The Gene Therapy Plan takes all these interactions into account. It is designed to help you combat the most prevalent and troubling diseases of our time, and it does so in the context of promoting overall health and well-being through weight control, stress reduction, and exercise.

I've based the recommendations of the Gene Therapy Plan on my nearly thirty years of broad clinical experience. After my fellowships in hematology and oncology, I became director of medical oncology at the Strang Cancer Prevention Center, where I continued the study of nutrient-gene interactions I'd begun at Rockefeller. I also continued my exploration of toxicogenomics, the study of how environmental toxins affect gene expression. What I found was that many of the same underlying cellular functions that play a role in cancer—inflammation, signaling proteins, transcription factors, hormone regulation, toxin metabolism, the immune response—were factors in a wide spectrum of other diseases as well. More to the point, these functions could be influenced at the cellular level by the strategic use of nutrients regardless of the disease in question. This is precisely how my practice began to expand in scope.

When I first began incorporating nutrigenetic concepts into patient care, nutrition was barely on the radar for most physicians. Most medical schools and residency programs offered a few lectures on nutritional deficiencies and their associated diseases, but that was about it.

So what I was doing was considered highly unorthodox, yet I was a cancer specialist with mainstream training—I even had an academic appointment at one of the country's best medical schools—so physicians began to refer patients to me, often those patients for whom traditional treatment methods had been exhausted. And because the results I was able to achieve through a nutrigenetic approach were often astonishing, the referrals increased and my practice grew.

Consider, for instance:

- The patient mentioned by Dr. Oz in the foreword to this book who approached him for a heart operation five years after the diagnosis of cancer that was supposed to have killed him within months. My nutrigenetic approach had brought about the complete remission of his disease.
- The dentist (who happened to be my father) who developed hepatitis C after accidently pricking himself with a needle. Before interferon therapy, at a time when there were no medical treatments for hep C, I treated him with a regimen of common Chinese herbs, seaweeds, and juices, and no trace of the virus remained or ever returned.
- The woman with melanoma I began to treat after her oncologist had directed her to hospice for end-of-life care. Her cancer, which had

started on her heel, had spread upward and the lesions became in-fected, making her left leg four times the diameter of her right. The disease had also metastasized to her lungs and abdomen. I treated her with low-dose chemotherapy, immune pharmacological therapy, green tea, and magnolia, and within three months she was in complete remission.[2]

- The young man from Turkey with autoimmune hepatitis and liver failure. The Mayo Clinic had put him on high-dose steroids and told him he needed to be on the list for a liver transplant. I put him on glutathione, resveratrol, turmeric, alpha lipoic acid, and omega-3 fatty acids and his liver function began to normalize. He regained all the weight he had lost and within three months he was back in school. His autoimmune hepatitis resolved and he never needed a transplant.

- The woman with stage IV pancreatic cancer whose oncologist told her she had four to six months to live. I put her on a dietary regime of cruciferous vegetables, supplements, and juices, combined with chemo, and she went into complete remission and has remained so for nearly twenty years.

- The woman with the rare dermatologic condition perforating collagenosis, which led her to leading academic medical centers throughout the world before she found her way to me. She had diffuse, severely painful red skin lesions all over her arms, legs, and back, and they were spreading despite large doses of steroids and ultraviolet light therapy. I treated her for underlying inflammation, allergies, and immune imbalance. Within a few months the skin lesions on her arms had resolved and those on her legs had improved by 80 percent.

- The twenty-three-year-old newlywed who developed severe psoriasis on her face and neck. She had been treated by several dermatologists with courses of prednisone, which temporarily helped, but the disease came back worse each time she was tapered off the drug and it was beginning to cause scarring. I treated her with targeted nutrition, and after one month all the lesions resolved, with no recurrence after five years.

- The sixty-one-year-old barber who gained a significant amount of weight after a knee injury and became diabetic. On my nutrigenetic diet plan he lost seventy pounds over one year and is now taking only a small dose of metformin rather than insulin.

Today I divide my time equally between Gaynor Integrative Oncology, a practice focused on treating cancer patients, and Gaynor Wellness, in which I apply the same ecogenetic principles to treating people with a variety of concerns, ranging from general health maintenance and disease prevention to weight loss, insomnia, chronic fatigue, dermatological diseases, and Parkinson's.

Both practices incorporate meditation, music therapy, guided imagery, and cognitive behavioral therapy in concert with activities such as restorative physical therapy, yoga, aerobic exercise, and qigong as well as nutritional counseling based on the same principles presented here in the Gene Therapy Plan. My aim is always to treat the entire person in a way that acknowledges the complex nature of chronic illness, and to work at every level of the body's healing processes—physiological, genetic, psychosocial, and spiritual—to create an optimal state of well-being.

The recommendations in this book, with their powerful and targeted ability to influence genetic expression, actually lead us to a new definition of what we mean by health. In this new view, we should see ourselves not as being merely "healthy" or "ill," but as being ecogenetically "well managed" or "poorly managed" across the life span. This is especially true as new developments in disease diagnostics make the distinction between being healthy and being sick no longer black and white, but more a shade of gray. In other words, we all have the seeds of illness within us. The question is whether that potential for disease will become active or will remain dormant.

Imaging technologies like MRIs and CAT scans, as well as more finely grained autopsy studies, show us that the more sensitive our instruments for detecting disease become, the more disease we will find, and at earlier stages. For a long while we have been finding these seeds of serious illness in the surprisingly young. For example, fully 45 percent of soldiers killed in action during the Korean War and 77 percent of those killed in the Vietnam War showed early signs of heart disease. Even children under three years old—sometimes even fetuses—can have these early indications. And the case is the same for almost any disease you choose to look at closely.

It is now plausibly estimated, for instance, that almost 100 percent of people, if they had their thyroids dissected for examination by the newest methods, would show signs of cancer or precancerous mutation. And no matter how finely you slice the tissue, there may always be smaller tumors that fit into the spaces between the slices. The same is true for prostate cancer. Almost 50 percent of men between sixty and seventy would show signs of the disease if examined in this way. Almost 40 percent of women between forty and fifty would show signs of breast cancer under the new microscopes.

The unsettling reality, once again, is that every one of us has these signs of illness in dormant or slow-moving precursor forms. But that doesn't make us passive victims. Not when we are able to exercise control over what we eat, and thereby significantly influence how our genes express themselves to affect our health. The fact is, for good or ill, we are all practicing gene therapy on ourselves all the time. We breathe in the smoke from a cigarette, we gulp down a soda, we train for a marathon. In each case, we are participating in a process that involves the regulation of our own genetic status.

Once we grasp the implications of being able to influence gene expression, and once we align that fact with the prevalence of disease precursors well before symptoms appear, the case for the Gene Therapy Plan becomes incredibly compelling.

All diets have their goals. Some are focused on losing weight, others on reducing risk of heart disease. Some have a vague wish to "detoxify," or purge the body of harmful toxic buildup from pollutants and metabolic waste.

The Gene Therapy Plan can achieve those objectives, but its purpose is much more basic and comprehensive. It is designed to keep dormant disease dormant, and to help active disease go back to being dormant. And it does so in an integrated way that keeps a multitude of health variables in proper balance.

Too many eating plans promote one kind of virtue (for example, weight loss) at the expense of others (such as cancer prevention). But it doesn't make much sense to slim down if in the process we incur a higher degree of total-body inflammation, which can lead to other problems. In the same way, it makes little sense to eat for heart health while ignoring the possibility of cancers. The Gene Therapy Plan weaves all these elements into a consciously holistic picture of total human wellness that also addresses all the microscopic dormant and precursor conditions that could, given the wrong ecogenetic influence, turn into illness.

By far the biggest causes of death in the United States are heart disease and cancer, accounting for around 50 percent of all deaths each year. Diabetes is another major killer. Obesity, systemic inflammation, and exposure to environmental toxicants are contributing factors to all these and many other disease conditions. Aging is a process we all undergo, and while its effects can't be avoided entirely, they can be managed in order to optimize quality of life.

Taken together, these conditions and processes are among the most significant obstacles to health and happiness. They are, therefore, necessarily the primary targets of ecogenetic nutrition and the Gene Therapy Plan.

The plan is designed to help you:

- resist cancer
- resist heart disease
- resist diabetes
- maintain a healthy weight
- reverse low immunity
- ameliorate the effects of aging
- remove toxins from the body
- promote energy

Anyone who wants to improve his or her health can benefit from the diet simply by following its general guidelines for better nutritional choices. There's no rigid formula. You don't have to sign on for a complicated program with steps and levels and layers. At the same time, though, anyone with specific concerns can follow the diet's more directed recommendations and use it *preventively* to lower the risk of a specific disease long before any symptoms become apparent. And those hoping to reverse specific disease processes can use the plan in an even more targeted and nuanced fashion. In postmenopausal women, for instance, vitamin D deficiency can lead to osteoporosis and a greater likelihood of fractures, so increasing supplemental and dietary intake of vitamin D will help most women decrease the risk for fractures. But not all women. Differences in genetic makeup mean that not every postmenopausal woman has the same vulnerability. So increasing the amount of vitamin D should not be a blanket recommendation for all women.

At this point I know that some of you are probably thinking, "But what if I'm concerned about several diseases? Will the Gene Therapy Plan help me if I want to lose weight, have a family history of cancer, and want to prevent wrinkles?" In a word, yes! That is what the Gene Therapy Plan is all about— preventing and treating diseases at the level of your genes. In the case mentioned above, I discuss how vitamin D can help prevent bone fractures in postmenopausal women. But in addition to strengthening bones, vitamin D has many other benefits: it fortifies immunity, improves brain and heart health, and protects against cancer. So as you read these recommendations, particularly in the disease-specific chapters, keep in mind that these nutrients have many benefits. The book is organized by health conditions (e.g., heart disease, cancer);

however, real-life medical problems are rarely so clean-cut. The nutrients presented here all have many bioactive substances whose healthful effects can be seen in the entire body. Good health begets good health: as you incorporate the advice laid out in the book, you'll be on your way to living a happier, healthier life.

In the first chapter, I lay out what I call the Basic Plan, the general nutrigenetic principles of healthful eating that apply to anyone and everyone.

With those comprehensive guidelines established, I then move on to address the specific ecogenetic approach to the five most pressing health concerns of our population—obesity, heart disease, cancer, diabetes, and aging—each addressed in one of five targeted chapters.

I then provide menu plans and recipes that easily guide you toward incorporating the basic nutrigenetics concepts into your daily regimen.

Many of the recipes in this book were adapted from those passed along to me by my mother, which can give you some idea of the depth of my lifelong personal commitment to developing and sharing this approach to targeted nutrition.

Even though it was not acknowledged at the time, my mother always suspected that her cancer had been triggered by the DES she'd been treated with during her first pregnancy. But then, years later, in an undergraduate biochemistry course, my professor declared emphatically that pharmacologic estrogen had been shown to cause cancer in animal studies and that this had been known for thirty years. And yet those findings had not been absorbed into clinical practice. This was the first time it occurred to me that my mother's life might have been spared if only existing knowledge had been acted upon.

Today we have vastly more knowledge about how substances affect gene expression, in ways both good and bad. It's this knowledge that I'm now pleased to pass along to you in *The Gene Therapy Plan*.

Part I

Targeting Disease with Gene Therapy

Chapter 1

The
Basic Plan

VIEWED FROM A NUTRIGENETIC PERSPECTIVE, the average American diet is not a pretty sight. In general, most Americans eat far too much food that is high in carbohydrates, high in saturated fat, and high in sugar. About 33 percent of calories in the average diet come from fat (around 11 percent in the form of saturated fat), about 15 percent from protein, and about 52 percent from carbs.

Having slightly more than half our calories come from carbs seems disproportionate in itself, but the picture is actually worse than that, because the average American's diet is all too often filled with the *worst* kind of carbs: simple, processed sugars, high-fructose corn syrup, milled white grains. Among the highest-calorie sources for the average adult are sugary pastries, bread, soda, pizza, pasta, and alcohol. This is not just disproportionate but extraordinarily skewed in a single ruinous direction, massively tilted toward foods that contribute mightily to the five conditions that concern us most: cancer, heart disease, inflammation, obesity, and premature aging.

The Basic Plan is what I propose as a first step in changing direction and regaining solid nutritional footing. It is a broad-based approach to eating rooted in very sophisticated science, but I've deliberately kept it simple and made it practical enough to work for real people in real life. After all, a diet does not have to be a cult. And if a diet is too extreme in its demands—if it requires too great or too eccentric a deviation from "normal" eating patterns—people will lose their motivation and begin to backslide.

That is why the Basic Plan is centered on just a few basic concepts, and why the concepts themselves are offered as *guidelines*, not ironclad behavioral *prescriptions*.

The fact is, even with the strictest dietary regimens, positive, measurable results can and do often follow from only partial compliance. In other words, you don't have to follow a diet perfectly in order to benefit from it.

Take, for example, the widely reported results of the yearlong 2007 Stanford study that compared weight reduction across four popular diets: Atkins, Zone, Ornish, and LEARN. As published in the *Journal of the American Medical Association*,[1] the study seemed to demonstrate that the Atkins diet produced the largest weight losses—about 10 pounds against a range of 2.5 pounds to 5.5 pounds measured in the others. But was it actually the Atkins diet that was being tested? If you look closer at the details of the study findings, you find that those in the Atkins group did not actually eat the diet they were supposed to. According to the Atkins recommendations, the dieters should have stuck to less than 20 grams of carbs daily for the first two months, and then less than 50 grams for the remainder of the study. But the researchers reported that the Atkins group averaged around 60 grams at two months into the diet, around 113 grams at six months, and nearly 140 grams at the study's end.

This is not to say that low-carbohydrate diets don't do what they claim—indeed the better weight loss results for Atkins in this study suggest that lowering carbs (which the dieters did successfully do in comparison with those on the other diets) can be effective. But the point is that no one in the study actually *did* the Atkins diet. Or at least we must question whether we would want to attribute the study's results to the eating plan that goes by the name "Atkins." Or "Zone" or "Ornish" or whatever.

For in fact no one actually "did" any of the other diets either. The Zone eaters never achieved their goal of a 40-30-30 breakdown across carbs, proteins, and fats. The closest they came was at two months, when they averaged 42 percent, 24 percent, and 35 percent respectively. Thereafter, like every other group in the study, they faded back toward baseline. The LEARN eaters never once hit their 55 percent to 60 percent target for carbs. The Ornish eaters never came close to eating less than 10 percent fat, as prescribed. Similar variances can be seen in many other studies, including an impressively comprehensive and long-running 2009 trial done at Harvard.[2]

The point is, all you can ask is that you do the best you can, by first empowering yourself with the best available information so you know that what you're committing yourself to is worthwhile. You then need to frame your choices in keeping with edible ecogenetic principles, so that you are reliably moving toward the bulk of the best benefits, without getting upset about a percentage point of difference here or there, or worried about being perfect in your compliance.

In keeping with the effort to be compliance-friendly, and to simplify and demystify the search for a more healthful diet, the Basic Plan is grounded first and foremost in what I call the Rule of One-Thirds.

Concept 1:
The Rule of One-Thirds

Flying in the face of the high-protein, low-carb, reduced-fat orthodoxy that has dominated dietary thinking for more than a generation, my Basic Plan suggests that you consume roughly one-third of your calories from each of the three major macronutrient groups of fats, carbs, and proteins. According to the latest science, there is simply no rationale for any one group of nutrients to be favored or marginalized.

After all, human beings evolved eating a remarkable mixture of foods, often available at different times in different quantities and proportions. And the effects of many foods are synergistic, while the effects of many others are still unknown. Artificially skewing the slate in one direction or another can rob us, in ways that aren't immediately apparent, of beneficial interactions between various elements.

An even distribution of nutrients allows you to benefit from the good qualities of each while avoiding the pitfalls of overdependence on any one thing. Too many carbs can lead to insulin insensitivity and inflammation. Too much fat deprives you of necessary fiber and phytochemicals. Too much protein is likely to be high in saturated fat, and in any case eating a high-protein diet is extremely difficult to maintain for long as it eliminates whole groups of foods that one's body needs and craves over time such as whole grains, fruits, vegetables, and dairy. The high-protein, low-carbohydrate diet is actually a high-fat, low-carbohydrate diet that often contains 55 percent to 60 percent of calories from fat, especially saturated fat. People are not obese because they consume carbohydrates. They are obese because they consume too many of the wrong types of carbohydrates, just as eating too many of the wrong fats or proteins can cause the body to lose calcium and become deficient in carotenoids, critical nutrients like tocotrienols, vitamin B6, magnesium, and fiber. Solid research supports the idea that breaking macronutrients roughly into thirds is a healthy foundation for eating, not least because of the way it can liberate the way you think about food. Again, there is no need to be obsessive about maintaining a precise balance every day or with every meal. Simply be mindful of the principles outlined in the following chapters and follow the meal, juicing, and targeted nutrient recommendations at the end of the chapters and in the final section of this book. Beyond that, let common sense be your guide. For instance, if you have pizza for dinner on Monday, don't continue the carbohydrate theme on Tuesday by having pancakes for breakfast.

To see more deeply into the rationale for the Rule of One-Thirds, let's look at each of these three food categories in turn.

Fats

Fats have gotten a bad rap in recent popular nutrition. In the 1980s, even the standard-bearing USDA zeroed in on fat as a public menace. In a context of rising obesity, some of this is understandable: fats are nutrient dense (they have 9 calories per gram, as opposed to the 4 calories per gram of carbohydrate and protein), so any diet that simply wants to maximize weight loss, and equates weight loss with fewer calories, will tend to limit fat. But as with everything else, the true picture is more complicated, which in this case means there are good fats and bad fats depending on your goals.

The Seven Countries Study, one of the classic nutrition studies, tracked more than twelve thousand men in the United States, Europe, and Japan beginning in 1958 and looked specifically at diet, lifestyle, and heart disease risks. Of all the populations studied, Greeks from the island of Crete had the lowest incidence of heart disease, the longest life expectancy, and among the *highest* levels of fat intake, at over 40 percent of calories. What this suggested was that fat by itself does not harm you. But more than that, as we've learned since 1958, fat in the right forms can do you a lot of good.

In the 1950s and 1960s the Cretan diet was rich in fruits, vegetables, legumes, and whole grains, and the preponderance of the fat they consumed was in the form of olive oil.

Olive oil is a mainly *monounsaturated* fat; along with *polyunsaturated* fats, it promotes good (HDL) cholesterol and reduces insulin sensitivity. The dangerous fats—those that may increase risks for both heart disease and cancer—are *saturated* fats and, especially, *trans* fats. Trans fats, formed by the hydrogenation of vegetable oil and used to make processed foods harder so as to extend their shelf life, are among the worst things you can put in your body. They raise bad (LDL) and suppress good (HDL) cholesterol levels, make the bad cholesterol even worse by miniaturizing its particles (meaning it can sneak into smaller spaces and do more damage), and promote inflammation (and therefore diabetes and a host of related ailments).

As just one example of the harm trans fats can cause, a 2008 study published in the *American Journal of Epidemiology* showed that women with the highest serum levels of these fats had up to a 75 percent increased risk of breast cancer.[3] Another study published in *Cancer Epidemiology, Biomarkers & Prevention* in 2008 found men with the highest serum levels of trans fats also had an increased risk of prostate cancer.[4]

The Four Fats

Fat Type	Ecogenetic Food Source	Effects
Monounsaturated	Olives, olive oil, almonds, cashews, avocados, lean red meat and low-fat dairy	Lowers LDL, raises HDL
Polyunsaturated	Fish, walnuts, sesame seeds, flaxseeds, sunflower seeds	Lowers LDL, raises HDL, stabilizes insulin sensitivity
Saturated	Red meat, whole milk, cheese, candy bars, cake	Raises LDL and HDL
Trans	Margarine, deep-fried fast foods (French fries, donuts), partially hydrogenated vegetable oil, shortening, and some commercial baked goods (crackers, cookies, cakes) that contain them	Raises LDL, lowers HDL, causes inflammation

So what the Basic Plan recommends in terms of fat consumption is straightforward: replace bad fats (excessive saturated fats, all trans fats) with good ones (monounsaturated and polyunsaturated fats). There is no need for the average person to limit all fats indiscriminately; the evidence is that good fats have good effects, and they also can usefully replace an overreliance on carbs.

If you're on a 2,000-calorie-a-day diet, just under 700 calories can come from dietary fat. Fat contains 9 calories per gram, so this translates to about 65 grams of fat a day. Aim for polyunsaturated fats to make up 10 percent of your calories, or about 22 grams each day if you follow a 2,000-calorie diet, and monounsaturated fats should make up the remaining fat in your daily allotment, adding up to 20 percent of calories, or about 45 grams per day. Good sources of polyunsaturated fats include fish, grapeseed oil, sunflower seeds, and soybeans. The best sources of monounsaturated fats include nuts, avocados, and olive oil.

Carbs

If anything, carbohydrates have been even more vilified recently than fats. "Low carb" has become almost as common an advertising ploy as "low fat." Store shelves are filled with "low-carb" snacks and treats, all purporting riskless and convenient satisfaction. Look out! If the big processed-food companies are telling you that a food sounds too good to be true, it almost certainly is. Most prepackaged synthetic foods are the result of exactly those dubious chemical processes that, for the sake of your genome, you want to avoid.

But some of the anticarb bias is well deserved. Modern diets worldwide, influenced by American patterns, tend to overemphasize carbs generally and many of the worst, highly processed carbs specifically. One important randomized study, the OmniHeart study,[5] separated participants into three groups, each consuming a heart-healthy diet, but one emphasizing high carb consumption, one protein consumption, and one fat consumption. The study showed that risk factors for heart disease could be significantly improved simply by replacing 10 percent of a standard high-carb diet (54 percent carbs) with either unsaturated fat or protein. In other words, lowering your intake of carbs can indeed make you healthier.

I mentioned above that one good reason not to restrict carbs too drastically is that you don't want to cut yourself off from all their beneficial micronutrients. Most carbohydrates break down into glucose—the main fuel source for all cells and the only type of nourishment your brain utilizes. And carbohydrate-rich fruits and vegetables are chockablock with vitamins and minerals. Spinach, broccoli, and kale provide vitamin K, which aids calcium regulation.

Citrus fruits like oranges and lemons provide vitamin C, a powerful antioxidant that also prevents scurvy.

But there are plenty of other reasons to change your carb habits. Since carbs are basically digested into sugars, they are the primary regulators of insulin, the body's sugar-shuttling hormone. Insulin, in turn, has a variety of crucial functions: not only moving sugar from the blood into the cells, but also signaling the body to store energy in the form of fat. Thus carbs can have a big impact on one of today's primary health concerns, obesity.

Nearly all foods, with the exception of meat, eggs, and seafood, contain some carbohydrates, so it is vitally important to be consuming *the right kind of carbs*. There is so much junk out there—and not only the fast food you buy on the run, but all the cheaply made, conveniently packaged, heavily sweetened and texturized products that are the staple of American eating. If it comes in a box or a wrapper or a bottle, feels unnaturally smooth and tastes too pleasantly sweet, and has a long list of unpronounceable ingredients, it's probably a processed carb that can do you almost nothing but harm. Even most bread and pasta, plain as it seems, has had most of the cancer-preventing, insulin-normalizing fiber stripped out of it. There's almost nothing left but the soft, sweet interior of the grain, which we were never intended to eat without all the other healthy stuff too.

For example, over 80 percent of vitamin E and magnesium are lost from wheat when it's processed. These nutrients are vital to insulin regulation, which is why it's not surprising that people diagnosed with diabetes are often vitamin E and magnesium deficient. Chromium and zinc are also important minerals lost when sugar is highly refined, yet these minerals are necessary for digesting and metabolizing carbohydrates.

What does the body do when it can't get necessary nutrients from food? For one, it constantly "feels" hungry. Then, as the body continues to be denied the nutrients it needs from food, it will start to deplete nutritional stores, leading to deficiencies.

Each gram of carbohydrate contains about 4 calories, so if you follow an average 2,000-calorie diet and you want one-third of those calories to come from carbs, you need about 180 grams of carbs per day. If you tend to stick to a 2,500-calorie diet, you'll need 225 grams of daily carbs. So a good rule of thumb is to have roughly 45 to 60 grams of carbs per meal and 15 to 30 grams for snacks.

For a good carbohydrate snack, I tell my patients to choose Swiss cheese, four 1-ounce slices of which contain about 4.5 grams of carbs along with 319 calories.

Nuts are another healthy carb snack that, like cheese, also contain a lot of calories. One ounce of dry-roasted almonds (about twenty-two nuts) contains a little over two grams of effective carbohydrate. One ounce of dry-roasted pecans contains about one gram of carbs.

Proteins

Americans typically get around 15 percent of their calories from protein, mainly from meat and milk products. These, as we've already discussed, are high in saturated fat, so the goal of one-third protein will require eating not only more protein, but ideally protein that is more nutritious. As with fat, one very good reason to eat more protein is simply to substitute it for excessive carbs.

There is some evidence that eating higher than typical—though not extremely high—levels of protein has a number of independent beneficial effects. Some studies have suggested that protein can protect against heart disease. The protein-based diet in the OmniHeart study lowered LDL cholesterol further than the carbohydrate-rich diet did, and it scored better on some lipid markers than the fat-substituting version of the diet.

Protein also tends to have a satiating effect—you feel fuller when you eat more protein, in part because it moves more slowly than carbs through your digestive system. Similarly, because its effect on insulin is muted, it also doesn't provoke the quick return of hunger after a meal. So protein can be particularly useful for weight maintenance. And because fighting obesity is such a crucial threshold for health, eating more protein can be considered an important part of the basic goal of resisting diabetes, cancer, heart disease, and the other nasty hallmarks of the self-perpetuating metabolic spirals.

A recent study demonstrated a way of maximizing the benefits of protein consumption by distributing your intake more evenly throughout the day. Researchers compared two groups of volunteers who consumed 90 grams of protein each day, primarily in the form of lean beef. One group ate 30 grams of protein at each meal, while the other group ate 10 grams at breakfast, 15 grams at lunch, and 65 grams at dinner. The volunteers who consumed the evenly distributed protein meals had a twenty-four-hour muscle protein synthesis 25 percent greater than those subjects who ate according to the skewed protein distribution pattern. Better muscle synthesis means a more efficient utilization of calories, and less protein being oxidized and ending up as glucose or fat. So balancing your protein intake throughout the day is key. Add an egg, a glass of mixed vegetable juice, Greek yogurt, or a handful of nuts to get closer to 30 grams of protein in the morning. Do something similar to get to 30 grams for your midday meal, and then consume no more than 30 grams of protein for dinner. Many of my patients are in the best shape of their lives after fifty by simply bringing back the balance that helps them shed the fat, build muscle, and look younger.[6]

Distributing your protein throughout the day is easier than you might think. Here are some suggested sources of protein and the amount each provides:

- Lentils contain 18 grams of protein per cup cooked. They are easier than other legumes because you do not need to soak them to cook in advance and they cook quickly.
- Whey or part-skim ricotta cheese contains 14 grams of protein per half cup. This is great to put on whole grain pancakes with honey for breakfast.
- Shrimp contain 12 grams of protein per 3 ounces.
- Eggs contained 6.3 grams of protein per large egg.
- Beef contains 30 grams of protein per 4-ounce serving. This 4-ounce serving also contains only 275 calories.
- Hempseeds contain 13 grams of protein per quarter cup. These are great to sprinkle on salads or other foods to add a crunchy texture.
- Edamame contains 8 grams of protein per cup (in the pod). You can buy these precooked in the frozen section of the supermarket.
- Greek yogurt (Fage 2 percent plain or Oikos traditional plain) contains 18 grams of protein per 6-ounce container or 24 grams of protein per cup. This is great with fruits, nuts, or honey.
- Light or 2 percent fat cottage cheese contains 21 grams of protein per 6 ounces. This is great with berries or walnuts.
- Quinoa contains 8 grams of protein per cup cooked. This is a great gluten-free choice for breakfast mixed with almond milk, banana, and honey.
- Almonds contain 5.9 grams of protein (and 169 calories) per ounce (roughly twenty-two nuts).
- Walnuts contain 4.3 grams of protein (and 184 calories) per ounce (roughly fourteen halves).

■ Cashews contain 4.3 grams of protein (and 163 calories) per ounce (roughly eighteen halves).

Concept 2:
No Fads, No Faux Foods

As I've tried to show with my Rule of One-Thirds, there is no single food group responsible for all our ills. Nor is there a single food group or nutrient that can put us on the path to health. Yet the popular culture continually throws up new dietary villains or saviors to capture our attention.

Can you ingest too much wheat? Of course you can, but you can also ingest too much water. Is gluten bad for you? It certainly is if you are among the 6 percent of our population that has a gluten sensitivity. But that leaves 94 percent of the population with no reason to avoid it. Meanwhile, the other nutrients in whole grains are essential to health. The *British Medical Journal* recently reported the results of a ten-year study of four thousand Americans showing that those who ate the most cereal fiber had a 27 percent lower mortality rate from heart attacks during the study period.[7]

Is sugar bad for you? My response is that all sugars are not the same, and some actually confer health benefits. So I don't ask my patients to adopt a total ban on sweets, but I do prefer that they rely on sweeteners derived from honey, maple syrup, coconut, or stevia, a sweet substance derived from a plant related to daisy and ragweed. These sweeteners have lower "glycemic indices" than refined cane sugar, meaning they require less insulin for them to be metabolized, thus avoiding the insulin imbalance that can lead to a number of chronic conditions, most notably diabetes.

My advice is to avoid extremes and avoid rushing to the dietary passion of the moment. It also pays to realize that we are subjected to billions of dollars in marketing money spent by the food industry each year to shape our thinking and our buying habits. For generations, convenience, packaging, and profits were the dominant considerations rather than health and nutrition. But then the same food industry discovered that they could build a new growth sector by promoting certain foods for their health and weight loss benefits. So knowing what's actually good for us—as opposed to what's good for the industry—becomes increasingly difficult. For instance, fat provides more than twice the amount of energy per gram than carbohydrates and proteins. Since fats contain more energy, and excess energy obtained from food is usually stored as fat, you can see how consuming too many calories precipitates weight problems.

Macronutrient	Calories/gram
carbohydrate	4
protein	4
fat	9

Here are a few examples of food "posers" that appear to be healthy on the surface, but a closer look reveals that they are surprisingly high in calories, the wrong kinds of fats and sugars, and salt:

- Whole ground turkey contains more fat than ground turkey breast or 97–99 percent lean turkey meat.
- Store-bought smoothies are likely to have little fiber and lots of the wrong kinds of sugar, so you end up feeling hungry faster after drinking them. Blend your own smoothies with real fruit to promote fullness (see Chapter 9 for my healthy recipes).
- Sports drinks contain electrolytes for people who need to replenish what they've lost after an intense workout, but they also contain lots of the wrong kinds of sugars. So my recommendation for the average person after an average workout: when you're thirsty, drink water—and that means tap water. "Enhanced" water contains minerals and vitamins, but you're probably already getting enough of these through your diet. Tap water is the most efficient and economical way to hydrate your body, although installation of a reverse osmosis water filter is a good idea if there is concern about your water quality.
- Granola bars and flavored yogurt may be your breakfast pick du jour for a rushed morning, but these foods are packed with refined sugar. Instead, try steel-cut oats with fruit or add fruit or nuts to low-fat plain yogurt.

Beyond the simple guidelines of the Basic Plan, there is no need to seek out exotic, specially crafted foods, as these may in fact do more harm than good. Along with lowering carb consumption while increasing good fats and protein, I recommend moving away from the oversweet, too easily digestible carbs that will spike insulin and inflammation as well as promote cholesterol and weight gain (and thereby obesity, diabetes, cancer, and the rest). I also recommend moving toward the kinds of carbs that contain fiber and all the micronutrients that are bioactively beneficial. I encourage you to eat fewer boxed, wrapped, sliced, or synthesized carbs, and more whole foods, whole grains, legumes, fruits, and vegetables, and to eat red meat and dairy in moderation. I also encourage you to rely on walnuts, almonds, and cashews as a healthful snack food in place of chips or energy bars. They are filled with protein and the good fats we explored above, and have been shown to reduce heart disease.

I find that many of my patients appreciate having simple yes/no choices set out for them, which makes compliance a no-brainer. So here is a bare-bones guide that reduces the Basic Plan to a summary that could almost fit on the back of a business card and can help you remain steadily on course as you navigate the maze of dietary fads and conflicting food claims:

Avoid	Target
■ Just about anything that is crunchy and comes in a box, that is loaded with preservatives like nitrites, or that has a shelf life of months rather than days. This includes processed lunch meats.	■ Organic food as much as possible
	■ Fermented or pickled foods
	■ Whole grains (not to be confused with "multigrain," which may or may not deliver the benefits you need)
■ White flour, refined sugar, and anything containing high-fructose corn syrup, which means commercial sauces, salad dressings, and of course sodas	■ Protein from lean meats, almonds, cashews, and walnuts
	■ Olive oil for raw foods and salads
■ Peanuts, peanut butter, and peanut oil (Peanuts, unlike tree nuts, grow underground where they become contaminated with *Aspergillus*, a toxin-containing fungus linked to cancer and developmental delays in children.)	■ Grapeseed oil, ghee, butter, or coconut oil for cooking, since these have higher heat coefficients and are therefore not damaged by high heat
	■ Raw fruits and vegetables
	■ Vegetables with rich colors to get the nutrients you need
■ Microwave popcorn treated with perfluorooctane sulfonate (PFOS) to keep the popcorn from sticking together; PFOS is an endocrine-disrupting chemical that has been linked to infertility, cancer, and thyroid disease	■ Natural sea salt, which is about 90 percent sodium chloride, plus critical trace minerals for healthy DNA function and repair
	■ Naturally sweet foods like fruit, honey, and maple syrup, as well as sugar substitutes like coconut crystals and stevia
■ Oils that have been subjected to high heat during the process of refining, which gives oils a long shelf life	■ Lamb, due to its smaller size than cows, bioaccumulates fewer toxins like dioxin
■ Tuna and swordfish, as these longer-living predator fish bioaccumulate mercury	■ Organic almond milk or organic hormone-free milk

Avoid	Target
■ Processed table salt, which is 98 percent sodium chloride, but also contains processing chemicals ■ Margarine, which is loaded with trans fats as well as solvents and chemical preservatives ■ Canned soups or vegetables, unless the label says "BPA-free" ■ Artificial sweeteners, which have been found to stimulate appetite, resulting in weight gain despite being "calorie-free"	■ Organic Greek yogurt with probiotic kefir cultures ■ A 3:1 ratio of omega-6 to omega-3 oils

Merely by following these simple guidelines—which incorporate the Rule of One-Thirds—you will be well on your way to a more healthful diet.

Concept 3:
Supplements Are Essential

The sad truth is that we are not living on the same planet that our grandparents lived on, where you could eat a reasonable diet, including a few servings of fruits and vegetables every day, and expect to be in good health. We're living in a heavily polluted world in which we're exposed to toxic chemicals—from BPA to dioxin to pesticides and herbicides to heavy metals—beginning while we are still in our mothers' wombs. All these substances affect gene expression, which necessarily means that some counterbalance is in order. Simply consuming a balanced diet will not provide adequate amounts of critical nutrients such as krill oil, biotin, or carnosine, which are necessary for ecogenetic health.

Throughout this book I'll be mentioning various supplements, and in Part II I'll provide a comprehensive, detailed analysis that correlates specific supplements with specific health concerns. But for now, a few thoughts on ensuring safety and value.

Supplements are a multimillion-dollar business not regulated by the Food and Drug Administration. They are not required to undergo rigorous clinical trials before being marketed to the public, and in most cases they are easily obtainable without a prescription. All of which means that your safety and assurance of value lies in being an informed and cautious consumer.

From time to time isolated problems with supplements have made head-lines, which has caused some commentators to be skeptical of supplements al-together. But dismissing supplements out of hand is like saying no one should drive because one model of car from one automaker had a safety issue.

However, sometimes the problem is with a study itself, when faulty conclu-sions are not based upon actual fact. In 2001, the journal *Science* published a paper showing that vitamin C had prooxidant effects on DNA,[8] which would mean that the vitamin had the potential to cause rather than protect against damage to our genes from "free radicals," those atoms and molecules with un-paired electrons that wreak havoc in our cells by trying to bind too freely with other molecules. Suddenly there was a hue and cry in the media claiming that taking any extra vitamin C was harmful, even though people had been con-suming it for decades without negative effects.

More to the point, this study was not conducted in the living cells of living people. Instead, the vitamin C was incubated in an artificial cell culture envi-ronment in the presence of oxidized fatty acids that are inherently unstable and that themselves form free radicals. These reacted with the vitamin C, caus-ing it to also break down into free radicals. But the natural environment of the human cell contains a wide variety of antioxidants that normally prevents the vitamin C from undergoing this transformation.

Public uneasiness grew in 2005 when a meta-analysis published in the *An-nals of Internal Medicine* found that "doses of vitamin E supplements greater than 400 units per day may increase all-cause mortality and should be avoided." But just as the vitamin C study isolated the one nutrient in an artificial envi-ronment, the vitamin E study used only one form of vitamin E called d-alpha-tocopherol, which was synthetically derived.[9] Vitamin E in food sources comes in eight different forms: alpha-, beta-, delta-, and gamma-tocotrienol and alpha-, beta-, delta-, and gamma-tocopherol. It's simply not valid to compare a synthetic form of vitamin E, in isolation, to the eight natural forms that have been demonstrated to have beneficial synergistic effects on cholesterol, cardio-vascular disease, and cancer prevention.

Similar studies done in smokers showed that those who took beta-carotene supplements actually had a higher incidence of lung cancer. But beta-carotene (a supplement I never recommend, by the way) is quite different from the carot-enoids found in nature. There are dozens of different carotenoids in whole foods and whole food extracts that are quite different from synthetic beta-carotene taken in high doses.

This is why I tell my patients to consume a diet rich in fruits and vegetables and use nutritional supplements derived from a variety of plant-based concentrates. This will avoid the prooxidant effect of taking a single antioxidant in large quantities. Nutrients, like the organs of the human body, were designed to work together to form a well-functioning homeostatic alliance. Do not be misled by studies like the ones just mentioned that, in my opinion, draw conclusions that are unwarranted based on their own data.

Here are some tips to consider before you start using any supplements:

- Always discuss your plan for supplemental nutrition with your physician before beginning any new regimen.
- Look for pharmaceutical-grade supplements. These tend to be of higher quality and they undergo testing in an independent lab to ensure that the nutrients will be absorbed into the body at levels deemed effective.
- Look for supplements that are made from plant-based foods or whole foods, because these contain additional compounds to provide you with antioxidant and anti-inflammatory coverage.
- Avoid supplements that give you more than you bargained for. Some may contain additives, allergens, and even contaminants such as lead or mercury.
- Read the label and look for an expiration date. Make sure that the ingredients are organic. And know the recommended doses for the nutrients you're shopping for.

Despite the need for caution, specific supplements are one of the most important ways of engaging with the cellular processes at the root of the diseases we're targeting, and I rely on them heavily with my patients.

Concept 4:
Whenever Possible, Go with the Whole Food

Bioactive phytochemicals—naturally occurring substances in plants that affect us right down into our genes—are a big part of what makes fruits and vegetables as good for us as they are. While many of these substances can be extracted and delivered in pills or supplements, they are much better accessed in their whole-plant form. Partly this is because rigorous processing often disrupts or kills the enzymes and substances that provide the benefit. Whole food is also fresher than a pill, and the nutrients survive better without being pulverized or heated.

Another major reason to look to whole foods is that we don't yet fully understand the exact mechanism by which many of these substances work. It may be the complex interactions of several of their properties working together that give the desirable effects. Or the health benefits we see may be due to elements in the plants that we haven't even identified for study. Out of the ten thousand or more phytochemicals that may be present in fruits and vegetables, only a relative handful have been researched in any depth. Since the benefit is high and well known, and because we are still pretty ignorant about the full range and mechanism of their bioactivity, the easiest and best course is simply to eat the whole plant.

Another beauty of eating whole fruits and vegetables, rather than taking supplements or extracts, is that there are no side effects. You can pretty much eat all you want, and yet their mixture of macronutrients, bulk, fiber, and water content will automatically keep you from consuming any single phytochemical in excess.

The list below contains the phytochemicals that you will find in the whole foods featured in the Gene Therapy Plan recipes in Part II. Knowing the scientific names is not important; the important thing is understanding the benefits the common sources of these nutrients can provide. These nutrients address recurring issues associated with disease, such as chronic inflammation and free radical damage. Operating at the level of fundamental cellular mechanism, they can:

- boost adiponectin, a protein that regulates sugar and fat
- kill unhealthy fat cells
- destroy cancer cells
- lower cancer-promoting molecules
- inhibit cancer-promoting enzymes
- promote anticancer hormones
- block new blood vessels that supply fat tissue and feed cancerous tumors
- support the function of mitochondria, the energy powerhouse of cells
- improve sugar metabolism
- trigger healthy aging effects

Phytochemical	Sources	Benefits
Ajoene	Garlic	Sulfur-containing compound with antimicrobial effects; anti-inflammatory and antioxidant
Apigenin	Apples, grapes, cherries, beans, broccoli, celery, onions, leeks, and tomatoes; also in wine and tea	Bioflavonoid with antioxidant, anticancer, and anti-inflammatory effects
Baicalein	Skullcap roots (*Scutellaria baicalensis* Georgi), thyme, mad-dog skullcap (*Scutellaria lateriflora* L.), and broken bones plant (*Oroxylum indicum*)	Flavonoid with anticancer and anti-inflammatory properties
Brassicasterol	Rapeseed oil	Anti-inflammatory effects that improve cardiovascular health, immunity; chemopreventive
Campesterol	Chili peppers, eggs, walnuts, potatoes, fava beans, and avocados	Plant sterol that reduces cholesterol absorption from the gut
CLA	Eggs, milk, cheese, butter, and beef (grass-fed ruminants usually contain higher amounts)	Unsaturated fatty acid with protective effects against cholesterol, breast cancer; promotes weight loss and enhances body mass
Coumestrol	Soybeans, red clover, alfalfa sprouts, peas, and brussels sprouts	Anti-inflammatory polyphenolic molecule that protects against neurodegenerative disease, cancer, bone disease
DHA	Coldwater fish (e.g., salmon), fish oil supplements, and seaweed	Omega-3 fatty acid in retina (although also found in the brain and sperm) that's crucial for vision; protects against Alzheimer's disease, heart disease, cancer, and advanced aging
Diosgenin	Legumes and yams	Phytoestrogen used to treat inflammation, asthma, high cholesterol
EGCG	Green tea	Polyphenolic antioxidant substance that protects against cognitive dysfunction, cancer, obesity, cardiovascular conditions

Phytochemical	Sources	Benefits
Fisetin	Strawberries	Flavonoid with anti-inflammatory effects; protects against cancer, neurodegenerative disease
Fucoxanthin	Brown seaweed	Pigment that gives seaweed and kelp its brown, olive green colors and is also found in marine animals like sea urchins; appetite suppressant; energy booster; anticancer compound
Genistein	Soybeans and soy milk	Isoflavone that protects against prostate, breast, and ovarian cancers; also helps with menopausal symptoms
Guggulsterone	Guggul plants (*Commiphora mukul*) and gum resin	Herb that promotes weight loss, improves thyroid function, regulates cholesterol levels, removes toxins
Hesperidin	Oranges, tangerines, grapefruits, and lemons	Bioflavonoid (highly concentrated in citrus fruit peels) with potent antioxidant and anti-inflammatory effects; also vasodilates blood vessels, which helps reduce hypertension
Kaempferol	Strawberries, grapes, broccoli, cabbage, kale, beans, endive, leeks, tomatoes, and tea	Antimicrobial, anti-inflammatory, cardioprotective, and neuroprotective effects; chemopreventive; improves bone strength
Luteolin	Green peppers, celery, thyme, and chamomile tea	Bioflavonoid that checks against cancer; also protects against free radical damage and proinflammatory molecules
Naringenin	Tomatoes (skin), oranges, and grapefruits	Bioflavonoid with anticancer antioxidant properties; cardioprotective and neuroprotective; improves blood glucose levels
Procyanidins	Red wine	Polyphenolic substance with anti-inflammatory, antioxidant properties; used mainly for its cardioprotective effects

Phytochemical	Sources	Benefits
Quercetin	Capers, apples, and onions	Potent antioxidant with anti-inflammatory and antihistamine properties; improves cholesterol profile; cardioprotective; chemopreventive
Resveratrol	Grapes, wine, and soy	Antimicrobial, anti-inflammatory, antioxidant polyphenolic substance that protects against heart disease, cancer, neurodegenerative diseases
Rutin	Lemons, limes, oranges, grapefruits, and cranberries	Bioflavonoid helpful in the prevention of strokes, cancer, osteoarthritis
Sitosterol	Soybeans, wheat germ, and rice bran	Phytosterol used to treat heart disease and high cholesterol; immune booster that prevents diseases from the common cold to colon cancer
Stanols	Fruits, vegetables, seeds, nuts, and legumes	Phytosterol that lowers cholesterol, improves immune function, protects against cancer
Stigmasterol	Soybeans and rapeseed oil	Phytosterol that prevents against osteoporosis, high cholesterol, and cancer
Xanthohumol	Hops and beer	Anti-inflammatory, antidiabetic, anticancer effects; promotes weight loss; regulates cholesterol levels; boosts immunity

Seeing the power in simple foods can help you to become an informed partner in the pursuit of genuine health.

But the ecogenetic approach to health is not just a collection of details. It is first and foremost an overarching point of view, which is that illness and health are not two diametrically opposed conditions. All of life occurs on a gradient between the two, and our objective should be to interact with our bodies in such a way that we're continuously tipping the balance away from illness and toward health—by consuming nutrients that prevent and attack disease.

Beneath the simplicity of my dietary recommendations, and beneath the appeal of the recipes I offer, these substances are the fundamental components of my plan. By virtue of its ecogenetic approach, the Gene Therapy Plan employs them throughout to help you achieve better health and live a longer, happier life.

In the chapters that follow, the Gene Therapy Plan will amplify and extend these basic recommendations, refining them for specific concerns and introducing you to more specific nutrients that can add power to the positive effects you're already achieving.

Chapter 2

Obesity

The Obesity Epidemic

If fighting obesity seems to be an obsession everywhere, that's not your imagi-
nation. Roughly 67 percent of adults and 32 percent of children today are either
overweight or obese. We want to bring weight down and avoid weight gain not
because our culture idealizes thinness as an aesthetic ideal, but because obesity
contributes to the incidence of the other conditions that concern us most: cancer, heart disease, diabetes, and premature aging.

"Obesity" itself is not so much a disease as a collection of influences,
propensities, and non-illness-specific processes—a cluster of effects that, taken
together, generate fat accumulation, insulin resistance, metabolic dysfunction,
and particular patterns of hormonal imbalance.

At the most basic level, though, obesity is simply a matter of having too
much body fat. What constitutes "too much" is usually determined by a measure called the body mass index (BMI), which correlates height and weight according to norms established by studying large populations and determining
the range of BMI values associated with good health. But there is an even sim-
pler definition that works perfectly well: you have too much fat when it begins
to impinge on other elements of your health.

Again, we're making a distinction between "weight" and body fat because, after all, a bulked-up bodybuilder could be said to be "overweight," but well-toned muscle has never been associated with health risks. But fat is very definitely a health risk, and not just because it weighs the body down.

Given popular images like the "saddlebag" or the "spare tire," it's easy to think of the fat on your body as being somehow separate from the rest of you, something that lies "outside" your "real" body, something that's merely an add-on. But fat tissue is not only an integrated part of who you are, it actually functions as if it were a separate organ, releasing hormones that contribute to the body's overall regulation. In other words, fat is not the inert substance it might appear to be, but something that causes systematic, disease-related harm. This complicates the issue of how much fat is too much, because these hormonal influences begin to affect the body's functioning right from the start, long before a term like "obesity" would ever seem appropriate. Which is why our comprehensive and integrated approach is so essential—so you can get in there and correct imbalances long before they appear as symptoms of pathology.

Success Story

Meet Allan. He's fifty-three years old. He's gregarious, ambitious, and successful. He's also fought a twenty-year battle with his weight, and it's a fight that he's been slowly losing. This despite the fact that he pays pretty close attention to his health and tries to follow the advice he picks up from various popular sources. He follows a fairly rigorous exercise regimen, churning along on an elliptical trainer four times a week for forty-five minutes. And he watches what he eats—serially, in fact, in the various contortionist ways that each of the many diet plans he's followed has recommended. But all to no avail.

When he came to see me for dietary advice, I could easily understand his frustration. "Doc," he said, "I think I'm just meant to have a spare tire my whole life. I mean, no matter what I do I'm stuck at 190."

In my practice, I see this all the time—patients who try their best, but for whom the standard diet and exercise prescriptions only trim a few pounds that are usually packed right back on. I told Allan, "It's never too late to bring back balance." After all, he did not lack motivation or intelligence. He simply lacked the proper mix of nutrients required for healthy gene expression.

So with Allan I performed the usual battery of tests to determine, among other things, his blood glucose and cholesterol levels. The test results revealed that Allan was vulnerable to three quite serious chronic diseases. The endocrine workup showed that he was not a diabetic, but he was in danger of developing diabetes because his hemoglobin A1c (HbA1c) value of 6.1 percent, a snapshot view of blood sugar levels in a six- to twelve-week period, was squarely within the "prediabetic" range, which is from 5.7 percent to 6.4 percent. Allan's risk of stroke and cardiovascular disease was also slightly elevated. We determined this by testing his C-reactive protein (CRP), a marker of inflammation strongly linked to these ills, as well as to diabetes. Whereas a CRP level less than 1.0 milligrams per liter is low risk, Allan's was high, at 3.2 milligrams per liter.

Given these vulnerabilities, as well as his tendency to put on weight, Allan needed a dramatic turnaround. Happily, we were able to put him on the right path with just a few simple changes. And you know what? After three months of diligent effort, Allan was at his ideal body weight of 165 pounds and his risk of diabetes, stroke, and cardiovascular disease was greatly reduced.

While much of the advice I gave him would apply to most patients—that is, follow the Rule of One-Thirds, consume a variety of fruits and vegetables daily, get adequate sleep and physical activity—it's important to recognize that the supplements I suggested were tailored just for him.

Let me emphasize once again that, before starting any supplements, making any dietary changes, or implementing an exercise routine yourself, you should discuss the specifics with your medical doctor. With that caveat in mind, here's what I recommended for Allan as his individualized health plan for targeting obesity:

- **Stop eating a skewed diet.** Allan had tried just about everything—by the time he came to see me he was eating a vegan diet—and it still wasn't helping. To make matters worse, his restrictions on meat and dairy had left him with several nutritional deficiencies, including protein, iron, and omega-3 fats. So I advised him to take a more moderate path and to incorporate the Rule of One-Thirds, to even out his intake of protein, carbs, and fat. This balanced approach avoids the perils of macronutrient-obsessed eating plans, which have unintended consequences. A high-carb diet can lead to insulin insensitivity, a high-fat diet lacks important nutrients and fiber, and a high-protein diet leads to the consumption of way too many saturated fats. I gave Allan the same recommendation that I offer in the Basic Plan: the most sensible path is to avoid specific regimens or fad diets and just focus on eating nutritious foods from a sustainably wide range of choices.

■ **Stay active, but mix it up.** Physical activity is essential to good health, but its greatest contribution to maintaining proper weight is the way it revs up your metabolism. All that time Allan put in on the elliptical trainer was admirable, but I suggested that he move to a more circuit-training style: eight minutes on either the elliptical trainer or rowing machine followed by three ten-minute cycles of toning, free weights, and weight machines. By working out in shorter intervals with increasing intensity he'd burn more calories and build endurance, and by varying his routine he'd make his workouts more enjoyable.

■ **Go green.** I advised Allan to consume fresh, raw vegetables with each meal and to add fruit to his diet each day. These foods are packed with various nutrients and phytochemicals that help you maintain or achieve a healthy weight. I told Allan to make it a habit to eat carrot, beet, or celery slices after each meal. These provide enzymes and fiber, digested by bacteria in the gut, that ultimately activate nerve cells in the brain to signal that you are full. I also suggested that he eat three apple, orange, or grapefruit slices before each meal, not only because it's a great-tasting way to incorporate important nutrients, but because it makes you feel fuller faster by controlling insulin and sugar surges.

■ **Supplement your way of life.** In Allan's plan I stressed the importance of getting nutrition primarily from a wide variety of the right kinds of foods (nuts, fruits, poultry, fish, beans, and more), but I also suggested that he take supplements with his meals, which not only give the system a boost, but also help control how many calories the body actually absorbs. The specific supplements I suggested to Allan were:

- Glucomannan—665 milligrams, one before each meal. Glucomannan slows down stomach emptying and prevents rapid carbohydrate absorption, which helps to avoid the fluctuations in blood sugar levels associated with diabetes.
- Garcinia—1.33 grams, twice daily. A plant commonly found in Asia, garcinia amplifies leptin, a hormone vital to the control of appetite.
- Berberine—200 milligrams, twice daily. Used in traditional Chinese medicine, berberine is an herb that fights fat by lowering the body's triglycerides and LDLs (the bad form of cholesterol), and by regulating fatty acid release to prevent fat buildup in the body.
- CLA—750 milligrams, twice daily. Similarly, CLA has been shown to reduce body fat and stabilize LDL and triglycerides.
- *Phaseolus vulgaris* extract—445 milligrams, one before each meal. This extract from common beans blocks enzymatic breakdown of carbs so they are not absorbed into the bloodstream as glucose.
- Green tea—2-3 cups daily. Green tea contains epigallocatechin gallate (EGCG), which has been shown in studies to help people lose weight and keep it off by increasing the body's basic metabolic rate, thereby burning more calories. It also blocks the enzymatic breakdown of fatty foods.

Again, these are not blanket recommendations. Supplements need to be chosen in consultation with your physician.

By faithfully following this plan, Allan was not only able to reach his optimal weight, but to enjoy the best *health* of his life. And this is the most vital consideration of all. Being in good health rather than just being in shape includes being released from all the stress, anxiety, compulsion, fad dieting, and sense of failure that so often accompanies the struggle against obesity.

What Causes Obesity?

The best way to win the battle against obesity is to never let those stores of fat get established in the first place. Once established, fat stores create a vicious and self-perpetuating cycle.

That's largely because fat accumulation is an issue of energy balance. The fat that is stored in the body—the kind that leads to obesity—is called adipose tissue. It is different from the kinds of fats you eat, which are broken down by digestion and may or may not ultimately become stored in your body.

It also helps to remember that adipose tissue has its purpose, which is to serve as a very efficient means of compressing and storing energy. Hibernating bears, migrating whales, incubating penguins—in each of these cases fat stores are what sustain the animals during prolonged periods of fasting. And during the long history of our species, the ability to store fat as an energy reserve helped our ancient ancestors survive hard times when food was scarce.

For humans living in the developed world today, where starvation is thankfully not a perennial threat, it is all too easy for this natural energy-storing system to get out of whack. When we take in more food than we need for the body's immediate functioning, the excess energy supplied by that food gets stored away for future use, mainly as adipose tissue. When this occurs too frequently, the result is obesity.

This simple explanation makes the solution to obesity sound equally simple: just keep the balance even between food intake and the body's energy demands, or perhaps tilted more toward immediate use rather than storage. But as we all know, keeping obesity in check is not nearly so simple in daily practice.

The problem is that our consumption of food—including overconsumption—does not occur in a vacuum. Eating occurs not only within a complex psychological and social context, but also within a series of biochemical feedback loops. Certain kinds of foods, and certain patterns of eating, actually prompt us to *want* to overeat. And once overeating causes adipose tissue to begin to accumulate, it changes the body's system for regulating the storage of fat going forward.

On the other side of the energy equation, issues arise about the signals that regulate how many calories we feel like we want to take in, and the way adipose tissue affects the rate at which we can *burn off* more of the fat stores we already have.

To find the solution that really works, we need to examine how adipose tissue operates, its cycle of birth and death, what it needs to survive, and how we can influence or alter these processes. In other words, what are the best ways to burn up fat energy? How do you kill fat cells?

Imagine it's been only an hour since your last big meal and you're feeling ravenous again. You know you shouldn't need to eat—maybe you had a big bowl of cereal for breakfast or a hamburger and fries for lunch—but your stomach is still saying "Feed me!" and you know exactly the kind of food you're craving: a bag of chips, an energy bar, a tall mocha latte from the coffee shop.

None of which makes sense—or is sensible—especially if you're trying to lose weight. Surely you have enough energy stored up to operate normally without taking in more. The trouble is, when the body tells your mind that it needs food, even when the mind knows better, the body always wins. What's going on here?

What's going on is that you are *hungry*, which is to say that your brain is receiving signals that motivate you to replenish the body's energy stores. But why would your body be calling for more food when you've just eaten? Or put another way, why is your appetite working to throw off your body's actual energy balance?

Appetite is a continuous tug-of-war between hunger and satiety. When the hunger signal is stronger in our brains, we experience it as the need to eat. When the satiety signal is stronger, we feel full. But this ebb and flow of signaling is not an automatic or immediate response to a literal condition of "hunger" or "fullness." Hunger and fullness themselves *are* the signals that trigger the feeling of the need to eat or not, regardless of the amount of food currently in your digestive system. What hunger means is that the brain is receiving hunger signals. Satiety is the reception of satiety signals. If the hunger signal was turned off entirely, you would starve. And if the satiety signal was canceled, you would gorge yourself to death.

These signals aren't just symbols, like the flash of a traffic light that tells you to stop. They are in fact chemicals—hunger hormones—that travel from cell to cell throughout the blood. Structurally, they are just like any other hormones—like the insulin that regulates blood sugar levels or the serotonin that influences mood and sleep (and also appetite). Their ebb and flow is one current within the great ocean of hormones that is continuously circulating through the body's many systems and thus allowing its various parts to communicate with one another.

The Illusions of Hunger

The crucial point to understand is that these hormone signals are strongly related to, but not identical to, the body's actual energy needs. That is, the signaling can be out of sync with the body's current energy balance. The body needs
to draw energy from its stores or to eat when those stores run low, but its only
way of knowing which source is appropriate is through the signals of its hormones. The discrepancy between actual energy needs and the hormonal signals that represent the needs is why hunger can be extremely variable, and why
things like medications and mood can so strongly affect appetite. Depression,
for example, can interfere with the hunger hormones, making you eat less or
more than you would otherwise.

And this brings us to the key issue in thinking about obesity. One of the
findings of recent science is that obesity itself can be considered a manifestation of out-of-sync hormonal signaling. The obese person has more than sufficient energy stored in his or her adipose tissue. But the signaling that *represents*
the energy condition to the brain may still be saying, *"Hunger!"*

Happily, this opens up an avenue for ecogenetic intervention. If we can
manipulate the signaling in the direction *we* choose, so that our brain's percep-
tion of our need to eat is more in line with our actual needs, we can hope to
steer our body's tendency to accumulate too much fat back toward a healthier
balance.

Ghrelin and Leptin

Two of the primary hormones involved in this dance of appetite are *ghrelin*,
which signals feelings of hunger, and *leptin*, which signals feelings of fullness.
But either of these signals can be knocked out of whack. Ghrelin is secreted by
cells in the stomach and the pancreas. It moves through the blood to the hypo-
thalamus in the brain, where it triggers the feeling that our energy stores are
low and that we need to eat. Ghrelin levels increase in the periods between
meals, especially during nighttime sleep, and drop immediately after eating.
Ghrelin also increases growth hormone and cortisol levels, additional hormones associated with increased food intake. One study looked at how the tim-
ing of food consumption might affect ghrelin.[1] Researchers used mice that are
active at night and separated these "nocturnal" mice into two groups. They fed
the first group a high-fat diet but provided the food only at night, when the
mice usually eat. They fed the second group the same high-fat diet but made

the food available both day and night. Despite having the same caloric intake, the group that was allowed to feed during the day—which is to say, outside their normal feeding hours—gained more weight.

The exact mechanism is not known, but the fact that the same caloric intake led to greater weight gain in mice simply because it was consumed at odd hours suggests one possible culprit for human weight gain. We humans often eat at odd hours—when we're stressed, depressed, or lonely—and it may be that this dysregulated eating dysregulates ghrelin's ability to serve as a barometer for energy stores and to send the signal for more intake—also known as appetite—at the right moment.

The main culprit in upsetting leptin's primary function, which is to signal fullness or satiety, seems to be an excess supply of the hormone, which leads to insensitivity. Leptin is produced by our fat tissues, with the fat cells releasing the hormone at a fairly constant rate. This means that the more fat a person carries, the more leptin will be produced. In people with a normal level of body fat, this is a self-correcting system: if the number of fat cells increases, so does leptin production, which inhibits appetite, thereby keeping fat stores at a constant level.

But for those with high levels of body fat, and thus great numbers of fat cells churning out leptin, a chronic excess of the hormone overloads the receptors in the brain, which reduces their sensitivity so that they no longer respond to normal signaling levels. This, unfortunately, leads to a negative feedback loop in which increasing leptin insensitivity leads to an increase in appetite, which in turn incites more feeding, more fat accumulation, and more leptin production in a self-destructive cycle.

Gene Therapy Fact: Green Coffee

Green coffee, as you may know, is unroasted coffee, which studies have shown helps to control impaired glucose regulation in the body. You may also know that poor blood sugar levels lead to conditions such as type 2 diabetes, obesity, and metabolic syndrome, a condition marked by high blood pressure, obesity, elevated blood sugar, and abnormal cholesterol. Green coffee bean extract contains phenolic substances, such as chlorogenic acid and ferulic acid, that enhance weight loss. These antioxidant compounds up-regulate two genes (AMPK and PPAR) that control glucose and lipid levels in part via leptin regulation.

Researchers conducted a twenty-two-week study in which they evaluated the effects of green coffee bean extracts in sixteen over-weight adults. All of the study participants were given a high-dose of green coffee bean extract for six weeks, a lower dose of green cof-fee extract for six weeks, and a placebo for six weeks. Between each phase, the study participants underwent a two-week washout period to minimize the effects of the preceding treatment. During the high- and low-dose chlorogenic acid phases, the participants had signifi-cantly greater reductions in body weight and fat and BMI.[2] Most important, the study participants all worked out regularly and ate a healthy diet, which demonstrates the importance of a well-rounded approach toward maintaining an appropriate weight.

The Federal Trade Commission (FTC) filed a complaint against the marketers of GCA™, which is the green coffee bean extract product cited in this twenty-two-week study. While study design flaws, such as a small sample size, were among the complaints cited by the FTC, this study shows that green coffee bean extract is prom-ising. As a supplemental weight management option, other studies demonstrate the potential efficacy of green coffee bean extract.

1. One study evaluated the effects of green coffee bean extract in mice; the research showed that genes involved in fat synthesis and proinflammation were downregulated by the extract;[3]
2. In another study, researchers found that mice fed green coffee bean extract had a reduction in visceral fat and body weight;[4]
3. A meta-analysis found that studies show green coffee bean extract intake promotes weight loss but indicated a need for more rigorous trials.[5]

Although studies exploring the effects of green coffee bean ex-tract have some limitations, the findings on the use of the extract as a turnkey option for weight management remain optimistic.

There are various ways to benefit from the effects of green coffee beans. One way is to order lightly roasted coffee; you'll get about 92 milligrams of chlorogenic acid for each cup of java. But you can almost double this amount (to 172 milligrams) with just one cup of polyphenolic-retaining coffee, which is made by adding chlorogenic acid back into the coffee after it has been roasted. If you're not the morning joe type, then opt for green coffee bean extracts, which are readily accessible. Most people can maintain adequate glucose control (and weight loss) by taking 200 milligrams of the extract before most meals. But for those of you who struggle with maintaining normal blood glucose levels, 400 milligrams should be taken before meals. (It's likely that those with glycemic problems will have to take the extract before all their meals.)

Restoring the Balance

The first task of anyone who is obese should be to rectify eating patterns that are triggering this kind of hormonal dysregulation and disrupting the ability to keep food intake in line with the body's genuine needs. Unfortunately, it seems as if the typical American diet was *designed* to promote unbalance.

The key player in balancing energy and appetite is the hormone insulin, a potent activator of energy *storage*. High insulin levels signal the body to put the brakes on energy use and to ramp up energy hoarding—to absorb glucose and fat from the blood, to stop breaking down stored glucose (glycogen) and fat, and to initiate additional glucose and fat synthesis and storage. Thus insulin makes fat energy harder to release and easier to accumulate.

Insulin also has an indirect role in triggering hunger. When we eat an easily digested meal, blood glucose spikes and insulin rushes in to shuttle the recently consumed, easily metabolized sugars into the cells. This in turn dramatically reduces blood sugar, as it should, but the effect of the big relative drop in levels is that you soon feel hungry again. We call this state of low blood sugar hypoglycemia. It triggers feelings of hunger to prompt us to eat in order to restore blood sugar to its previous (high) equilibrium.

It's the sugar rush followed by the blood sugar drop that makes simple, high-glycemic, highly processed, highly palatable, easily digested carbs a primary culprit in fat accumulation and obesity. A diet full of cheap carbs routinely floods the body with insulin, which, if it becomes chronic, may lead to fat gain that does not reverse itself.

Simply following the broad guidelines set out in the Basic Plan will put you on the path to better balance with regard to leptin, ghrelin, and insulin. But here are some additional tips:

- Eat foods that contain fiber to keep you fuller longer, avoid sugary snacks, and incorporate plenty of plant-based foods for their anti-inflammatory and antioxidative effects. Simple carbohydrates are quick energy sources that lack fiber and nutrients that your body needs. Complex carbohydrates are better because they provide you with energy as well as nutrients and fiber, and greater satiety.
  - *Seeds are the best source of starch, since 70 percent of their weight is composed of complex carbs.*
  - *Beans and peas are the second best source of complex carbs, as they are made up of 40 percent starch by weight.*
  - *Tubers, which come in third, include many foods that are particularly popular in non-Western cultures, such as cassava and yams.*
- Drink green tea for its EGCG, a catechin that prevents fat buildup in the liver and keeps the liver healthy.
- Eat avocados, which help to detoxify the liver and are loaded with unsaturated fats. They also contain a lot of fiber, which helps to keep your hunger in check.
- Eat nutrient-dense—not calorie-rich—food like nuts (walnuts, almonds), vegetables (broccoli, kale, spinach), fruit (oranges, strawberries, blueberries), and coldwater fish (salmon, cod). By eating a healthy assortment of carbohydrates, proteins, and fats, your body will maintain adequate energy stores and your hunger pangs will be kept at bay too.
- Exercise portion control. If you eat three ecogenetically balanced meals a day and snack on healthy foods, then you'll be more energized and healthy. So avoid piling too much food onto your plate. For perspective on what is meant by a "serving" throughout the book, here's what I consider an optimal serving of several food items:
  - *cheese: 1 slice, 1-inch cube, 1 ounce*
  - *nuts (never peanuts): 2 teaspoons nut spreads, almonds (eight), cashews (six)*

- *oils: 2 teaspoons*
- *salad dressing: 2 tablespoons olive oil and balsamic vinegar or lemon juice*
- *seeds: 2 tablespoons pumpkin seeds*
- *flaxseed: 2 tablespoons, ground*
- *soy nuts: 2 tablespoons*
- *berries: 1 cup*
- *yogurt: 8 ounces*
- *vegetables: 1 cup raw, ½ cup cooked*

There are many other factors to consider in bringing the whole system into a fuller, wider, health-reinforcing balance, but certainly one of the most crucial factors for targeting obesity is to take control of your insulin response to food.

Of all the easily digested carbs fueling our current epidemic of obesity, perhaps the most pervasive—and the most dangerous—is *refined fructose*. In nature, fructose appears mainly in fruits, berries, corn, and root vegetables, including cane sugar and beets. But in our diets, fructose all too often appears in the form of refined table sugar or in the form of high-fructose corn syrup, which, in its most common configuration, is 55 percent fructose and 43 percent glucose.

To see how insidious concentrated fructose can be, we need only look back to the role of ghrelin and leptin in turning on and then turning off our feelings of hunger. The fact is, these hormones respond differently to fructose than to the simple glucose that most carbohydrates break down into. A study comparing ghrelin and leptin levels after glucose-rich or fructose-rich meals found that, in comparison, the fructose doses both decreased leptin (the "off" signal) and increased ghrelin (the "on" signal), creating a double whammy that decouples hunger signals from actual energy needs.[6]

Fructose is more "lipogenetic" than glucose, meaning the body converts fructose into fat more easily than it does glucose. This means that fructose is an especially potent driver of insulin resistance and, by desensitizing the body to insulin, it promotes fat accumulation and obesity. In particular, fructose promotes storage of fat in the liver, which can result in nonalcoholic fatty liver disease (NAFLD), which in turn is strongly correlated with insulin resistance.[7]

In one recent study, mice were brought into a state of insulin insensitivity by being fed a high-fructose diet. However, when a specific gene (PGC-1b) responsible for accumulating fat in the liver was disabled, the mice were protected from developing insulin resistance.[8] They had become, in effect, "fructose-proof." Scientists were able to determine that a single fructose-activated gene was the linchpin in a cascading series of other fat-accumulating genes. Blocking the ability of fructose to initiate that epigenetic domino chain meant, for these mice, avoiding insulin resistance and obesity. This is the kind of effect we're trying to have with our epigenetic approach to food choices.

Given the specific effects of fructose on hunger and insulin resistance, it's no wonder that the rise in high-fructose corn syrup consumption has so closely paralleled the rise in obesity rates. High-fructose corn syrup is everywhere, adding not only to our sugar consumption but adding extra calories to all the foods it is used in—in sodas, snack foods, commercial or bottled salad dressings, and so on. The average American now consumes almost *forty pounds* of high-fructose corn syrup each year.

Taken together, these points are a powerful argument in favor of seriously minimizing artificially concentrated fructose in your diet. I do, however, recommend consuming fruits, berries, and root vegetables, all of which contain some fructose. Again, it's the glycemic index of carbohydrates that affects gene expression and disease risk.

Sleep and Hunger

As I mentioned earlier, ghrelin (the "on" signal for appetite) rises during night-time sleep. But, curiously, in one study dramatic sleep deprivation was associated with increases in ghrelin production and with declines in the production of leptin (the "off" signal). As ghrelin rose and leptin fell, participants in the study not only felt hungrier but also found their food more palatable. Just as significant, after sleep deprivation these study subjects had a special craving for calorie-dense carbohydrates like sweets, snack foods, and starches.[9]

As we previously discussed, these are just the foods most likely to lead to insulin spikes, and thus to storing more energy as fat. So failing to sleep well is not unlike starvation: it puts the body into a state of perceived hunger crisis that it tries to rectify in the most efficient way, which, unfortunately, is also the least healthful way.

So another aspect of our epigenetic approach to overall health—including avoiding obesity—is to try to regularize your sleep patterns so that you achieve the typical requirement of seven to eight hours each night. Getting the appropriate amount of sleep not only combats obesity, it improves mood, improves concentration, and contributes to higher energy levels. And as we will continue to see over and over, many of these health conditions are subtly interlinked. By affecting mood, sleep in turn affects energy and eating patterns, which can circle back to affect how much we sleep. Health is an integrated system that needs to be approached on many fronts simultaneously.

Protein

Another well-established way to curb your appetite is by eating protein. As we've seen, protein itself produces a feeling of fullness. And because protein does not affect blood sugar or insulin levels, you will not feel hungry soon after eating a protein-rich meal. So adding protein is a good thing and, by the same token, subtracting protein can be bad.

If you restrict protein too much when dieting, you may actually end up overeating because the body tries to compensate via appetite for the depletion of protein levels in what is known as the protein leverage effect. In one study, men and women whose protein intake fell below 10 percent tended to eat more carbs and fatty foods, resulting in weight gain. The researchers suggested that keeping total protein intake between 15 and 25 percent helped to curb weight gain.[10]

One of the best studies of its kind, the Diogenes study showed that a higher protein intake allowed people to maintain weight loss after completing a diet.[11] The study results emphasized that a long-term healthy diet is one in which basal metabolic rate is increased (see below) and hunger is diminished. The study participants accomplished this with a good variety of protein-rich foods, including beans, dairy, lean meats, and fish, while at the same time limiting processed sugar and flour.

As you've already seen, a source of protein I strongly recommend (for multiple purposes) is nuts, especially unpeeled raw almonds, hazelnuts, and walnuts. These have been shown to raise the levels of serotonin in people diagnosed with metabolic syndrome. Serotonin functions to maintain energy levels and regulate metabolism in the body by transmitting nerve impulses to the brain that signal satiety. It also helps to control glucose balance, one of the primary challenges for those with diabetes, and indeed for the many prediabetic and preobese people who struggle with insulin insensitivity.[12]

It also takes about twice as many calories to digest protein as it does fats or carbs. Keep in mind that digesting your ecogenetic food alone accounts for one-tenth of the calories that your body burns daily. And almost one-third of the calories in protein are burned just via digestion!

Following the same principle, I also recommend building muscle through exercise—a pound of muscle burns about 6 calories per day, whereas a pound of fat burns only 2.

The Ecogenetics of Eliminating Fat

We have discussed the first half of the energy equation: how eating, as medi-ated by appetite, can cause us to take in more energy than we actually need to function. Now we will look at the second half of the equation: how we can en-courage our bodies to burn off or otherwise get rid of excessive fat energy stores we already have.

Raise Basal Metabolism

Probably the most direct way to eliminate excess fat is to raise metabolism. Your basal metabolic rate (BMR) is the number of calories that you burn at rest, which means the amount of energy your body uses to carry out its essen-tial functions, such as thinking, breathing, maintaining skeletal muscle, and keeping the heart pumping. The higher your BMR, the more calories you burn, including calories from fat stores, just by existing. These are in effect "free" expenditures, since they require no special effort or decision on your part. They are also the largest portion of energy use—BMR accounts for around 70 per-cent of the calories we burn during a typical day. Another 20 percent is used in exercise, and the remaining 10 percent goes to digestion of food. You inherit much of your BMR with your genes, but in true ecogenetic fashion, you can also take steps to increase it by changing your behavior.

The first thing to mention is that leptin, in addition to its role in govern-ing appetite, also has specific effects on fat metabolism. In general, these track the appetite effects: leptin up-regulates metabolism when you are energy satis-fied and down-regulates metabolism when you are energy deprived. This is one part of the self-balancing system I described—fat burning increases when you have excess energy, thus bringing the system back down to balance, and de-creases when you don't have enough energy, thus saving or "defending" fat stores in case of extended deprivation. But just as they do with hormonal bal-ances, leptin insensitivity and obesity mix up this metabolic process. The body gets used to high circulating levels of leptin (from its substantial fat stores) and treats a drop in these levels as starvation, which it then fights by slowing me-tabolism. This is a primary reason why losing weight, once you have accumu-lated a lot of fat tissue, is so difficult. The body interprets normalizing fat levels as life-threatening.

So the first point of business is to get a handle on the hunger hormones, as described above, which will in turn indirectly push metabolism in the right direction. After this, the simplest way to raise your basal metabolic rate is to increase your muscle mass through exercise. As I suggested above, lean body mass burns much more energy than fat. By reducing fat, through the strategies outlined here, and also by building muscle, you can multiply your antifat metabolic advantage. Even a modest weight training program—about half an hour three days a week—can substantially improve your "free" fat burning power.

Starve Fat Cells

It is estimated that each pound of fat requires almost a *mile* of blood vessels for support. Blood vessels are created through a process called angiogenesis, and knowledge of that process gives us another point of access for moderating weight gain.

The study of cancer has taught us a great deal about the role of angiogenesis in fat tissue accumulation. Cancer cells thrive in an oxygen-rich environment because they need oxygen and nutrients provided by the blood in order to grow. Blood vessels also serve as a conduit by which cancer cells travel to other areas of the body, a process called metastasis. Some novel anticancer therapies exploit this dependency; the basic idea is that by destroying the biological context in which cancer cells live, we can indirectly eliminate the cancer itself. And this indirect approach has in fact proved a fruitful tactic in treating a number of cancers.

Applying similar conceptual models—laying siege rather than attempting a full frontal assault—researchers have begun to test whether noncancer cells can similarly be "decontextualized." Using mice treated with agents that block the growth of blood vessels, scientists have reported a reduction in vascularization of adipose tissue and subsequent death of fat cells.[13] So the model seems to hold true for fat as well: by indirectly targeting fat cells through their dependence on blood supply, we can actually "starve" them to death.

Another study set out to produce a quantitative model for angiogenesis in adipose tissue. The researchers implanted immature fat cells beneath the skin of mice. Over two to three weeks, these nascent cells developed into fat pads with all the characteristics of normal subcutaneous fat tissue. But the really interesting finding was that blood vessels began to grow in and around the new cells within five days of implantation. This microvasculature appeared to spread out from larger blood vessels in the surrounding area.[14]

Yet another study tested the siege hypothesis from the other direction, to see whether existing fat tissue could be destroyed. Researchers fed two groups of mice an agent that blocks angiogenesis. One of the groups was made up of mice fed a high-calorie diet. The other group consisted of obese mice that lacked leptin, the appetite's "off" switch. In both cases, the mice either slowed the rate of weight gain or lost weight. The researchers even reported increased insulin sensitivity in the mice. So it appears that blocking angiogenesis in fat tissue not only destroys fat cells and prevents their further formation, but also helps to straighten out the very complex entanglement of hormones that is part and parcel of the diseases of fat—obesity, metabolic syndrome, type 2 diabetes, and so on.[15]

So how can we take advantage of this strategy and actively target the blood supplies of our fat cells? One promising approach is the use of curcumin, the chemical element that provides the yellow color in the spice turmeric, a member of the ginger family native to South Asia. Curcumin appears to affect the expression of vascular endothelial growth factor (VEGF) and its receptor VEGFR-2, which is involved in angiogenesis. Mice placed on a high-fat diet supplemented with curcumin not only did not gain weight, they lost fat. The spice also lowered cholesterol levels and other important genetic components involved in the development of fat cells.[16]

Because most American families don't cook with turmeric, I suggest using turmeric supplements to deliver a consistent, daily dose of fat-fighting nutrients. For those who prefer to cook with the spice itself, I suggest using turmeric root or powder rather than a pure form of curcumin, because whole turmeric provides additional nutrients and targets inflammatory conditions better than curcumin alone.

Fat Cell Death

In the human organism, billions of cells die off and are neatly disposed of each and every day. The cell death that occurs as part of the planned life cycle of an organism is called apoptosis. This is "programmed" cell death that is beneficial for the organism, as opposed to necrosis, which is unplanned tissue death as a result of injury or infection.

Apoptosis is a well-coordinated element of the body's continuous housecleaning operations. In a sense, apoptosis is the opposite of cancer: cancer is uncontrolled cell division and unnatural cell longevity; apoptosis is the routine limitation of cell activity within a useful life span.

Given this rough context for cell life, it makes sense that an appealing pathway for targeting obesity would be fat cell apoptosis. If we could consciously encourage fat cells to die their natural deaths, we could theoretically reduce fat tissue from the inside out—not just burn it off, but actually kill it through its own internal mechanisms.

This is an ongoing area of research, but preliminary evidence suggests that certain compounds can indeed encourage apoptosis in fat cells. Happily, the foods involved are healthful in other ways as well.

One of these is garlic, which contains a sulfur-containing compound called ajoene that has been shown to induce cell death in fat cells through the activation of hydrogen peroxide. This operates at the genetic level by encouraging many of the typical activities of apoptosis: fragmenting DNA, stimulating mitogen-activated protein kinases (protein kinases that are involved in triggering apoptosis and other regulatory functions), and migrating apoptosis-inducing factor (AIF) from the mitochondria to the nucleus.[17] Garlic is good for you in so many other ways that adding it to your regular diet is a no-brainer for both fat-related and general health.

Scientists have also reported that the active compound of a gum resin called guggulsterone, which is commonly used in the traditional medicine of India, induces fat cell death and blocks the formation of fat cells.[18] Piperine, a major component of black pepper, appears to block the development of new fat cells.[19]

And genistein, which is an estrogen-like compound found in plants such as fava beans and soybeans, has also been shown to induce apoptosis in fat cells. However, the apoptotic effects appear to be magnified by the addition of vitamin D3. In fact, the combination of vitamin D3 and genistein is 200 percent more productive than using genistein alone.[20]

Exercise

The to-do list for people hoping to reduce fat almost always includes exercise. I think it's important to remember that the goal is not to rival the performance of a professional, but to reap the rewards of a generally active life. The same perspective should apply in the context of weight loss. Exercise becomes much more palatable when it is not some dreaded chore we have to perform in the hope of trimming our bellies, but rather a pleasant part of life that makes us feel more alive.

In this context, it may be advisable to make smaller adjustments to the activities we are already doing than to try to introduce new, time-consuming, and perhaps daunting practices.

Rather than trying to commit to doing a weekly track session, then, with sprints and carefully timed recovery intervals, or an all-out two-hour weight training routine, try walking to the office three times a week, or taking the stairs rather than the escalators for part of your morning route, or getting off the bus a stop or two earlier to walk the rest of the way, or even just standing during some subway rides rather than always sitting.

Once activity becomes the default condition instead of a costly add-on, you can expand into exercise that is more sports or training based. If you already enjoy sports or physical activities, all the better. But for many people who have too much fat and too much inactivity, the real challenge—the one that will make the biggest difference—is making the mental shift from seeing activity as performance to seeing activity as the basic context for healthy living.

The fact is, the human organism requires regular moderate physical activity in order to function correctly. We evolved on the move, hunting and gathering food, finding shelter, following seasonal opportunities, defending ourselves from attack, and so on. When we become sedentary, we deprive the body of a fundamental component of its normal ecogenetic environment. Activity *is* the base state, the baseline for health. So rather than thinking about how to add activity to your inactive life, think about limiting the dose of inactivity in a life that needs to be active.

Ideas for Actions

Research has shown that working out in the morning helps to start your day off on the right track. Morning exercisers adhere better to their fitness regimen because it's the first thing they do—it's a routine. Studies have also shown that working out in the morning helps people sleep better. In particular, one study reported that overweight women who exercised at least four hours a week in the morning slept better than women who exercised less.[21] Interestingly, in this study the women who exercised in the evening and worked out for at least four hours a week still reported that they had trouble falling asleep.

A key aspect of the sleep-food-exercise connection is that hormones (such as serotonin) that control appetite are influenced by your body's internal clock. And exercise, especially a morning routine, is part of this paradigm because it helps to normalize your body's rhythm. So exercising in the morning not only helps you sleep well, it also controls hormones that help you eat better.

Exercise has benefits beyond controlling weight. It enhances mood and gives us an energy boost that can be transferred to work or play. Yoga, in particular, not only helps people keep their weight down, it also raises body awareness, which prompts people to stop eating when they're full.

The Antiobesity Attitude

Of all the culprits we can implicate in our epidemic of obesity, perhaps the most fundamental is our twenty-first-century drive to simultaneously *live hard* (stress out, lose sleep) and *live easy* (ride the train of convenience).

So the ecogenetic shift you need to make begins in changing how you think. Changing years of ecogenetically harmful habits—eating cheap carbs, eating too much sugar, overdosing on late nights, and inactivity—will take time, practice, patience, and persistence. While it may not be a simple fix to reverse the bad habits that are compounding obesity, taking the time to commit to these changes will benefit you in the long run because you'll not only lose weight, you'll keep it off.

The first thing I tell my patients is to think long term about weight loss. It's not about seeing that magical number when you step on a scale or fitting into a specific dress size. Because once those goals are achieved, most people will notice a slow creeping back of the pounds. And before they know it they've gained all the weight back and then some.

Achieving and maintaining a healthy weight begins with recognizing that a slow, steady pace wins the race. Wake up each day committed to instituting a healthier set of patterns until they become a part of your daily routine: enjoy a directed, varied, balanced diet as described in Chapter 1; break the carb and sugar addiction by avoiding foods that spike appetite; target the particular foods that have been shown to help eliminate fat; embrace your body's natural expectation of system-preserving sleep and frequent moderate activity. Perhaps no one of these items will make the difference for you. But taken together, they are a robust recipe for a better, leaner life.

Even so, the program outlined here is no quick fix—following these recommendations won't completely reverse obesity in a month or two (although you will start moving things in the right direction as soon as you start implementing them). But it provides something much more valuable: the blueprint for an antiobesity attitude.

They say that the first thing you should do when you find yourself in a hole is to stop digging. Similarly, the first thing we need to do is halt the slide toward the disease of fat. Then you can begin to consolidate the good habits that will be the substance of lifelong leanness. And that is what is crucial: the change in yourself that comes from changing how you think about yourself. No quick fix could ever really work—this is work that *you* have to do. By knowing how to target yourself for health, and then making the changes to do so, you are already a different person. It's the extraordinary ecogenetic opportunity we always have in front of us: to make ourselves, by following our bodies' guidance, more fully who we wish to be.

Targeted Supplements

Targeted Ecogenetic Juice for Weight Management

The following juice recipe is for those who are concerned about weight control. But don't feel as though you have to drink this specific juice every day. Shake things up! I've included several juicing recipes after the disease-specific chapter's section. The ecogenetic juices listed are general recipes that focus on using wholesome ingredients and organically grown produce that have beneficial effects on many body systems. So you don't have to worry about sticking to any specific drink. My patients usually drink one or two ecogenetic juices daily. Mix up the juices you drink to broaden your intake of bioactive nutrients on a weekly basis. If you have a specific health concern, increase your intake of that recommended ecogenetic drink.

> 2 celery stalks
> 1 beet
> ¼ cup freshly squeezed lime juice
> ½ cup brewed green tea
> 1 tablespoon whey protein powder
> ¼ cup blueberries
> 1 peeled lemon, including seeds
>
> Juice the celery and beet. Blend with the other ingredients for 15 to 20 seconds on low. Drink and enjoy.

Targeted Ecogenetic Supplements for Weight Management

The supplements listed below are recommended for achieving and maintaining a healthy weight. Don't get overwhelmed and feel that you have to take every supplement listed. Remember: everyone is unique. The supplement list is in no particular order. I recommend them all equally to my patients because each one has benefits in weight management. Many of my patients start off by taking one supplement to determine how well they are tolerating it. Then they add other supplements as needed. When taking supplements, the focus should be to maintain good health. Don't worry about whether you should be taking five, ten, or fifteen supplements. That is not the intent of the supplement list. Do what you can. And take your time in figuring out what works for you: good health isn't a destination; it's a lifelong practice. And supplements are a small part of attaining a healthy lifestyle. Supplements are meant to be an addition to—not a replacement for—eating a healthy diet, getting adequate sleep, and improving your level of physical activity.

The supplements below are among the most important ones I give to many of my patients. Because every person is different, certain supplements may be more important than others for a given individual.

- Bladder wrack (brown seaweed extract)—150 milligrams, twice daily
- Jarrow-Dophilus (probiotic)—once daily
- Green coffee bean (*Coffea arabica*, contains 5 percent chlorogenic acid)—500 milligrams, once daily
- Glucomannan—665 milligrams, one before each meal
- Guggul extract—500 milligrams, twice daily
- Kyolic Cardiovascular (deodorized garlic)—600 milligrams, twice daily
- Forskohlii root (*Coleus forskohlii*, contains 10 percent forskohlii)—350 milligrams, once daily
- L-tyrosine—500 milligrams, once daily
- Gingerroot extract—30 milligrams, once daily
- CLA—750 milligrams, twice daily
- Apple pectin—500 milligrams, one before meals
- Resveratrol—100 milligrams, once daily
- Meriva-SR (slow-release turmeric root extract)—500 milligrams, twice daily
- Black pepper fruit extract (*Piper nigrum*), contains 95 percent piperine—20 milligrams, once daily
- *Phaseolus vulgaris* seed extract—445 milligrams, one before each meal

Chapter 3

Heart Disease

HEART DISEASE IS THE NUMBER ONE KILLER IN DEVELOPED COUNTRIES. If you combine heart disease and stroke (both of which are largely related to blood vessel blockages), it is also the number one cause of death in poorer countries. But this sobering fact counts only *deaths*. The toll from disability is much greater. In the United States alone, there are more than one million heart attacks each year and eight hundred thousand strokes.

Heart disease comes in many forms. These include heart failure—when the heart muscle is simply too weak to keep up with its workload—valve problems, and the problem of irregular heartbeat known as arrhythmia. Yet the most significant category is disease of the blood vessels, or cardiovascular disease (CVD). When blood vessels to the heart become acutely clogged, the result is a heart attack; when the blocked blood vessels involved are those feeding the brain, it is a stroke. It is projected that, by 2030, almost 40 percent of Americans will suffer from some form of active cardiovascular disease.

But just because CVD is already more deadly than starvation, AIDS, malaria, or war, that doesn't mean we are powerless to stop it. In fact, the opposite is true. Once again, it is never too late to bring back balance. You see, the same ecogenetic combination of inflammation, toxins, and processed foods sow the seeds for heart disease just as they do for obesity.

Success Story

Meet Heidi. She's a forty-six-year-old nurse who came to see me for a second opinion. She had been diagnosed with stage IV breast cancer and heart failure, the latter of which developed as a result of two medications—Herceptin and Adriamycin—prescribed to treat her cancer. I agreed with her oncologist about continuing the Herceptin, which was essential for the cancer, but only if her heart function improved. So I started her on intravenous taurine (an amino acid critical to heart function) and intravenous glutathione (a tripeptide for cellular repair). I prescribed the supplements PQQ, CoQ10, and carnosine for mitochondrial support. As part of an ecogenetic diet targeted for the heart, I prescribed Enada (reduced NADH), acetyl-L-carnitine, fish oil, and Y.S. Eco Bee Farms' Triple Bee Complex (royal jelly, bee pollen, and bee propolis). Finally, I provided her with a recipe for a daily shake:

> 1 teaspoon D-ribose
> 1 teaspoon Thorne Amino Complex powder
> 1 tablespoon acai berry powder
> 3 drops vitamin D3 (3,000 IU)
> 1 tablespoon MetaCore cacao powder
> 1 tablespoon magnesium powder
> 1 tablespoon black raspberry powder

Mix all ingredients with 6 ounces almond milk and blend on low for 15 seconds.

Over a six-week period, Heidi's heart function returned to normal, and she was able to resume Herceptin treatment for her breast cancer.

The process by which arteries become clogged is called *atherosclerosis*, which means "gruel-filled lesion." That's a fairly gross description of what is in fact a pretty disgusting development: the arteries literally being pimpled over with inflamed, oozing sores. You may think of narrowing of the arteries or hardening of the arteries as an old person's disease. And it's true that heart attacks and strokes occur more frequently in older adults. But this tendency masks an enormously important truth: that we are all almost certainly atherosclerotic to some degree. I've already mentioned the appearance of heart disease in young military casualties. In another study, 99 percent of the children examined, who were all two to fifteen, showed some evidence of atherosclerotic disease.[1] Heart disease usually manifests later in life only because it takes that long to build up to something that grabs our attention, usually once it's become life-threatening.

So what can we do to protect ourselves? First, we need to know the *environments* in which the disease manifests so that we can identify where and how we can manipulate these environmental factors for the better. Once you begin to assess the landscape, you see that atherosclerosis occurs in a fairly narrow and predictable range of circumstances.

The Environments of Heart Disease

The Tree of Life

There are over sixty thousand miles of veins and arteries twisting and turning in the average human body. They start at the heart and fan up, out, and down. The aorta is the main outward channel and is about an inch thick. From that beginning, the vessels spread to the fingers and the toes, passing into every nook and cranny in between, in order to bring nourishment to the cells. As they go, they branch off into smaller and smaller side channels and tributaries, which is why the whole system is sometimes called the arterial tree.

One of the marked aspects of atherosclerotic buildups—and one that we need to consider if we're going to get to the bottom of the causes of cardiovascular disease—is that they are much likelier to occur at the branching and bending points along the vessels.

A River of Blood

If you've ever gone canoeing on a fast river, you already know what tends to happen when the flooded river rounds a corner: all the force and momentum of the water rushes forward to the *outside* of the bend. Meanwhile, on the inside of the bend, away from the full current, calmer water and eddies appear, and sometimes there are even reverse eddies, in which the water begins to flow backward against itself in irregular, turbulent loops.

This is exactly what happens in your vascular system. The pumping blood courses through the arteries, speeding down the straightaways and hurtling into the bends and branches where the arterial tree curves and divides. Over time, in those inner-bend areas where the blood tends to stagnate, the irregular flow of the fluid pushes both debris and pressure eddies into the arterial banks. This irritates the vessel walls at those spots and makes them vulnerable to abrasion and penetration by various drifting stuff, most significantly by particles of low-density lipoproteins, also known as "bad" cholesterol. In response to the damage, and also because they can sense the weakened flow, the vessel cells send out an alarm. This leads to an inflammatory reaction, with white blood cells arriving on the scene. In pursuit of the unwelcome cholesterol, they penetrate the arterial wall, and the result, when combined with some of the other trash deposits left by the stagnating blood, may be a new atherosclerotic lesion.

The Endothelial Wall

The innermost layer of cells—those closest to the blood—that make up the structure of the arteries is called the *endothelium*. The endothelial cells are long and thin in order to provide both shape and flexibility to the snaking blood tubes. They are also extremely smooth and slippery in order to speed the blood plasma flowing by. Unlike most other kinds of connective cells, they do not overlap; they fit end to end like row upon row of paving stones. With no overlapping edges to collect debris, and also very little depth for particles to work their way in against, these cells are highly resistant to mechanical penetration.

Nonetheless, despite the beautiful design, the endothelium is regularly breached, with "leaky" junctions occurring at spots on the wall where endothelial cells are dying or being replaced. One assault comes from high blood pressure, which makes the endothelium stretch and become thinner and more permeable, like a balloon blown too full of air. Over time the lining material begins to break down, and eventually it may spring a leak. If the blood has a high concentration of LDL particles in it, the pressure gradient across the artery surface encourages LDL to move through the holes in the barrier, to equalize the pressure. Once it passes through the weak spot, LDL can be retained in the interior of the artery wall for days and weeks, where a variety of bad things can happen. Other LDL particles may join it; it may begin to oxidize and break down; over long periods and under the right conditions large pools of cholesterol may collect; and, as mentioned above, when the body attacks these waste deposits in order to remove them, you have the beginnings of an atherosclerotic plaque, the waste product that most dangerously narrows the arteries.

But the critical point to remember is that while the shape of the vessel affects the blood flow dynamics, the nature of the blood flow helps to determine the shape of the vessel. The blood vessels are not merely a passive plumbing system, shuttling energy and nutrients where they need to go. They are in fact active participants in regulating the blood flow and in responding to it.

The endothelial cells are able to detect the pressure of the blood's flow rate, and in response to high-flow environments they can suppress a variety of inflammatory responses.

This has a whole range of good effects. Typically, among the first triggered inflammation responses is the call for adhesion molecules—that is, the activated endothelial cells become "stickier" in order to attract various healing agents. Blood and other kinds of cells rolling down the artery walls literally get stuck on the inflaming endothelial tar patch. These add-on healer cells actually exacerbate the problem by inflating the size of the plaque and eventually becoming part of the dangerous mass of a heart attack–inducing blood clot. By silencing the call to become sticky, the strong flow helps to keep the vessel walls smooth and trash-free; scum doesn't accumulate on the artery lining, and the chances of irritation and damage are much reduced.

There are other good effects too. High flow encourages the expression of antioxidant defense genes that help to reduce the damages of rancid, oxidizing LDL. And when they detect the strong flow, the endothelial cells can actually send signals to expand the diameter of the arteries, through the release of nitric oxide, so that any narrowing by lesions and plaques is offset by natural vessel widening.

Yet all of these benefits are reversed in the low-flow areas: inflammation gene processes are heightened, the smooth paving stone wall becomes sticky and begins to catch flotsam from the blood, the LDL particles that enter the wall induce further rounds of inflammation and thus exacerbate autoimmune attack, the wall begins to break down from the inside out, more damaging repair work ensues—and this, in short, is the sad cycle of heart disease.

Gene Therapy Fact: Can Care

The thought of a hot bowl of soup is comforting, especially during the winter months. But before you crack open a can, consider this. Volunteers in a study were divided into two groups. Both ate soup for five days, one from cans and the other from fresh ingredients. BPA levels measured in the urine at the end of the study were 12 times higher in the canned soup group.[2] BPA has been linked to diabetes, heart disease, and cancer.

What the Blood Bears

So the arteries present a very particular determining environment for athero-sclerosis. Simply by virtue of its shape, the arterial tree has a set of mechanical weak spots where blood flow tends to be slower and irregular. Under the wrong conditions, this hemodynamic setting triggers a series of detrimental reactions by the vessel walls: unsuppressed inflammation, silenced protective genes, arterial hardening rather than relaxing and expanding, coagulation, and trash accumulating.

But once again, biological environments affect and change one another. In the case of the endothelium, it not only responds to the flow quality, whether smooth and strong or disrupted and slow, it also responds to the content of the blood. Another way of saying this is that what the blood bears helps to determine how the arteries react. The arterial structure shapes how the blood content moves through it, but the content also shapes how the structure does its shaping.

During your entire life, your arteries are in constant contact with blood. Day after day, year after year, the blood courses along, pumping through in its steady, inexorable rhythm. And that blood is full of a mind-boggling array of particles, cells, and information. White blood cells are patrolling for infections; tiny platelet cells stream along in case of leaks, which they plug; and, like the constant foot traffic in a city, the red blood cells are endlessly circulating in their great, revolving duty to bring the breath of life to every nook and cranny in the body.

For our purposes, however, the most important of these particles are the LDL packages: the low-density lipoprotein containers that transport cholesterol and other fats around the body. The LDLs are considered the "bad" cholesterols because they are the ones that breach the endothelium, get trapped, oxidize, and then set off the atherosclerotic reactions. But no cholesterol is really bad in itself—all cells need it to survive, notably for use in constructing the cell membranes that provide their structural integrity.

The problem occurs when there is too much of a necessary thing. Lots of small, dense LDLs are like grains of rice in a colander—inevitably, some are going to sneak through the holes. This is a crucial point because LDL has other effects. It turns out that LDL, just like the endothelial cells or the fat cells, is not a passive but a powerfully active agent in the environment it helps to create. We said that the endothelium makes itself sticky in response to sluggish and irregular blood flow. Blood and other particles drifting along the vessel get attracted to the site of inflammation—sort of like rubbernecking at a highway accident. LDL provokes the same response simply by its presence in the blood, by changing gene expression, which then sets off a domino chain that ends by (once again) making the endothelial cells stickier and more attractive to clotting agents. Other studies have linked LDL levels to suppression of endothelial nitric oxide signals and thus suppression of the arteries' ability to dilate—the same process triggered by blood flow rates.[3]

We are beginning to assemble a good picture of the environments involved in atherosclerosis. Low blood flow combined with high LDL concentrations are mutually exacerbating conditions, and they exacerbate many of the *same* responses. In effect, their combination is a doubling of the double whammy: mechanically, both conditions set the stage for heart disease, and these same conditions trigger further changes in genetic expression (via epigenetic changes in the vessel walls) that intensify the risks. In this sense, the environment of heart disease is quite specific and identifiable—those curving areas where flow is low, where the vessel walls are sensitive and often stickier, and where mobs of LDLs further inflame, deform, and then crowd through the walls they have helped to break up.

The Epigenetic Environment

Once again, the environments in which the body operates—whether these are external geographical ones or internal physiological ones—have an enormous influence on gene expression.

So, when you look ever more closely, it makes sense that flow rates would either suppress or excite inflammation by activating or silencing helpful or detrimental genes. Or that what makes disturbed, sluggish flow *dangerous* is not that it's slow—the body doesn't care about any of this one way or the other—but in part that the slowness silences the messages of antioxidant genes that could combat the damaging oxidation of LDL. The *effect* of this slowness is to make changes in the epigenome and hence in the activated genome that make atherosclerosis more likely. *That's* what's bad about it.

One powerful epigenetic effect involves an amino acid called *homocysteine,* a by-product of protein metabolism and DNA methylation. DNA methylation is a crucial epigenetic process that influences gene activity. Folic acid and B vitamins help to convert homocysteine to methionine, which is necessary for DNA methylation. Without adequate amounts of fruits and leafy green vegetables, the body does not have enough vitamins to convert homocysteine. Not only do large amounts of homocysteine block DNA methylation, but this has been linked to kidney disease, colon cancer, brittle bones, and heart disease.

So how exactly does homocysteine affect the cardiovascular system? The particular *environment* that homocysteine occurs in and helps to create dictates its ecogenetic effects. Researchers have found, for example, that homocysteine corrodes some of the structural elements of the blood vessels.[4] High levels break down the arteries' collagen and elastin—the very same connective tissue proteins that give shape and tone to your lips and skin. Such corrosion contributes to the weakness and permeability of the endothelium—the innermost layer of blood vessels. The loss of endothelial integrity creates those leaky junctions, which allows LDLs to cross from the lumen into the blood vessel wall and form arterial plaques. These plaques lead to cardiovascular diseases such as heart attacks and strokes.

The Ecogenetic Way

We have seen how individual aspects of the environments in our bodies affect one another back and forth—how, for example, the vessels' shape determines blood flow and, conversely, how blood flow determines vessel wall responses. This kind of reciprocity or overlap is also the case when we think about how to act in order to tilt the environments back in our favor.

For instance, many of the actions that help our vessels stay strong will also keep our cholesterol levels lower. And eating to keep cholesterol in check will also ordinarily suppress inflammation. This is one of the secrets of universal good health: just as the double whammy of high LDL and low flow will suck your health down the drain, so adding good nutrition to physical activity and proper supplementation will stack your benefits many times higher.

In a way, this doubling down on the good stuff is using disease against itself. Disease processes typically reinforce one another—that's why in this book you will repeatedly encounter phenomena such as inflammation or obesity or a sedentary lifestyle. Diseases "use" all these contexts in order to advance their states, whether it's heart disease or cancer or diabetes. Your job is to reclaim these same elements, turn the tables on unhealth, and replace a confluence of disability with a synergy of well-being.

Go with the Flow

One of the best and simplest things you can do for your blood vessels is to ramp up the flow rate. As we saw, there are a number of positive effects from higher flows: more nitric oxide, less inflammation, less scum accumulation, more flexible and nicely widened vessels, and activated antioxidant gene expression. And low flow is bad in all the reverse ways. In patients with serious heart disease, blood flow may be as much as 40 percent slower throughout the body! That is a seriously stagnant river of blood.

So, what can you do?

Move!

When your heart beats faster, it's pumping the blood faster, which means the flow is increased. The endothelial cells are stimulated to release more nitric oxide, which is the chemical messenger that tells the artery to relax and let the blood flow freely. Studies have shown that even quite moderate exercise, when done consistently, can dramatically increase average flow rates and the diameter of arteries.[5] I recommend approximately thirty minutes of aerobic exercise daily to significantly improve your chances of avoiding serious heart trouble. In this context, "aerobic" means that you are breathing more heavily than normal, but you don't have to be completely out of breath and covered with sweat. So while a jog around the park might be a great thing, a brisk walk will also do you a world of good.

On the downside, a sedentary lifestyle will certainly slow down your flow. The arteries are just like any other muscle in your body: they need to be used and challenged to remain strong. When they are allowed to weaken through too much disuse, they do what all out-of-shape tissues do: they lose their flexibility, they respond to changes more slowly, and they become more prone to injury. Because we are all slowly (or quickly) accumulating cholesterol in our vessel walls, it's crucial that we don't allow ourselves to become passive.

A+ Fats

When it comes to human behavior, type Bs are supposed to be the nice guys. They're the ones who get along, the easygoing types. Type As are hard-charging, self-interested, and always on the verge of running someone over.

In the world of lipoproteins, however, these roles are reversed.[6] What researchers call phenotype A is the larger, softer, more genial side of cholesterol. It's characterized by large and relatively fewer LDL particles. Phenotype B, on the other hand, is tougher, faster, and much more dangerous. It has more of the smaller, denser LDLs and more particles overall. In this world, if you had a choice, you'd definitely want to be an A.[7]

Similar to personality types, these phenotypes are the general *styles* different individuals have of generating blood fats.

LDL levels that fall below 130 milligrams per deciliter are ideal. For people at risk for heart disease, LDL levels should fall below 100 milligrams per deciliter. Unfortunately, these values are just the tip of the iceberg. The real issue lies in the size of cholesterol particles. Take two patients, for instance, who have the same cholesterol number of 100 milligrams per deciliter. One patient suffered a heart attack, the other patient didn't. With all health parameters being equal, the cholesterol particle size is the missing piece of data needed to understand why one was predisposed to heart disease and not the other. The heart attack patient's LDL particle size is phenotype B—small, numerous, dense LDL particles. These small, fatty particles can move into the blood vessel wall more readily and thus are more likely to form arterial plaques than the buoyant phenotype A particles.

The A pattern includes not only larger LDLs but also lower triglycerides (another basic form of blood-borne fat energy) and higher HDL (the "good" cholesterol), which usually improve the LDL cholesterol profile. The B pattern clusters the opposite traits: more LDL particles in total, lower HDL, and higher counts of triglycerides. When it comes to our health, the bottom line is quite direct: how do we move from B to A, and what are the behaviors that encourage staying at A?

I want to be clear: all the evidence points to smaller and denser LDL, as major causes of arterial plaque. As it turns out, triglycerides are an especially helpful marker here.

Triglycerides do not seem to cause atherosclerosis in quite the same way that LDL does (although in the form of very low-density lipoproteins, or VLDLs, they are also atherosclerotic). But they do have a set of very useful relationships to the other members of the phenotype constellation. Triglycerides have a strong *inverse* relationship to HDL and a strong *positive* relationship to LDL particle number.[8] Thus they serve as a "pointer" for what's inside the LDL measurement. When triglyceride is low, the LDL reading will tend to be more benign, or A-like: low triglyceride is telling you that there are fewer particles per level of LDL. And when triglyceride is high, the LDL score will be more worrisomely B-like: high triglyceride is warning you that each LDL level has a lot of particles in it. In effect, triglyceride is the flag that tells you if you're A or B.

Gene Therapy Fact: Olive Oil

Olive oil is a monounsaturated fat that helps to keep cholesterol problems in check. Among its long list of healthful effects is that it lowers LDL cholesterol. Use it for dressing salads or for Mediterranean-style dipping of hearty breads and vegetables—but not for cooking. (Heating destroys its healthful properties, so use coconut oil instead.) Shopping for olive oil can be quite dizzying. Simplify your life by always choosing extra-virgin olive oil, because it undergoes the least processing.

Now that we know how to read the pattern of our phenotype, what can we do to push it in the right direction? Again, your triglyceride level (Trig) provides a useful handle by which to take hold of the problem. Although the ultimate aim is to lower LDL, doing the things that lower your triglyceride level will put you in the position of having done what's good for LDL and HDL too. Fortunately, your triglyceride level (and by extension LDL) is eminently treatable. Here are the basic steps to turning yourself into a bona fide phenotype A personality:

1. Avoid Processed and Easily Digested Carbs
One of the most potent means of reducing your triglyceride level is to reduce bad carbs. This has been demonstrated in a wide range of studies, and is one of the hallmark effects of low-carb diets. White bread, pasta, pastries, cookies,

crackers, pizza, sugary drinks—many of the things that Americans eat most are precisely those that raise triglycerides and bring on heart disease. Based on an impressively comprehensive review of the scientific literature, the American Heart Association estimates that for each 1 percent of total calories that you switch from carbs to good fats, you lower your triglyceride level by 1 to 2 percent.[9] So a 10 percent reduction in cheap carbs, when replaced with healthy fats, could yield a full 20 percent drop in triglyceride level.

2. Avoid Trans Fats
Trans fats are the hydrogenated oils that some restaurants and food companies use to crisp, flavor, and preserve their products. Fast-fried food is a major source, as are some margarines. In whatever form, trans fats are bad news. In a major Nurses' Health Study that tracked women for over two decades, those with the highest intake of trans fat were 50 percent likelier to develop cardiovascular disease. Those with the lowest intake were up to 70 percent less likely.[10] My advice? Just say no.

3. Embrace Good Fats Rather Than Low-Fat
Low-fat diets, while they sound commonsensical for heart disease, have never been shown to be especially good at lowering triglyceride levels and hence at getting at the nasty core of LDL counts. Indeed, low-fat diets, when they are correspondingly high in carbs, can lower LDL while *raising* triglyceride levels. On the other hand, Mediterranean-style diets, which are high in mono- and polyunsaturated fats, are proven to lower triglycerides by around 10 to 15 percent.

- Primary sources of healthy monounsaturated fats include: olive oil, almonds, pecans, sesame seeds, pumpkin seeds.
- For polyunsaturated fats, walnuts, sunflower seeds, flax, and sesame seeds are good sources.

4. Take a Fish Oil Supplement
Fish oils contain an especially potent form of omega-3 fats that deserve special mention all by themselves. The American Heart Association estimates that each gram of these polyunsaturated fats can lower triglycerides by 5 to 10 percent. And they're good for the heart in other ways too—for example, in regularizing the rhythm of the heartbeat. Don't overdo it, though; too much can prevent blood clotting. Three grams or less is plenty.

Gene Therapy Fact:
Omega-3 and Heart Health

Increasing omega-3 fats in your diet can lower cholesterol, blood pressure, and the risk of forming blood clots in the arteries. Omega-3 has such a widespread effect on cardiovascular disease that researchers often call it the "poly pill." People with the highest levels of EPA (one of the omega-3 fats) have a 50 percent lower risk of developing congestive heart failure. Chances of surviving congestive heart failure are 35 percent greater for those with the highest omega-3 consumption.

In 2013, a scientific paper made headlines by reporting that men with a higher blood concentration of omega-3 fats had a higher risk for developing prostate cancer.[11] However, the method of analysis that allowed the scientists to arrive at that conclusion was highly flawed, and the results were widely misinterpreted. Bottom line: the benefits of omega-3 fats far outweigh any risk.

Soothe Your Aching Vessels

It is no exaggeration to say that atherosclerosis is a disease of inflammation. Low blood flow, LDL-induced stickiness in the endothelium, and the cascade of follow-on inflammatory reactions to LDL's breaching the vessel walls are hallmarks of the disease's progression.

In light of this, it obviously makes sense to focus on reducing inflammation. This is generally the case for good health, since inflammation, wherever it occurs in the body, does many of the same bad things: sensitizes tissues to overreacting, incubates cell growth (particularly bad for cancer), and gums up the works with excessive coagulation and adhesion.

Just how big a problem is inflammation? Well, seven of the top ten causes of death in the United States are caused in large part by chronic, low-level inflammation:

1. Heart disease
2. Cancer
3. Respiratory disease

4. Stroke
5. Alzheimer's disease
6. Diabetes
7. Kidney disease

A particularly potent antioxidant and anti-inflammatory substance is sulforaphane, which has been shown to work directly on the same inflammation-signaling pathways that are activated by low blood flows. But whereas low flow silences the soothing response, sulforaphane calls it forth. It "frees up" the potent antioxidant enabler Nrf2 to activate a series of inflammation-calming gene expressions. By suppressing the protein that usually suppresses Nrf2, sulforaphane indirectly gets the good genes going.[12]

Sulforaphane is found in abundance in the cruciferous vegetables, a large and commonly accessible family of plants: bok choy, broccoli, brussels sprouts, cabbage, cauliflower, collard greens, kale, kohlrabi, radishes, rutabaga, turnips, and watercress; broccoli sprouts are the highest-potency form. There are so many beneficial bioactive effects from this class of vegetables—antioxidant, anti-inflammatory, satiating, and so on—that I recommend making them staples of your diet. Cruciferous vegetables all contain compounds called glucosinolates, which form small amounts of goitrin, which is metabolized into a hormone-like substance that in high doses interferes with the synthesis of thyroid hormones. It has been noted that animals that consume large amounts of cruciferous vegetables rarely develop hypothyroidism. This is not found commonly in humans, however. I recommend my patients have at least one serving, but not more than three servings, of cruciferous vegetables daily. Also loaded with potent heart-healthy, anti-inflammatory anthocyanins are acai berries, blueberries, strawberries, and black raspberries. You really can't eat too many of these fruits!

Oil Your DNA

If your DNA (not to mention your histones and all the other crucial methyl-mediated functions in your body) can't methylate, it can't properly respond to the changes and demands of all the environments outside of it and in which it is realized. Which is to say, it can't do its most essential work: answering the call of your life. It's important to understand that this is an enormously changeable and dynamic operation. The DNA, at whatever individual spots along the miles of helical threads in your cells, isn't either methylated or demethylated once and for all. The genes are dynamically being methylated, demethylated, and remethylated throughout your life. In order to keep this methylation engine humming, you need to supply it with the raw materials for the process— namely, a steady supply of usable methyl groups. The primary nutrient that provides methyl-groups is methionine. Methionine-rich foods include: eggs, sesame seeds, Brazil nuts, chicken, fish, oats, almonds, lentils, and brown rice. It's this flexibility to respond to whatever life throws at you—a little more here, a little less there, to keep the overall methylation pattern in balance—that defines the work of the epigenome.

So how do you oil your methylation engine? Normally, sufficient methionine is consumed in the diet to provide plenty of SAM (s-adenosylmethionine), which serves as a methyl donor for homocysteine. This is the other side of the cycle that's sometimes problematic. Methionine is essential for the production of cysteine, which in turn protects your liver from fatty degeneration, also known as fatty liver. Methionine deficiency can also increase atherosclerosis by allowing free radicals to damage lipids throughout the body. However, excessive amounts of methionine increase the levels of homocysteine, which may result in atherosclerosis as well. While nutritional deficiencies are often linked to poor health, this exemplifies that an overabundance of a nutrient may adversely affect gene expression and health.

Ecogenetics and Aging

The world expert on ecogenetic aging factors is the queen honeybee. She lives forty times as long as the other bees in the hive, yet she is genetically identical. The only difference is the queen alone eats the royal jelly. Scientists have found that there is a reduction in DNA methylation caused by micronutrients in the royal jelly, thus causing genes associated with longevity to be activated. This is why I recommend it so highly to patients.

Part of homocysteine's link to cardiovascular disease may be that it retards and dysregulates aspects of DNA methylation, but we just don't know for sure. Methylation is a very potent process to manipulate directly; when you do, you are literally stirring the mix of your basic being. As always seems to play out in such cases, it is likely that we will want to maintain methylation resources (including methionine and folate) within a band of "normal" functioning. We don't want excessive homocysteine, but we also don't want excessive folate. I routinely measure levels of B12, homocysteine, and folate on my patients. For now, being careful to avoid folate and B12 deficiencies is a very good idea, and those with high homo-cysteine may want to discuss with their doctors supplementing with folate and B12 and following blood levels of all three. This should keep the epigenetic machine running smoothly, without burning it out by running it too hard.

Gene Therapy Fact: Right Cooking Oils

The best oil sources for baking and cooking are organic butter, palm oil, coconut oil, and grapeseed oil. Virgin coconut oil is highly stable, resistant to oxidation, and can be stored for longer periods. It's a healthy saturated fat that contains about 50 percent lauric acid, which is a medium-chain fatty acid that is also found in breast milk and has ecogenetically mediated antimicrobial and immune functions. Coconut oil also contains tocopherol (vitamin E), a potent antioxidant that's important for preventing the oil from turning rancid. Because coconut oil is mainly composed of medium-chain triglycerides (MCTs), once it enters the body it is shuttled directly toward the liver, where it's used for energy rather than being stored as fat. Studies have shown that MCTs help to burn calories, control body weight, and balance satiety.

Coconut oil is also loaded with minerals like magnesium, calcium, phosphorus, and iodine. While it contains saturated fat, the benefits outweigh the risks. Lauric acid is the dominant fatty acid and is critical for immune function through epigenetic mechanisms. In fact, coconut oil is a natural warehouse of lauric acid. It's no wonder that Thailand, a country with one of the highest per capita consumptions of coconut, has one of the lowest cancer rates! Many studies have confirmed that people who consume coconut oil experience increased fat burning as well as weight loss.[13] Since coconut oil can be used to make energy within the mitochondria, the powerhouse for cellular energy, cooking with it can help to bolster your metabolism and energy.

The oils to avoid are peanut, sesame, canola, safflower, corn, sunflower, cottonseed, and soybean. These oils are sensitive to heat-induced free radical formation and contain an excess of omega-6 fatty acids.

The Ecogenetic Way: Heart Summary

Here's a quick review of the essential steps you can take to improve your heart disease environments:

- **Go with the flow.**
  - *Move! Work your vessels out to keep them strong, limber, and scruff- and inflammation-free. Try to get at least two to three hours of aerobic exercise each week. This can be of moderate exertion—steady breathing, but not breathless. A good walking pace is ideal. Keep each session going for at least twenty to thirty minutes to get the full benefit.*
- **Adopt a type A personality.**
  - *Eliminate all trans fats. These are especially present in fast-fried foods, margarines, many frozen pies, and packaged baked goods. Get in the habit of reading the nutrition labels.*
  - *Avoid cheap carbs. These include all the processed, man-made stuff that comes in plastic wrapping or cardboard boxes.*
  - *Embrace good fats. The good fats are monounsaturated and polyunsaturated fats, found in olive oil, avocados, flax seeds, and more.*
  - *Take a fish oil supplement. Aim for 3 grams or less of these omega-3 fats. Make sure you get a supplement that has been filtered of all impurities and toxins.*
- **Soothe your aching vessels.**
  - *Eat plenty of cruciferous vegetables for sulforaphane. Broccoli, cauliflower, cabbage, and brussels sprouts are potent inflammation fighters.*
- **Oil your DNA.**
  - *Get enough folic acid and vitamin B12. These will help keep homocysteine from clogging up the DNA methylation works.*

Targeted Nutrition for the Heart

By making these structural shifts in your eating style, you give yourself the best chance of remaining heart-healthy for the long term. As I will keep repeating, the most important change is in your *attitude*. Change your mind and the rest will follow. If you know what to do and you believe in doing it, then making the change in practice will follow naturally from your decision to change your mind-set.

The goal is to assemble a basket of options from which you can reliably choose foods that will be both tasty and healthful. Once you've got the menu of options, the question of "making hard choices" or "dieting" per se essentially vanishes. You are simply accepting as good and reasonable whatever is on your list. And you're not considering (or weighing, or negotiating with yourself over, or balancing, or making trade-offs with, etc.) what's not on the list, because you've already made those decisions. What's on the list is good, what's not on the list has already been ruled out, and that's that.

Of course, you'll always be adjusting your lists of healthy foods—adding some things and dropping others—as you learn more and as you gain a better sense of how your body responds to the new nutritional environments you'll be putting it in. Adopting a new eating routine is not necessarily easy at first— there's the law of inertia to overcome—but it can be made a lot easier by taking the time to compile a generous list of appealing, healthful options.

That's what this section offers: a series of recommendations for filling up your basket. These items by no means exhaust the possibilities. Once you begin to get comfortable in your adjustments, feel free to try out other foods that share the basic characteristics of these good choices. When your mind and your eyes are educated—when you're confident about the shape of the environments you're trying to occupy—you'll be leading yourself in the right direction automatically.

A note on not fixating on the "exact right" amounts of these foods to eat. The idea is not to nail down the precise "nutritional dosage" of this or that substance, but to enrich your nutritional environment *in general*. You want to *live* this new food attitude, not be obligated to optimize its outcomes at every meal. So don't get hung up on the exact amounts of plum juice or tea to drink. Concentrate on including *all* of these foods in your basket of staples. When you want a caffeinated drink, choose tea (black or green) or coffee for an antioxidant kick. If you're looking for a shot of something sweet, try pomegranate or grape juice. And for a treat, nibble on a square of dark chocolate. The idea is to align your activity with your health—and by doing so consciously recontextualize your genes.

Eat Natural, Fresh Food

Food consumed in the Western diet is processed and composed of atherogenic substances like refined carbs, preservatives, and other chemicals. As the food works its way through the gut, it is broken down by many compounds, enzymes, and microbes. Our gut is inhabited by between three hundred and a thousand different bacterial species, which influence digestion as well as immunity, considering that over two-thirds of the body's immune system is located in the gut.

Cultivate healthy gut bacteria by eating fresh, natural foods, and avoiding (as always) processed foods. Also eat fermented foods, such as yogurt, tempeh, kefir, and kombucha, to nurture healthy gut bacteria, which is crucial for disease prevention, including heart disease. Probiotic supplements, such as lactobacillus, can also help to improve the gut's healthy microflora.

You'll also keep your digestive environment healthy by consuming foods that are high in fiber, like beans and seeds. High-fiber foods pull in toxins from the gut and prevent them from getting absorbed into and destroying the intestinal lining.

Red meat has been vilified by some as being unhealthy, yet research has shown that the ecogenetic balance in the diet rather than any single component, determines whether or not it promotes health. For instance, red meat contains L-carnitine, a nutrient produced naturally by the body and which can be healthy, but when it is converted to a compound called trimethylamine-N-oxide (TMAO)—a process that may occur if it's digested by detrimental intestinal bacterial—it may become unhealthy. A study published in 2013[14] found that some intestinal bacteria metabolized L-carnitine found in red meat to TMAO, which has been shown to produce atherosclerotic plaque in mice. The researchers discovered that if this bacteria were suppressed with antibiotics, feeding the mice L-carnitine supplements no longer caused accelerated heart disease. However, these findings are not an indictment of either moderate red meat consumption or carnitine supplementation. Many studies have demonstrated that carnitine helps resist cardiovascular disease.[15] In addition, a meta-analysis of over 1.2 million people found that consumption of processed meats, but not red meats, was associated with an increased incidence of heart disease and diabetes. The 2013 study does confirm that the balance of bacteria in your gut is a key factor for ecogenetic balance.

So what should omnivores do? Again, ecogenetic balance is the answer. Avoid processed flour, sugar, and oil. These have been found to result in dysbiosis or an unhealthy population of gut bacteria.[16]

Reducing the acidity in the gut by eating more alkaline foods like leafy green vegetables enhances a healthy gut microbiome. Adding lime or lemon to your water or squeezing a wedge of lemon or lime over your salad in lieu of dressing will help to create an alkaline environment in the gut. (And don't get confused by the citric acid found in lemon or lime; these fruits are indeed alkaline.) Consume fiber when you consume meat, as it traps toxins in the gut so they are excreted rather than absorbed.

Studies have shown that people who consume more saturated fat like red meat and avoid healthy carbohydrates like vegetables are at an increased risk for developing heart disease.[17] Since most carbohydrates consumed in a Western diet are processed and refined,[18] this is not a surprising finding.

Moreover, a recent study showed that the major cause of rapid weight loss observed after gastric bypass surgery was due to the restructuring of the gut microbiome created by the surgical procedure.[19]

Choose high-quality meat when you shop. I always tell my patients to buy hormone-free organic meats.

Whole Grains

Eating a higher proportion of whole grains, and especially replacing processed grains with whole grains, has repeatedly been shown to improve heart health. In a Harvard-based study, women who consumed two to three servings of whole grains a day were 30 percent less likely to experience a heart attack or die from cardiovascular disease over a ten-year period.[20]

Grain's Anatomy
A whole grain is composed of three layers: the bran (outer), the endosperm (middle), and the germ (inner). The bran layer is packed with B vitamins and minerals as well as fiber and proteins. The middle layer, the endosperm, is a bit starchy because it contains lots of carbohydrates, in addition to protein. The germ layer has healthy unsaturated fats and proteins. When food manufacturers process grains, all of the layers are removed except the starchy middle

layer. Removing the nutrient-rich outer and inner layers produces a minimally nutritious grain. Whole grains are nutritious in their natural form, so it makes sense to buy whole grains that contain 100 percent of the original kernel—bran, endosperm, and germ. How do you know if you're buying nutritious whole grains? Turn your attention to the terms on the front label of food packages:

- **Whole grains** are nutrient-dense foods that are packed with vitamins and minerals. These grains contain a lot of fiber, which helps promote satiety. If "whole grains" appears on your food package, it means that the kernels' three layers are intact.
- **Refined grains** are whole grains that have undergone a milling process. The milling process removes the bran and germ layers to improve the texture and extends the shelf life of the product. After the refining process, the grain becomes a carb-rich product. Some examples of refined grains include white bread, white flour, and white rice as well as many desserts and pastries.
- **Enriched grains** are grains in which nutrients that were lost during the refining process are added back into the grains. The final product contains more carbs and very little fiber.
- **Fortification** is the process of incorporating vitamins and minerals that are not naturally occurring in foods. Folic acid, for example, is added in cereals and other foods. Folic acid is the synthetic form of folate, a naturally occurring vitamin found in many grains, fruits, and vegetables. Fortifying food with folic acid prevents neural tube defects.

Choosing Healthy Grains

When shopping for whole grains, flip the food package over. The back label has important clues regarding the quality of the grain. Look for the word "whole"— it should be a part of the first ingredient (e.g., whole wheat, whole rye). Whole grain imposters assume various names: multigrain, cracked wheat, bran, stone-ground, seven grain, and so on. These types of grains are refined and do not contain the full nutritional value of whole grains.

Refined grains are usually white (e.g., white bread); however, some manufacturers may choose to change the color of their processed grains so that they appear brown. Again, check out the first ingredient on the back of the label. Don't stop there: evaluate other things like sugar and sodium content. Avoid products with ingredients such as high-fructose corn syrup, malt syrup, sucrose, and molasses. Too much sugar is an easy way to pack on extra calories. Packaged foods tend to sneak in a lot of salt. The recommended daily intake of sodium for Americans is 2,300 milligrams or less.

Incorporating whole grains into your diet is easy and a panoply of whole grains is readily available. You don't have to worry about limiting your options to brown rice and whole grain cereals. Here are some whole grains to consider:

- Amaranth
- Barley is a whole grain that is chock-full of vitamins B and E, antioxidants, and beta-glucan. Beta-glucan has been shown to reduce the risk of cardiovascular disease. Most of the barley found in a supermarket is "pearled" or polished to remove the outer bran layer as well as the hull. Therefore, pearled barley is a refined grain, but it is healthier than other refined grains because barley fiber is distributed throughout the kernel rather than just in the outer bran layers.
- Oats are a source of omega-3 fats, folate, potassium, and fiber. Eating oatmeal a couple of times a week has been shown to reduce LDL levels. Choose the less processed forms—for example, rolled or steel-cut oats rather than the instant varieties. The intact grain contains more fiber, is slower to digest and easier on blood glucose levels, and more filling. All good features!
- Buckwheat
- Bulgur is a quickly cooked form of cracked wheat.
- Flaxseed
- Millet
- Quinoa is full of nutrients like vitamin E and iron. In addition to helping reduce the risk of cardiovascular disease, it has also been linked to lowering the risk of obesity and diabetes.

Flavonoids

Flavonoids are a large family of plant-derived chemicals. *Flavus* is the Latin word for "yellow"; plants rich in flavonoids are typically yellow colored, although the range bleeds into oranges, reds, and even some blues, greens, and purples. Flavonoids are subdivided into other groups according to their particular chemical makeup. This can be confusing, since the names generally sound very similar: "flavanols" (with an *a*), "flavonols" (with an *o*), and "isoflavones" all refer to different types of flavonoids. But the main thing to remember is that almost all of these compounds have been shown to impart health benefits in one way or another. Indeed, as a group flavonoids have demonstrated an enormous range of benefits, including their antioxidant properties as well as their role in suppressing cell growth genes, encouraging appropriate cell death cycles, and inhibiting angiogenesis. Important for us here is that these effects include the by now familiar cluster of core heart-healthy processes: suppressing inflammation, quieting endothelial adhesion and stickiness, and increasing blood vessel relaxing. The bottom line: if it has "flav" in the name, it's probably good for you and your heart.

Flavanols

Flavanols are a subclass of flavonoids that include the catechins, which are found particularly in tea, chocolate, grapes, and berries. Epicatechin is the flavanol that appears to be responsible for the many health benefits in cocoa. Numerous studies have shown that eating or drinking cocoa lowers blood pressure and helps the endothelium's release of nitric oxide.[21] Similar results have come from daily intakes of black tea or grape juice.

Gene Therapy Fact: Chocolate Nugget

There are many studies that suggest eating chocolate is good for your health.[22] But you want to pay attention to the quality of the chocolate you're using. Dark chocolate, with at least 60 to 70 percent real cocoa, will provide the best flavonoid concentrations. Milk chocolate, on the other hand, contains lots of dairy and sugar, both of which have been shown to dampen cocoa's benefits. And remember that even the best dark chocolate, healthy as it is, contains plenty of calories. In order to keep your chocolate nutritious and indulgent, keep these rules in mind:

- Eat only one square of dark chocolate daily.
- Avoid chocolate whose labels include the words "partially hydrogenated" or "trans fat."

Flavonols

Flavonols are another class of flavonoids that have well-researched health benefits. Sources include yellow onions, kale, scallions, broccoli, apples, and berries. The most prominent flavonol is quercetin, which is found in a wide range of foods: kale, watercress, red onion, purple plums, blueberries, cranberries, and others. Quercetin can lower blood pressure, improve endothelial function and nitric oxide release, and fight LDL oxidation. Higher intakes of flavonols in large-scale diet trials are linked with fewer problems related to cardiovascular disease.[23]

More Flavonoid Foods

There are a great many fruits and vegetables that contain healthful flavonoids. I've reported on only some of the most prominent and well-researched ones above. But scientists are constantly learning more about the phytochemical components of plants, and the more we learn, the longer and richer and more potentially beneficial the list of foods becomes:

- Pomegranate appears to be a particularly potent antioxidant and anti-inflammatory, packed with polyphenols that are good for your heart. In some studies, it has outperformed other flavonoid-containing foods in the "virtuous suite" of CVD benefits: enhancing nitric oxide production, reducing LDL oxidation, keeping the endothelium smooth and the blood flow undisturbed. In another study, participants who consumed 330 milliliters of pomegranate juice daily compared with those who didn't experienced a significant decline in their blood pressure.[24]
- Red cabbage contains, in addition to the potent anti-inflammatory sulforaphane, dozens of anthocyanins, another subclass of flavonoids that has proven anticancer and anti-CVD effects.
- Like most red, purple, or blue fruits and vegetables, cherries are full of anthocyanins too. So are raspberries, blackberries, blackcurrants, cranberries, blood oranges, and purple corn—look for the deep red or purplish colors as a guide.

Tomatoes

Lycopene is another phytochemical with demonstrated heart-protective effects. Like the flavonoids, lycopene suppresses inflammation, and also seems to reduce LDL oxidation especially well. Part of this may be due to its interfering with the body's synthesis of cholesterol, thus turning down excess LDL production at the source.[25]

Tomatoes and tomato products like juice and ketchup are the best sources of lycopene. Importantly, tomatoes also include beta-carotene and loads of other phytochemicals—these seem to account for some of the benefits that can't be attributed solely to lycopene content. So, as with all the fruits and vegetables recommended here, eating the whole tomato is the best bet. When you do, you're not only absorbing protective chemicals in an extremely safe form, you're also hedging yourself against the limits of science. In ten or twenty years, what we will know about these foods will make your decisions now seem even wiser.

Antioxidants

Because oxidation of the LDL entrapped in the endothelium is fundamental to atherosclerosis, antioxidants are a special concern for heart health. Researchers have developed a concept called total antioxidant capacity (TAC), which is the sum of the many varied antioxidant effects of the things you eat. Measuring TAC is tricky because individual antioxidants act differently alone and in combination with others, including others within the same food item. Current understanding puts those in the table below at the top of the list.[26]

Foods with High Total Antioxidant Capacity (TAC)

Berry	Vegetable	Fruit	Beverage
gooseberry	artichoke	pomegranate	espresso
bilberry	pepper	prune	coffee
crowberry	spinach	olive	pomegranate juice
black currant	red cabbage	plum	green tea
strawberry	beet	orange	black tea
blackberry	mushroom	cherry	red wine
blueberry	arugula	pineapple	red vinegar
goji berry	brussels sprouts	kiwi	grape juice
cranberry	broccoli	lemon	prune juice

Other foods of note: walnuts, pecans, and sunflower seeds are very high in antioxidants, as are many herbs and spices and many dried forms of fruits and vegetables. In certain cases, the more "condensed" the food, like dried apricots or espresso coffee, the higher its TAC. In most other cases, though, fresh foods—not dried or otherwise reduced—not only have the higher total antioxidant content but are also the most natural and the least processed. Thus, for example, wild strawberries have a much higher TAC than those bought in the store, canned, or jammed; and chestnuts eaten from the shell with the pellicle (the thin membrane surrounding the meat) are much higher than shelled and roasted in a can.

It is also worth noting the *worst* places to look for a boost to your antioxidant capacity: not surprisingly, in the kinds of fast foods you'd get from McDonald's, Burger King, Pizza Hut, KFC, and all their ilk.

Gene Therapy Fact: Olive Leaf

Oleuropein is a bioactive compound found in olive leaf extract that has been found to reduce blood pressure. In a double-blind, controlled clinical trial, oleuropein and captopril (an antihypertensive drug)[27] reduced systolic and diastolic blood pressure by an average, respectively, of 11.5 and 4.8 millimeters of mercury, a measure of pressure. While olive oil is a widely touted healthy fat, oleuropein is a major component of the olive leaf, which has various vascular health benefits. Oleuropein also targets hardened arteries by reducing arterial resistance and stiffness as well as enhancing endothelial function to decrease blood pressure. Its cardiovascular health benefits stem from its ability to control calcium channel flow.

Nuts and Seeds

A large and growing body of research has demonstrated the benefits of eating nuts and seeds. For instance, a meta-analysis of four large epidemiological studies showed that the highest intakes of tree nuts were associated with about a 35 percent reduction in coronary heart disease.[28] And in another study, participants who consumed a diet rich in plant sterols, combined with fiber, soy, and almonds, fared much better in reducing cholesterol than those who were given cholesterol-reducing medications.[29]

Pine Nuts

Pine nuts are the edible seeds from pines; there are about twenty-four pine species that produce seeds big enough to be eaten as major components of the diet. These seeds are packed with all twenty of the amino acids needed to sustain human life, as well as vitamins A (aids in night vision) and C (immune system booster). High in mono- and polyunsaturated fats, they are also heart-healthy.

Chia

Chia, the edible seed of *Salvia hispanica,* a plant in the mint family, contains even more omega-3 fatty acids than flaxseed, which makes it a great nutrigenetic choice for preventing inflammatory diseases. Chia is also very convenient—chia seeds don't need to be ground to release their nutritive components, which include fiber, calcium, phosphorus, magnesium, iron, and other minerals.

Tree Nuts

Tree nuts are a great source of fiber and healthy fats. Walnuts, almonds, pistachios, and macadamias are packed with mono- and polyunsaturated fats. One study reported that eating more than a 5-ounce serving of nuts each week reduced the risk of developing a heart attack by about 35 percent.[30] Another study showed that individuals who ate about an ounce of tree nuts daily had fewer risk factors for heart disease (as well as for diabetes and metabolic syndrome). Walnuts are anti-inflammatory, lower blood pressure, and reduce cholesterol. Pistachios and almonds are also on the list.[31] Pistachio nuts contain 29 grams of monounsaturated fat and 17 grams of polyunsaturated fat but no cholesterol. They do contain phytosterols that lower levels of plaque producing LDL.

Gene Therapy Fact:
The Raw and the Cooked

At least 20 percent of your vegetables, fruits, and nuts should be consumed raw. This can include salads, soups, smoothies, and sauces. Cooking destroys most enzymes (though, significantly, not all vitamins and phytochemicals) that are a big boost to health.

Another way to ensure that you're consuming these good enzymes is to allow seed (and that includes beans and some grains) to germinate—for example, chia, chickpea, lentil, barley, or sunflower. As the seeds sprout, the enzyme inhibitors are neutralized and your body can absorb the unlocked nutrients. Note that irradiated seeds will not sprout.

I recommend juicing to all my patients because it's a great way to boost your consumption of raw fruits and vegetables and to retain the full nutritional value that is often diminished in store-bought juices. And the health benefits of raw juices are many. Here's a sample:

One study showed that the consumption of juices such as orange and blackcurrant compared with placebo were shown to improve inflammatory conditions in patients with peripheral arterial disease.[32]

Another study evaluated the effects of fruit and vegetable juice powder concentrate on inflammation. The results showed that sixty days of consuming the concentrate led to significant reductions of different inflammatory biomarkers.[33]

Tomato juice, which contains nutrients such as lycopene and vitamin C, has been shown to reduce C-reactive protein (CRP), a marker of inflammation linked to many chronic diseases.[34]

Vitamins, Minerals, and Supplements

Vitamin D

A Harvard study evaluated the effects, over twenty years, of vitamin D intake on approximately seventy-three thousand women and forty-five thousand men.[35] Men who met the dietary intake of vitamin D (at least 600 IU per day) experienced a 16 percent lower risk for cardiovascular disease than men with a daily intake of less than 100 IU per day.

Magnesium

Researchers reported an inverse relationship between the levels of magnesium in the diet and stroke risk.[36] For older adults, every 100 milligrams of magnesium reduced the risk of atherosclerosis-induced stroke by 9 percent. And the same dose reduced the risk for any type of stroke by 8 percent. Dietary sources that provide 100 milligrams of magnesium include: an ounce of almonds or cashew nuts, one cup of brown rice or beans, three-quarters of a cup of cooked spinach, or one cup of cooked oat bran cereal.

CoQ10

Coenzyme Q10 (CoQ10) is a powerful, natural, fat-soluble antioxidant found in the majority of cells in the body. It helps to soothe the endothelium by blocking oxidation stresses that interfere with nitric oxide production. A CoQ10 meta-analysis found a very consistent reduction in blood pressure across all studies: an average decrease in systolic and diastolic readings of, respectively, 17 and 10 millimeters of mercury.[37] Daily doses of around 150 milligrams were sufficient to be effective in patients with coronary artery disease.

L-Carnitine

Researchers reported that the supplementation of L-carnitine for three months lowered the inflammatory marker CRP and IL-6 (proinflammatory cytokine) in patients on hemodialysis.[38]

Grapeseed Extract

Grapeseed extract greatly reduced C-reactive protein among patients with type 2 diabetes. Lyophilized grape powder, consisting of 92 percent carbohydrate and enriched with bioactive substances such as resveratrol, quercetin, anthocyanins, flavans, kaempferol, and myricetin, was administered to pre- and postmenopausal women. The researchers found that the lyophilized grape powder lowered TNF-alpha, which is a marker for inflammation in the body.[39]

Targeted Supplements

Targeted Ecogenetic Juice for Heart Health

The following juice recipe is for those who are concerned about heart disease. But don't feel as though you have to drink this specific juice every day. Shake things up! I've included several juicing recipes in the recipes chapter. The ecogenetic juices listed are general recipes that focus on using wholesome ingredients and organically grown produce that have beneficial effects on many body systems. So you don't have to worry about sticking to any specific drink. My patients usually drink one or two ecogenetic juices daily. Mix up the juices you drink to broaden your intake of bioactive nutrients on a weekly basis. If you have a specific health concern, increase your intake of that recommended eco-genetic drink. And most important, enjoy!

½ cup unsweetened almond milk
1 teaspoon Barlean's olive leaf extract
1 tablespoon black raspberry powder
1 tablespoon hempseed oil
½ teaspoon fresh ginger
3 tablespoons raw cacao powder
1 teaspoon pomegranate powder

Blend for 15 to 20 seconds on low. Drink and enjoy.

Targeted Ecogenetic Supplements for Heart Health

The supplements listed below are recommended for achieving and maintaining a healthy heart. Don't get overwhelmed and feel that you have to take every supplement listed. Remember: everyone is unique. The supplement list is in no particular order. I recommend them all equally to my patients because each one has benefits in heart health. Many of my patients start off by taking one supplement to determine how well they are tolerating it. Then they add other supplements as needed. When taking supplements, the focus should be to maintain good health. Don't worry about whether you should be taking 5, 10, or 15 supplements. That is not the intent of the supplement list. Do what you can. And take your time in figuring out what works for you: good health isn't a destination; it's a lifelong practice. And supplements are a small part of attaining a healthy lifestyle. Supplements are meant to be an addition to not a replacement for eating a healthy diet, getting adequate sleep, and improving your level of physical activity.

The supplements below are among the most important ones I give to many of my patients. Because every person is different, certain supplements may be more important than others for a given individual.

- Carnosine—500 milligrams, once daily
- Grapeseed extract—300 milligrams, once daily
- Sytrinol—150 milligrams, once daily
- Taurine—500 milligrams, once daily
- P5P50 (activated pyridoxine)—50 milligrams, once daily

- L-carnitine—250 milligrams, once daily
- CoQ10—100 milligrams, once daily
- PQQ—20 milligrams, once daily
- L-citrulline—500 milligrams, once daily
- Magnesium glycinate—120 milligrams, twice daily
- Alpha lipoic acid—300 milligrams, twice daily
- Pterostilbene—50 milligrams, once daily
- Quercetin—250 milligrams, once daily

Chapter 4

Cancer

CANCER IS THE SECOND BIGGEST KILLER OF AMERICANS, following heart disease. In the United States, about one in four people will die from it. But cancer is very much a disease of developed civilizations. In richer countries, lung, colorectal, and breast cancers are all among the top ten causes of death. In poorer or middle-income countries, no cancer even makes it onto the list.

Physiologically, cancer is bewildering. Each tissue of the body can develop cancer—often multiple types—and there are more than two hundred different forms of cancer. But in developed countries the greatest number of cases cluster in a much narrower range. For American men, the most common cancers are prostate (28 percent of total new cases, 10 percent of deaths), lung (14 percent, 28 percent), and colorectal (9 percent, 9 percent), together accounting for about half of all new occurrences. For women, they are breast cancer (29 percent, 14 percent), lung (14 percent, 26 percent), and colorectal (9 percent, 9 percent), also combining for about half of all new cases.

Cancer is also bewildering in terms of its origins. The question I am most commonly asked by my cancer patients is: "How did I get it?" The causes and sources of cardiovascular disease, obesity, and diabetes are fairly intuitive, but cancer seems different. Often it appears to be more like a mysterious evil *force*. But cancer is no such thing. It does not have a will of its own. It's not out to get you. And most important, it can be defeated . . . Or better yet, prevented.

Cancer, like heart disease and obesity, is due to multiple imbalances. The same ecogenetic dictum for heart disease and obesity applies to cancer as well: *It is never too late to bring back balance.* Even if you've already had or have cancer. Even if you've smoked for twenty years and have been overweight for thirty.

Success Story

Gordon is a fifty-year-old man who came to see me fifteen years ago along with his three brothers. Their father had developed prostate cancer at age forty-eight and died from it at fifty-one. Each of his three brothers had been diagnosed and treated for early-stage disease. Each underwent surgery to have his prostate removed and received radiation therapy to ensure that the cancer cells were eradicated. Gordon was desperate to avoid the family disease, and to help his brothers: "I need to know what my options are because I need to beat this thing."

After meeting with them, I started the siblings on my gene therapy plan, which included nutrients and lifestyle changes to target the progression of cancer in those who had been diagnosed with the disease and medically treated, as well as to prevent it from developing in Gordon. Their regimen included the following:

- Metformin slow release—500 milligrams, once daily. Originally derived from the French herb lilac, it is an antidiabetic drug with proven anticancer effects because of its ability to activate tumor suppressor genes as well as lower levels of IGF-1, a tumor-prompting chemical made in the liver.
- Aspirin—81 milligrams, three times a week (Monday, Wednesday, and Friday). A dose of 81 milligrams is often given daily to people at risk for heart attack or stroke, but it also prevents cancer and blocks the spread of cancer cells.
- Ecogenetic morning shake:

    1 tablespoon black raspberry powder—an antioxidant-containing phytonutrient, it kills cancer cells and activates tumor suppressor genes

1 tablespoon pomegranate powder—slows cancer cell growth

1 teaspoon fruit anthocyanin liquid concentrate—blocks cancer cell proliferation by inhibiting genes that code for the cancer growth factors NF-kB and AP-1

1 teaspoon turmeric powder—prevents cancer development and proliferation by at least 20 different mechanisms

1 tablespoon broccoli sprout powder—a cruciferous vegetable with sulforaphane, a potent cancer-preventive and anti-inflammatory compound

Mix all ingredients in 1 cup of soy milk and blend for 15 seconds.

- Rule of One-Thirds macronutrient diet (a third each protein, carbohydrate, fat). A diet balanced with healthy servings from all three macronutrient groups builds the body's antioxidant resources and maintains adequate energy levels.
- Fish oil—1,000 milligrams, once daily (ProOmega). Contains antioxidants and activates detoxifying enzymes.
- Deodorized garlic—500 milligrams, twice daily. Contains ajoene, a compound that inhibits cancer cell growth and cancer metastasis.
- Meriva-SR—500 mg, twice daily. A cancer-killing supplement that combines phosphatidylcholine (compound found in soybeans and eggs that is a necessary part of every cell membrane in the body) and curcumin (strong anti-inflammatory and antioxidant compound in turmeric).
- Rosemary extract—500 milligrams, once daily. Suppresses cancer growth at various steps of cancer development.
- Broccoli sprout extract—500 mg, twice daily. Contains antioxidant compounds such as sulforaphane and glucosinolates that are found in cruciferous vegetables, targeting cancer proliferation and migration.
- Coconut milk powder—1 tablespoon, once daily. Interrupts cancer blood vessel formation.

- Magnolia extract—200 milligrams, twice daily. Contains honokiol, a compound from magnolia bark with multiple anticancer functions, including tumor cell death.
- Conjugated linoleic acid—750 milligrams, twice daily. Unlike
other omega-6 fatty acids, CLA, which is sometimes referred
to as an omega-9 fatty acid, lowers the risk of cancer by promoting lean muscle mass and lowering body fat.
- Skullcap extract—400 milligrams, three times daily. Contains
baicalin, a flavonoid used in Chinese herbal medicine to treat
anxiety, inflammation, and hypersensitivity. Baicalin also
blocks the growth of prostate cancer cells by triggering cell
death.[1]

I'm happy to report that fifteen years after I treated these brothers they all remain disease free.

Genetic Errors

In trying to unravel the mystery of cancer, one factor we can quickly put into
perspective is genetics. Cancer is decidedly *not* a disease we typically inherit
from our parents. Only about 5 percent of cancer cases are strongly inherited
from a mutation in a parent's gene. Even the well-known BRCA genes, which
predispose women to breast cancer, account for only around 5 to 10 percent of
breast cancer cases, and for much less than 1 percent of cancer cases in the
general population.

Cancer is primarily an *environmental* disease. It comes about through the
individual's experience over the course of a normal human life span.

And yet, looked at another way, cancer is certainly a genetic disease in the
sense that it acts upon the genome, disturbing the workings of cells as they
read, activate, and copy genetic information.

Much of what goes on in the nucleus of the cell could be compared to the
activity inside a supercharged copy center in a big office building. Each of the
genes lined up along each strand of DNA has one very specific job to do, which
is to copy the instructions for making one specific gene product, most often a
single protein. It does this by transferring the instructions onto a copy-tape

molecule called RNA, which then carries the message out to other regions of the cell, where the protein is assembled and combined with other substances to get on with the business of life.

The copy center in the nucleus of our cells is under the simplest kind of management. It is run by "go" genes that initiate the copying, and "stop" genes that limit this activity to the making of new proteins that the body actually needs and no more.

The "go" genes are called *proto-oncogenes*. They have the special power to initiate cell division, and they are normally dormant after the organism has matured and no longer needs the superfast expansion of embryonic development.

The "stop" genes are called *tumor suppressor genes*. They have additional functions as error checkers and fixers to ensure that the copying of instructions for making the new cells is accurate.

And on a good day, it's as simple as that.

But as you might imagine, in any big copy center that cranks out thousands or even millions of replicas each day, errors can creep in. A machine might jam, or the pages might get shuffled, or the toner might be running out, or a computer might throw in some text that was supposed to be in a document that was copied last week.

In the world of genes and cells, these kinds of errors are called mutations, and they occur entirely by chance—simply because over time, and over thousands of replications, freakish little things go wrong.

Most mutations are benign, and they are easily cleared out of the system by the tumor suppressor genes. Sometimes they cause precancerous or benign changes such as polyps, skin flaps, spots, or lumps. These kinds of changes are not yet cancer. We live with these kinds of changes all the time.

But sometimes the errors pile up and overwhelm the system in a catastrophe that's comparable to every copy machine in the building going haywire at the same time, getting stuck in the "on" position, and after hours when everyone who's supposed to be watching out for mistakes is gone for the day.

It takes just this kind of overwhelming cascade of errors, a tide of errors that overrides all manner of safeguards, for a mutation to become cancer.

We give the name "carcinogens" to substances originating outside the body that have the ability, on exceedingly rare occasions, to overwhelm the system and create the mutations that cause cancer. They include: UV radiation from sunlight, other kinds of radiation (such as X-rays), naturally occurring chemicals like arsenic or asbestos, smoking, certain viruses like hepatitis B, and an increasingly large range of man-made chemicals such as vinyl chloride or BPA. It's also possible to think of certain cancer-promoting foods as carcinogens: meat cooked at high temperatures, excessive fat, or aflatoxins in some nut butters.

There are also cancer-inducing behavioral states that can be thought of as carcinogens. These include lack of exercise, lack of sufficient sleep, and chronic stress, each of which has been shown to contribute to cancer formation. Carcinogens are the origin of all the cancer risks we think of as "environmental." And since this is by far the greatest proportion of cancers, avoiding exposure to carcinogens and the mutational errors they cause is a crucial first step for cancer prevention.

Gene Therapy Fact: BPA and Toxins

Bisphenol A (BPA) is a carcinogenic substance that is found in a lot of the products that we use every day (e.g., baby bottles, water bottles, canned food, eyeglass lenses, toys, paper). Follow these tips to reduce your BPA exposure:

- **Buy fresh or frozen food!** Food in contact with either a can lining or plastic wrap allows BPA and other toxins to seep into it.
- **Use microwave-safe containers.** Heating food in plastics allows harmful poisons to creep into it.
- **Pack it up safely!** Store leftovers in glass or stainless steel containers. Don't give your food a chance to marinate in BPA or other toxins.

Some mutations are simple errors in copying sections of DNA during cell replication. Bits of the gene's sequence can be cut off, extra copies of certain bits can be added in, whole genes can be copied too many times or fail to be copied at all. Many of these errors result from earlier kinds of damage or mutation to other areas of DNA. If the genes that regulate the copying work—the *tumor suppressor* genes that serve as proofreaders—are themselves damaged or mutated, then significant errors may not be caught or repaired and may become part of the daughter cells' genome.

There are also changes that force an abnormal expression in the underlying DNA. These include methyl groups being added to or subtracted from the DNA, and histone proteins curling tighter or looser to expose more or fewer of the DNA strands to regulation. These epimutations can be just as cancer promoting as physical mutations in the DNA sequences, interfering with the "stop" signal being sent to the copiers and allowing basic errors to pass through uncorrected.

Once a cell has acquired enough mutations, by way of either out-of-control copiers or damaged tumor suppressor genes, it is essentially free to multiply without limit. This multiplication run rampant is what generates the cancerous tumor. The tumor itself is simply a collection of cells multiplying out of control.

Theoretically, tumors could expand forever, but they don't. That's because the nascent tumor has to be able to survive in the larger environment of the organism. As it develops, the tumor becomes a little ecosystem, with a series of interrelations with the tissues surrounding it, and with certain internal relations to its own processes. This is what scientists call the microenvironment of the tumor: the set of conditions that maintains the tumor's independent life in the context of the rest of the body.

The most basic conditions a tumor requires are oxygen and nutrients, which also requires a network of new blood vessels to shuttle these resources into the tumor cells. Otherwise, tumors could grow no larger than about two or three millimeters—about the size of the tip of a pin.

Angiogenesis, the rapid production of new blood vessels, involves creating new branches from the existing blood vessels that feed normal, healthy tissues.

Gene Therapy Fact:
Cancer Cells and Energy Consumption

Gene expression of normal cells favors protective mechanisms by increasing cellular maintenance and energy-conserving responses. Cancer cells favor energy expenditure by promoting cell growth and division, which is a pattern of cellular activity that is targeted by chemotherapeutic drugs. Decreasing high-glycemic foods reduces the fuel that cancer cells use for energy such as glucose. So the effects of reducing high-glycemic foods on cancer cells is twofold: it reduces energy sources and helps cancer drugs selectively target dividing cells. One study showed that short-term fasting sensitizes cancer cells to chemotherapy and protects normal cells.[2] Another study found that older adults with cancer who fasted the evening prior to chemotherapy treatment experienced fewer side effects such as fatigue and gastrointestinal problems.[3]

A better alternative to fasting is caloric balance, using the Rule of One-Thirds. The following are some of the ways in which caloric balance "targets" cancer:

- slows down mitotic activity and cell proliferation
- boosts and extends immune response
- starves precancerous cells
- blocks cancer-promoting hormones, chemicals, and receptors
- fixes and regulates DNA damage
- regulates oncogene or proto-oncogene expression
- promotes growth inhibition by raising glucocorticoid levels

Unfortunately, part of the body's own healing system—inflammation—becomes subverted during cancer growth and helps the tumor thrive in its microenvironment.

Inflammation is the body's response to injury. We're familiar with it in the form of redness, warmth, pus, and perhaps swelling as the body deploys its healing agents to tend to the damaged tissues.

The body's first responders—the pus and yellowish discolorations on wound sites—are the white blood cells that have rushed to the scene to sweep it clean of immediate danger. Once the area has been secured and sanitized, the damage must be repaired, which calls for the replacement of the dead or broken tissues with new tissue. This means that the body must enter a special growth mode as new cells of the appropriate type—skin, blood vessel, and so on—are activated, copied, and moved into place.

Inflammation is all about speed; it needs to get the job done fast. It stops the bleeding as fast as possible, it sterilizes the wound site as fast as possible, and it begins to repair and grow back the damaged tissue as fast as possible.

All of this is good and necessary—our lives depend on this normal, healthy process of repair. But problems arise when the emergency condition lasts too long, when inflammation becomes *chronic*.

In the interest of rapid healing, many of the substances involved in the inflammatory response are endowed with special growth-promoting powers. This is what makes inflammation especially pernicious in relation to cancer.

Some of the products of inflammation—the cytokines, growth factors, COX-2—activate proteins that are simultaneously involved in two independent processes: 1) activating the "go" signals called oncogenes, and 2) further activating the inflammation products themselves. So the two branches of the process begin to feed each other. Inflammation produces growth factors, growth factors trigger the transcription proteins, in one direction the proteins activate certain oncogenes, in another direction the proteins help to activate more growth factors, the additional growth factors trigger more transcription proteins, and the whole cycle becomes a feed-forward loop. The copier is stuck on "go" and the body's normal growth processes speed up.

The ecogenetic way of dealing with cancer is to anticipate how cancer wants to inhabit each of its preferred environments and then to systematically reshape those environments in our own favor.

Gene Therapy Fact:
Aspirin Protects Against Cancer

In line with the American Heart Association, low-dose aspirin is recommended for individuals with a high risk of heart attack or stroke. Yet there's also a compelling body of evidence that demonstrates that aspirin is effective in helping to prevent certain cancers, especially prostate and colorectal. Not only have I prescribed it to many of my patients, I take my daily dose of aspirin too.

In a population-based cohort study, participants with cancers (e.g., colorectal, lung, prostate, and breast cancer) who were taking low-dose aspirin before they were diagnosed with cancer had a lower risk for lung and colorectal cancers.[4] A 2014 meta-analysis published in the *Journal of the National Cancer Institute* showed daily use of low-dose aspirin was associated with up to a 34 percent reduced risk of developing ovarian cancer.[5] Through observational and cohort studies, researchers have found that aspirin also helps to minimize metastasis, which occurs when cancer spreads from its site of origin to other places in the body.[6]

Because aspirin can have serious side effects, the prophylactic or therapeutic use of aspirin in cancer requires the purview of a medical specialist.

Take the Long View and Take It Now

One of the most remarkable developments in cancer research over the past two decades is the emerging view of cancer as a time-based phenomenon. For centuries, and certainly for most of the twentieth-century, cancer was regarded as a strange and sudden irruption of misguided cell proliferation. "Cancer" simply appeared and the main problem seemed to be how to deal with the damage.

But now we understand cancer to be a side effect of your properly functioning life, an echo of the clock of life ticking along. The epigenetic mind-set acknowledges that life itself is the ultimate environment of cancer, and that the ordinary processes of going on living are the same ones that generate the cancers and precancers in us. But its very ordinariness is enormously empowering, because if you take the long view now, and act accordingly, you will be able to put yourself years ahead in the cancer prevention game.

Here's one powerful example: Colon cancer typically takes at least *three decades* to progress through all the mutations and stages of growth necessary for full-blown malignant disease. But it is only metastatic and hence directly life-threatening for the last *three* of those years. If you wait until those last years to think and act about cancer, you have already lost most of your opportunity for life-saving measures. You are seeing and responding to the tip of the iceberg, never noticing the twenty-seven years of slow-paced growth beneath the surface.

Slow the Cancer Clock

Cancer begins with mutations and epimutations—errors in gene function that make it through the gauntlet of checks and balances on cell proliferation. If we want to remain free of active cancer for as long as possible, we need to slow down the pace of these mutations.

How do we do that? The first step is to avoid those environmental triggers that cause the damage that leads to bad genetic copying, the carcinogens we've previously discussed, ranging from asbestos and radiation to chronic lack of sleep.

The *Report on Carcinogens,* produced by the U.S. Department of Health and Human Services, is a biannual compilation of all known or suspected carcinogens. The 2011 report, available online, lists 240 different substances that have demonstrated carcinogenic effects, although only 54 of the 240 profiles are for substances "known to be" human carcinogens.[7] Getting bogged down in the possible carcinogenicity of every substance you may come into contact with is a recipe for paranoia and paralysis. The appropriate middle course is to identify the main risks, keep up-to-date with new developments, and then orient your daily living habits to minimize the environments of primary threat and maximize the environments of greatest benefit.

Gene Therapy Fact:
Toxins Around the House

Common products in your home such as plastics, vinyl flooring, and personal care products can make your children sick. Plastic and other products contain chemicals called diethyl phthalate (DEP) and butylbenzyl phthalate (BBzP), which have been associated with an increased risk for the development of airway inflammation linked to asthma. While phthalates can enter the body through skin absorption, ingestion, and inhalation, these specific chemicals have been shown to enter the body via the airway. A study showed that children had high levels of phthalates in their urine and nitric oxide (measured by exhaled breath). Nitric oxide, a marker for inflammation in the airway, was reportedly highest among children who wheezed, a common symptom associated with asthma.[8] The key is to eliminate these chemicals. They are known to affect the endocrine system, and early exposure causes not only asthma, but neurological, behavioral, and reproductive problems.

Among those "known" carcinogens, here are some of the most prevalent—those that should be taken special note of, whether because of their widespread presence in the environment or because of their particular potency.

Aflatoxins

Aflatoxins are a group of substances produced by certain mold-producing fungi that grow in warm climates, including the warm temperate areas of the southern United States. Exposure is mostly through contaminated food—the fungi can grow on corn and other grains, peanuts, tree nuts, and cottonseed meal. Aflatoxins are mostly associated with liver cancer, although a few other cancers have been linked in laboratory animals. The greatest potential risk for Americans is probably in peanut butter, since we eat so much of it. Although the FDA tests peanut butters with special care, I suggest that you avoid peanut butter altogether. Opt, instead, for healthier nut spreads like almond butter or cashew butter. If you buy nuts in bulk from health food stores, make sure the stock is regularly refreshed. Don't store nuts for long periods, especially in hot or humid conditions. Throw out nuts of any kind that develop mold.

Alcohol

While limited intake of red wine has health benefits, chronic high levels of alcohol consumption are definitely linked to cancers of the mouth, pharynx, larynx, and esophagus. The more you drink, the higher the risk, and if you add smoking to the mix, the risk goes up exponentially.

Gene Therapy Fact: Air Pollution

Despite major efforts to improve air quality, tighter regulations of fossil fuel power plants, cement plants, and other industries are warranted to minimize the release of toxic chemicals into our atmosphere. Poisons such as soot, coal, and heavy metals can pose serious threats when emitted in large quantities into the air. These poisons are released during combustion, which is a process in which waste is formed due to the burning of fossil fuels. The table below includes commonly found wastes in the atmosphere and how they affect both your health and the environment.

Air Pollutants	Source	Environmental Effects	Health Effects
Fine particulate matter (PM)	Fossil fuel combustion	Haze; settles on ground or in water; deposits may stain or ruin stone, statues, monuments	Respiratory symptoms: exacerbates asthma, triggers coughing, affects breathing Heart problems: irregular heart beat, heart attack
Nitrous oxide	Number one ozone-depleting emission via natural sources (livestock manure, certain bacteria) and man-made sources (fuel combustion, byproduct of synthetic commercial fertilizers, motor vehicle emissions, and waste management)	Greenhouse gases; contributes to smog; acid rain formation	Respiratory symptoms: chest pain, cough, dyspnea (difficulty breathing), increased risk of respiratory infections
Volatile organic compounds (VOCs)	Fossil fuel combustion; contained in paints, glues, and solvents (VOCs change from liquids to gases on air exposure)	Greenhouse gases; contributes to smog; acid rain formation	Carcinogenic
Sulfur oxides (SOx)	Fossil fuel combustion	Acid rain formation; destroys plants and pollutes water	Respiratory complications: shortness of breath, wheezing

Arsenic and Asbestos

These are two well-known carcinogens. Arsenic was used as a pesticide up to the mid-twentieth century, in some medicines in the 1970s, and currently almost exclusively in wood preservation. Asbestos is a naturally occurring mineral that was widely used as an insulator and in many other products, including as a cement additive, in paper, and in some plastics. Arsenic exposure was mostly through drinking water; the Clean Air and Clean Water Acts of the 1970s dramatically reduced Americans' intake. Since 1985, there has been no domestic production of arsenic. Asbestos had a similarly high-profile flameout; production was banned in 1978, and currently only very limited applications are allowed (for instance, in some cements).

I include these two mainly as examples of why it is important to remain alert and informed about emerging carcinogens. Both arsenic and asbestos were popular because we mostly didn't know better. You can't predict the future, you can't know what may turn out to have been carcinogenic all along, but orienting yourself *away* from industrial processing in general, whether in building materials or in food, will put you on the right side of the probabilities.

Estrogens and Xenoestrogens

Estrogen is the primary female sex hormone, produced mainly by the ovaries and expressed throughout the body in the circulating blood. It occurs naturally in three forms: estrone (most prominent during menopause), estradiol (highest during the reproductive years), and estriol (during pregnancy). Estrogen is a very powerful growth hormone—its purpose is to drive female sexual development and then, during the reproductive years, to prepare monthly for the possible advent of pregnancy. It performs these functions by binding to estrogen receptors along the DNA and thus by activating the genes that in turn drive the various processes of female sexual growth.

It is not hard to understand how estrogen is related to cancer. The growth programs of the cells are repeatedly stimulated by inflowing estrogen; as the pace of cell division and replacement increases, the chance for gene copying errors also increases. The more estrogen-fueled growth a woman is subject to in her lifetime, the higher the risk that the errors will accumulate as mutations or that the growth programs will themselves be hijacked for cancerous proliferation. This is why events that decrease a woman's exposure to estrogen spikes are anticancerous: later onset of first period; early menopause; pregnancy and child-bearing, including breast-feeding.

An increasing problem is the prevalence of nonsteroidal estrogens, essentially man-made substances that mimic the shape of natural estrogens and hence are called xenoestrogens. These fake estrogens can also bind to the estrogen receptor sites along the DNA and thus activate the same growth programs, but to no purpose. BPA, the synthetic compound found in some baby bottles and in many other products, is, among other bad properties, a xenoestrogen. Estrogen replacement therapy is another form of xenoestrogen; it was withdrawn as a standard treatment for menopause for exactly this reason.

Gene Therapy Fact:
Saturated Fat and Breast Cancer

Most studies show a decreased survival in patients with breast cancer who eat a high-saturated-fat diet. One study in the *Journal of the National Cancer Institute* showed that when women were put on a low-fat diet, their levels of estradiol dropped 17 percent over a two-year period, which would imply a decline in breast cancer risk.[9] Another study, involving more than ninety thousand premenopausal women, showed that the women who had high-saturated-fat diets had an elevated breast cancer risk as compared with women who ate the lowest amount of these fats.[10]

Estrogens promote the growth that can lead to breast cancer; they also feed the growth of developing cancerous tumors. By far the majority—around 80 percent—of breast cancers depend on estrogen for continued growth once they are established. Excess estrogen is therefore another kind of double whammy, helping both to incubate and then to inflame cancer.

Breast cancer is very treatable when discovered early. Mammography is an example of trading ionizing radiation for better chances at survival. Because many more lives are saved through early detection by mammograms than are lost due to radiation exposure, mammography is still the preferred preventive test to detect tumors at an early stage. Do not be misled by the recent study picked up by the media suggesting mammograms were no longer beneficial.[11] That study was flawed, as it studied women in the 1980s, when the mammogram imaging technology was far inferior to that available today. Early detection is key and yearly mammograms for women over forty save lives.

Success Story

Anne, a successful, thirty-seven-year-old saleswoman for a major corporation, came in to see me for an evaluation. "My sister passed away at age forty-three of breast cancer," she told me, "and now I found a lump in my breast."

I ordered some diagnostic and imaging tests, which determined that the lump was a benign fibroadenoma (a noncancerous tumor). Because of Anne's family history, though, I also performed a screen for the breast cancer genes BRCA1 and BRCA2. Fortunately, she was not a carrier. Although Anne didn't have cancer, she was worried about getting it. Since she worked in a stressful, demanding job, I started her treatment regimen with stress management techniques.

Anne's lab tests revealed that she was deficient in vitamin E, which is a powerful antioxidant, as well as in 25-hydroxy vitamin D (a blood marker of vitamin D3 in the body). Antioxidants fight free radicals that damage tissues and can lead to cancerous copy errors. Vitamin E is also crucial in maintaining a healthy balance between progesterone and estradiol. I advised Anne to take a daily mixed tocotrienol/mixed tocopherol supplement (containing alpha, beta, gamma, and delta tocopherols and tocotrienols each with distinct but synergistic activities, extracted from rice bran oil), as well as magnolia extract (200 milligrams, twice daily) and vitamin D3 (5,000 IU daily). I also advised Anne to take daily supplements of selenium (200 micrograms) and CoQ10 (100 milligrams). A March 2014 meta-analysis published in *Anticancer Research*[12] showed that women diagnosed with breast cancer with high blood levels of 25-hydroxy vitamin D had half the risk of dying as women with low levels. A previous study[13] showed women with low levels of this vitamin D3 metabolite when diagnosed with breast cancer had an almost 90 percent greater likelihood of developing metastatic disease.

I gave Anne information on how to eat and snack in order to slant her ecogenetic profile toward health. Her busy schedule and the travel requirements of her job meant that she had little time to prepare home-cooked meals. I recommended that even on the road she should strive to eat lots of leafy green vegetables, fish, whole grains, and wheat germ. For snacks, I told her to carry almonds or Brazil nuts, healthy high-energy foods that would keep her satisfied between meals. I encouraged her to continue these healthy eating habits when she was at home too, and I recommended that she cook with grapeseed oil.

Six months after starting my gene therapy plan, Anne now says, "I feel incredible!" There is no sign of cancer and there has also been a significant decrease in the size of the fibrocystic lump in her breast.

Hepatitis B and C Viruses
The two hepatitis viruses are leading causes of liver cancer. In the case of hepatitis B, chronic infection over decades leads to an assortment of genetic malfunctions. The virus multiplies itself in order to survive; as the viral DNA contaminates the host DNA, this proliferative tendency can activate oncogenes in the host. The patient's gene copying gets dysregulated, often by sections of genes being mistakenly transferred out of order to other sites. The cancer clock is on fast-forward, the mutations pile up year by year, and active malignancy becomes much likelier.

Hepatitis is contracted from infected blood and other body fluids, which means that sex is a major avenue of transmission. So rule number one in combating hepatitis is to use safe sex practices; if you are in a longer-term sexual relationship, both partners should get tested. Intravenous drug use is also a risk among those who share needles, especially for hepatitis C.

Importantly, infection with the hepatitis virus does not always lead to the chronic stage of disease. Infants are *much* more susceptible to developing the chronic form after infection: over 70 percent of children under age one, versus only around 5 to 10 percent of adults, will become chronic. It is therefore imperative that infants be immunized with the available and effective vaccines.

UV Radiation
The sun is by far the most prevalent source of UV radiation. At high exposures, it damages the genes, which increases the burden on DNA repair work. If and

when repair fails, sometimes because of direct damage to the repair genes themselves, mistakes during copying increase the rate of mutation.

Try to avoid spending too much time in direct sunlight, especially if you are fair skinned. Definitely avoid sunbeds, sunlamps, or tanning salons, which hasten all the bad effects of direct sunlight without any of the benefits of enjoying the outdoors. If you're an outdoors lover, take sensible precautions to reduce your exposure to UV radiation. Don't exercise in the heat of the day. Use sunscreen faithfully. However, pick ones that are free of pthalates, phenoxyethanol, parabens, and oxybenzone. These can interfere with endocrine and neurologic functions. I recommend sunscreen lotions and sprays with zinc oxide such as Badger or Raw Elements.

Ionizing Radiation

This category includes forms of radiation that cause damage in the body by ripping electrons away from atoms. This is the violent, high-energy radiation we associate with nuclear bomb testing and with nuclear power accidents. The most prevalent forms of exposure are X-ray and gamma radiation, as well as radon. Paradoxically, then, most people's exposure to X-ray and gamma radiation is either diagnostically in CAT scans or as part of the regimen for combating leukemia, lung, and other cancers. If your doctor says you need to use radiation in order to get better, you will have to accept a trade-off. Don't boycott measures that could save or lengthen your life, but do voice your concerns and preferences. If you encounter a doctor who is unwilling to help you minimize your exposure, you can always find another doctor.

About half the average person's total ionizing exposure comes from radon gas, which occurs as a background emission from uranium and thorium embedded in the rocks of the earth. When inhaled in stronger concentrations, the gas can trigger damage leading to lung cancer. After tobacco use, radon inhalation is lung cancer's second most common cause, and it is first among nonsmokers. The primary danger is from accumulation in homes—as a heavy gas, radon can accumulate in the basements and lower levels of poorly ventilated structures. It can even contaminate groundwater supplies.

Although the radon-causing elements are inherent in the earth, concentrations vary markedly by region and locale. So the key is to learn whether you are living in a higher-risk area or house, and then, if you are, to take measures to mitigate the risk. Fortunately, radon testing is now simple and cheap, with kits available in many home improvement stores; in fact, testing and monitoring are mandatory in some high-radon states and cities. Before buying a new home, you should certainly have it checked for radon concentration levels. If you already live in a home with high radon, you can mitigate the buildup by sealing the foundation against leaks or by redirecting the flow of underground gas to an exit point away from the house. There are many radon mitigation contractors who specialize in this kind of work.

Gene Therapy Fact:
Limit Radiation Exposure

As an oncologist, I try to limit my patients' risk of exposure to radiation caused by diagnostic scans. The scans are necessary—they help not only to diagnose but also to pinpoint the area affected by a tumor. But there is a risk of stimulating cancer with every exposure to radiation. And as one study showed, children are the most vulnerable to these exposures. Researchers in Great Britain evaluated the records of patients without any cancer diagnosis. For those younger than twenty-two, they found a correlation between leukemia and brain tumors and radiation dose from CT scans.[14] Specifically, the researchers found that a dose between 50 and 60 milligrays (a measure of absorbed radiation) increased the risk of leukemia or brain cancer by up to three times.

Tobacco

Tobacco use is the reason why lung cancer is the leading cancer in the United States, both in terms of number of cases and overwhelmingly in terms of number of deaths. Here and worldwide, smoking is the single biggest source of preventable cancers. The very best thing you can do for your health, if you smoke now, is to stop smoking. Substances in the smoke cause the range of genetic damage, including mutation and chromosomal irregularity, mainly in the lungs but also in the mouth and many other tissues. Please remember that although smoking may *appear* relatively harmless in the present (aside from the coughing, asthma, high blood pressure, and stink), this is an illusion, since what you are actually *doing*—with every puff you take—is systematically speeding up your cancer clock. If you can't be motivated to stop for the sake of your current health, think about the health of yourself twenty years from now. Try to save *that* person's well-being.

Industrial Chemicals

According to the Environmental Protection Agency, the United States either generates or imports seventy-four billion pounds of chemicals each day. Some chemicals are extremely toxic and should be absolutely shunned, with benzene and mustard gas leading the list. Many others are mostly benign and help us to live pleasurable, satisfied modern lives. We simply can't know in advance which will ultimately fall in which category, so there is no hard and fast rule about how to handle all the run-of-the-mill chemicals we encounter daily. It is revealing, however, that each successive *Report on Carcinogens* keeps getting longer mainly because the list of "reasonably anticipated" carcinogens keeps growing to include more and more man-made chemicals. So my basic advice is to be conservative but reasonable. Avoid chemical exposures if you can. When you have a choice, take the route that is chemically less loaded. The best way to do this is not by systematic avoidance (a posture of fear), but by proactively choosing relatively untouched products for your life. Eat more organic foods and fewer processed foods. Buy green, nontoxic cleaning products. Choose arsenic-free, pressure-treated lumber. Simple choices like this, performed out of a well-informed but nonparanoid understanding, add up to big lifetime benefits.

Get Out of the Inflammation Hothouse!

As we have seen, inflammation initiates a vicious cycle of bad effects for cancer. Inflammation aggravates the cell in ways that initiate the copier oncogene "go" programs and simultaneously catalyze further irritants to further inflammation. This is one of those double-whammy conditions you really want to do your best to get under control.

Stepping out of the inflammation hothouse, into the cooler air of normal cell functioning, begins with your diet. By now many of my recommendations will be familiar:

Reverse the Western Diet

Here's a simple way of thinking about it. All those hydrogenated, trans, and added fats that make processed foods smooth, crispy, and energy dense? Give them up for mostly mono- and polyunsaturated fats—the good fats in olive oil, nuts and seeds eaten whole, avocado, and so on. All those added sugars, high-fructose corn syrup, "evaporated cane juice," enormous sweetened drinks, energy bars and energy drinks all sweetened to make them irresistible? Give them up for real fruits, dark chocolate, nuts, all the inflammation-soothing goodness of the cruciferous vegetables, and virtually all of the brightly colored vegetables. A diet high in cheap carbs, particularly one high in processed grains, is inherently inflammatory.

Take a Daily Fish Oil Supplement
This is one of the simplest, most effective ways to reduce inflammation. The omega-3 fatty acids in fish oil help to disrupt the pathways by which COX-2 acts. COX-2 is a linchpin in the cell's inflammation response, so by cutting it off fish oil suppresses the chain reaction that leads straight to the hothouse. It's like installing an air conditioner in your cells.[15]

Use Extra-Virgin Olive Oil as Your Primary Fat
Substances in olive oil act on many of the same principles as ibuprofen in silencing inflammation signaling by the COX enzymes. But olive oil is good for you in other ways as well and is considerably safer than supplementing with either aspirin or ibuprofen, both of which can have intestinal and ulcerative side effects and can cause liver or kidney damage. And make sure to choose extra-virgin olive oil; the inflammation-fighting substance is much more potent in that form.

Take a Daily Probiotic
Look for lactobacillus, acidophilus, or bifidobacterium probiotics containing at least one billion colony-forming units (CFU) per gram. Probiotics are a beneficial kind of bacteria commonly found in yogurt, certain beverages, and even supplements. Gastroenterologists recommend probiotics to help improve many gut conditions such as irritable bowel syndrome and Crohn's disease. Probiotics also play a role in the treatment and prevention of vaginal and urinary infections as well as the development of certain allergies in children. Choose coated capsules to protect the probiotics from stomach acid, and take them on an empty stomach.

Take Prebiotics
Prebiotics are not digestible compounds but simply enhancers of probiotics that serve to ensure the growth of these beneficial bacteria. Prebiotics work symbiotically with our cells to maintain good health by facilitating normal digestion, inhibiting intestinal inflammation, fighting infection, enhancing

immunity, and inhibiting deleterious bacteria. Here's a quick list of prebiotic foods you can begin incorporating into your diet:

- Jicama (*yacón*), Jerusalem artichoke, beets, and chicory root all contain inulin (no, not insulin), which is a form of prebiotic fiber that breaks down in the gut to acetate, which turns off hunger centers in the brain
- Dandelion greens, a leafy green vegetable made up of 25 percent prebiotic fiber
- Allium vegetables such as garlic, onion, leeks, chives, scallions (adding to food raw rather than cooked will provide the best source of prebiotics)
- Whole grain and sprouted-grain breads
- Wheat germ, whole wheat berries
- Avocados
- Peas, soybeans (e.g., edamame), chickpeas
- Potato skins
- Apple cider vinegar (organic)

Gene Therapy Fact: Choosing Fats for Cancer

The polyunsaturated fats come in three forms: omega-3, omega-6, and omega-9 fatty acids. The omega-3s are found in coldwater fish like salmon, sardines, halibut, cod, and tuna as well as nut-derived foods like hempseed, walnut oil, and flaxseed. One of the main constituents of flaxseed is alpha-linolenic acid. One study showed that breast cancer patients with low levels of alpha-linolenic acid in breast tissue had an increased risk of developing metastatic disease.[16]

Another study reported that women who developed breast cancer had significantly lower levels of EPA and DHA, the two omega-3 fatty acids in fish.[17] Omega-3 fatty acids are beneficial in decreasing the activity of the COX-2 enzyme, which promotes inflammation, and they have been found to decrease estrogen stimulation of breast cell growth. Flaxseeds contain the highest levels of omega-3 fatty acids of any vegetarian source.

Can an omega-3 fatty acid fish oil supplement increase tissue levels in humans? Can the supplements actually suppress the inflammatory COX-2 enzyme in humans? The answer, according to an April 2008 study, is a resounding yes![18] Researchers studied patients with Barrett's esophagus (a condition caused by acid reflux in which the lining of the esophagus shows precancerous changes). Half of the patients were given 1,500 milligrams of the omega-3 (EPA) supplement, and the other half were not provided with the pills. The results showed that the EPA-treated group had higher omega-3 fatty acid in their cells, as well as significantly decreased COX-2 protein in their tissues. Fish oil omega-3 fatty acids have also been shown to decrease cell proliferation in patients with precancerous colonic polyps.[19]

Tuna, shark, mackerel, and swordfish may contain excess levels of methyl mercury, which is toxic to the nervous and immune systems. Farmed (or Atlantic) salmon may contain obesity-triggering toxins such as mercury, PCBs, and dioxins. Thinking about tilapia for dinner? Think again! Tilapia is fattened with soy, which reduces the amount of healthy omega-3s found in fish. Even the American Heart Association urges people to abstain from tilapia because of the way in which it's processed. Go with wild salmon, haddock, anchovies, cod, and sardines.

Find Your Zen

Like every other type of human experience, cancer is affected by mood, with stress being one of the inputs that can lead to inflammation's vicious "feed-forward" loop.

Cancer itself can be its own source of major stress, and thus having cancer can to some degree contribute to the progress of the cancer. Cancer can also lead to general feelings of helplessness, which might lead you to not take actions for your own benefit.

This is yet another reason why it is so important to recast our view of cancer. If we think of the disease as an alien invader or as the body "betraying" us, we set ourselves up for a kind of emotional intimidation and surrender. But when we accept cancer as part of what the body naturally does—we all have precancerous miscopying going on within us right now—and above all see it as the expression of processes that we can redirect by changing our environments, we are more apt to stay in the game emotionally.

When cancer irrupts in open manifestation, it is scary and it can shake our perspective on everything. But our body with cancer is still *us*, and we're still living in the mix of health-sickness we had when we considered ourselves "healthy." It will take more focus and attention and work to try to get these dysregulated processes back under control. But it is still us, and because it is us we can do something about it.

Success Story

Emily worked as a saleswoman for a textile manufacturer in the garment district, where one of her clients, a young man named Carlos, always stood out because of his long, flowing brown hair. One day he dropped by her shop, and while he still had a certain hippie style, his long brown hair was gone. In fact, he was nearly bald.

When Emily asked about the sudden change, he answered with one word: "Chemotherapy."

Emily was saddened, of course, to learn that her friend was going through a health crisis, but she also couldn't help thinking how surprisingly healthy he looked. Like most people, Emily associated cancer therapy with a gray pallor and a generally miserable countenance that made the cure seem worse than the disease. But Carlos seemed flush with vitality.

When Emily pressed him for details, Carlos explained that he was being treated at my practice through a combination of traditional cancer treatments and "alternative" therapies such as meditation and dietary supplementation. Emily filed the thought away.

A few months later, she went in for a routine checkup with her OB/GYN. Years earlier, tests had revealed a small, benign growth on Emily's thymus, a small organ that resides behind the breastbone. So now the OB/GYN ordered a CAT scan, just to be sure. When the results came back, the news was not good. Emily had a series of metastatic tumors on her thymus called thymomas. Emily was now, like Carlos, a cancer patient.

Although Emily knew that her life was about to become much more difficult, she was determined to survive. Remembering her encounter with Carlos, she contacted me for a consultation.

To eradicate the cancer from her body, Emily would be treated with chemotherapy, radiation, and surgery. These measures are effective, but they are generally very taxing, and each is associated with its own range of debilitating side effects, such as nausea, vomiting, fatigue, and pain. That's why, in my integrative practice, I focus on spiritual development as well as physical well-being.

I prescribed nearly fifty dietary supplements and put Emily in touch with a nutritionist and an herbalist. To support and perhaps even improve her mental health, I introduced her to a guided meditation program and she began regular visits with a mental health counselor. Among the supplements she took, Emily noted that probiotics and IV glutathione seemed to produce the most immediate and dramatic effects. Probiotics improved her digestive health almost immediately, while glutathione improved the appearance of her skin and gave her abundant energy. Based on the advice of her nutritionist, Emily eliminated gluten from her diet, which over time helped to resolve a number of physical symptoms that had up to that point been of unknown origin.

Due to her multifaceted treatment plan, Emily experienced few of the side effects generally associated with chemotherapy, radiation, and surgery. Better yet, she soon found herself in remission. Emily was so happy for her new lifestyle and the return of her health that she decided to let the changes she'd made during her treatment direct her toward healthier living overall. She continued to meditate and to see a therapist because, as she expressed it, "Your mind is the most important part of your body." But most dramatic among the reforms she made was that Emily quit her job, which had always been inordinately stressful and physically exhausting. Instead, she began to pursue her passion, which was interior design.

Emily, like many of my patients, continues under my care long after her cancer treatment has ended. I serve not only as her doctor, but also as a friend and a mentor throughout the ups and downs of her remission.

Not only did Emily survive her fight with a frightening disease, but the men and women who helped her get through it changed her life in a number of ways. Her meditation practice resulted in a "spiritual awakening," which she believes improved her relationships with her husband and her daughters; meditation has given her the ability to handle stressful situations with a sense of calm and grace that she had not known previously. Although Emily acknowledges that her diagnosis led to the most terrifying and uncertain time of her life, she is grateful to have gone through the whole experience. She now says that cancer was the gift that allowed her a thousand years of growth in only a few years of life.

The Ecogenetic Way: Cancer Summary

Here's a quick review of the essential steps you can take to improve your cancer environments:

- **Take the long view and take it now.**
  - *Cancer is a disease of life and therefore of time. The mutations that lead to active cancer require years to accumulate. The key is to treat your dormant cancer cells proactively so that they remain dormant. If you have active cancer, use all available means to move it back to being dormant. Do this now!*
- **Slow the cancer clock.**
  - *Mutations are simple clocks marking the rate of random change in cells as they copy themselves, divide, and age. In this sense, the cancer genome is a histogram of your progressing life. If you live too fast, with lots of cancer-promoting behaviors and exposures, your cancer clock speeds up. Slow it back down by avoiding the most prevalent sources of damage and mutation.*

- **Eliminate toxins.**
    - *The place to start slowing your clock is at the beginning—at those triggering exposures that set mutation on its course.*
- Minimize unnecessary medical radiation. Protect yourself from the sun. Test your house for radon.
- Stop smoking. Don't drink alcohol in excess.
- Get immunized for hepatitis and HPV; be sure to immunize your children.
- Beware of xenoestrogens in the environment. Avoid products with BPA.
- Keep up-to-date on emerging carcinogens; the facts are always changing with the science.
- Orient yourself away from industrial chemicals.
- **Get out of the inflammation hothouse!**
    - *Avoiding toxins like those above will also reduce their inflammatory effects.*
    - *Take a fish oil supplement.*
    - *Use olive oil on salads, as a condiment, or for low-temp cooking.*
    - *Avoid cheap, highly processed, easily digestible carbs.*

Gene Therapy Fact: Conjugated Linoleic Acids

Unlike other omega-6 fatty acids, conjugated linoleic acids, or CLAs, lower the risk of breast cancer by reducing estrogen as well as promoting lean muscle mass and lower body fat. Since fat cells produce estrogen, then more muscle translates into less fat, which lowers estrogenic initiation of cancer. In addition, a 2000 study showed that women with the highest CLA levels had significantly lower rates of breast cancer.[20] CLAs are found so minimally in our diet that supplements are necessary to benefit from these fats.

CLA comes from a common omega-6 fatty acid called linolenic acid. So, if linolenic acid is so common, then why is CLA so rare? Because only ruminate animals, like cows, have the ability to convert linolenic acid to CLA. This is why it is found in small amounts in beef and dairy but more abundantly in a clarified (and concentrated) butter called ghee, which is used in Indian cooking. Clearly the Indians are on to something. CLA has been found to inhibit colon, prostate, and breast cancer cell growth; it also induces apoptosis (normal cell death) in these cells. This happens on an ecogenetically sensible level, which explains why mice with breast cancer that spread to the lung had regression of the metastasis in direct proportion to the amount of CLA they were fed.[21]

When it comes to choosing what type of meat you should eat, go green. Grass-fed beef is leaner and healthier than conventionally raised livestock. Not only does grass-fed meat have less fat, it also contains more nutrients like CLA and omega-3. And one study has shown that free-range chicken eggs have higher amounts of omega-3s, less bad fat, and fewer calories.[22]

Targeted Nutrition for Cancer

There is a great range of foods that have been shown to help in disrupting or reducing the progress of cancer. As always, the goal is not to try to optimize your dosage of this or that nutrient, but rather to live a flexible life in which, over the long term that cancer operates, you are generally influencing your body's environments away from cancer and toward better health.

Happily, the things you do to tilt the cancer environments in your favor will, typically, also tilt the heart disease environments in your favor, as well as those for obesity, and so on. Disease builds on disease, but health also builds on health.

Drink Up!

Coffee, tea, and wine all contain important nutrients that have been shown to prevent cancer. However, I prefer my patients limit alcohol consumption to no more than 4 ounces of wine or beer per day.

Coffee
A study reports that the consumption of three cups of caffeinated coffee a day resulted in a reduced risk of developing basal cell carcinoma by 21 percent in women and 10 percent men.[23] Drinking four or more cups of coffee daily has been shown to reduce colon cancer by 15 percent.[24]

Tea

Tea has many favorable health benefits:

- EGCG from green tea has been shown to activate cancer-inhibiting genes (e.g., p16, p65, and p70).
- Quercetin, an antioxidant compound found in certain teas (especially apple and chamomile teas), prevents free radical formations and inhibits cancer cell proliferation. It is also found in onions and red wine.
- The regular consumption of black tea among nonsmoking women lowered lung cancer risk by about 31 percent.[25]
- Polyphenols, which are antioxidants found in white, green, black, and red teas, were found to block anti-apoptotic proteins in prostatic cancer cells.[26] Some studies suggest it is best not to add milk to your tea as it can diminish the absorption of the beneficial polyphenols[27]. Try lemon, mint, or honey as an alternative.

Wine

One study has shown that the antioxidant compound resveratrol, found in red wine, sensitizes prostate tumor cells to radiation treatments, and that perforin and granzyme B were at particularly low levels in prostate tumor cells. Why is this important? Because these two proteins work together to kill cells, but it appears that prostate tumor cells keep these proteins from being expressed in the high amounts needed for apoptosis. Resveratrol, however, significantly increases the activity of perforin and granzyme B. After resveratrol was added and radiation treatment followed, about 97 percent of the prostate tumor cells were killed (this amount was even greater than if radiation had been administered alone).[28]

And men who consume one glass of red wine per day have 50 percent less prostate cancer, studies have shown.[29] Resveratrol inhibits the gene that makes aromatase and the enzyme that controls estrogen production. Resveratrol acts against several genes that promote and cause prostate cancer. It inhibits COX-2 expression (thus inhibiting the ability of cells to make new blood vessels in angiogenesis); plus it activates the tumor suppressor gene p53 and deactivates protein kinase expression.

Gene Therapy Fact: Coconut Power

I recommend that all my patients include coconut milk or its powder as part of their diet. Coconut milk is very rich in lauric acid and is associated with a low risk of breast cancer. As coconuts are a staple of Thai cuisine, it should come as no surprise that Thailand also has the lowest incidence of breast cancer worldwide!

- Add coconut milk powder to coffee instead of your usual creamer.
- Substitute it for cow's milk in recipes such as curries and desserts.
- Whip up a healthy, refreshing piña colada beverage using coconut milk.

Spices

Fenugreek

As a medicinal herb fenugreek made its mark in ancient Egypt, where it was first described as a remedy for digestive problems and menopausal symptoms. Centuries later, fenugreek is used as an appetite suppressant, antidiabetic antidote, and lactation stimulator. The herb is indigenous to the Mediterranean region. Although its seeds and leaves are used to spice up dishes, the herb has also been shown to fight prostate cancer.[30] Researchers have also shown that fenugreek kills breast and pancreatic cancer cells, but is selective enough to avoid normal cells.

Turmeric

Spice up your meals with curry because the curcumin in turmeric, which gives curry powder its yellow color, selectively targets cancer stem cells. (The same is true for piperine, found in black pepper.) A study showed that while cancer stem cells were targeted, normal breast tissue cells were unaffected by these compounds.[31] Turmeric is a strong antioxidant, anti-inflammatory, and chemotherapeutic agent. It has also been shown that curcumin slows down the growth of tumor cells and keeps cancer cells from replicating.[32] In addition, studies are under way to explore the ability of curcumin to cut off the oxygen supply to tumor cells.

Gene Therapy Fact:
Curcumin Targets Cancer

There are at least twenty ways in which curcumin suppresses pre-cancerous lesions and tumor cell lines. Here are some of its anti-cancer activities:

- blocks nuclear factor–kappa B (NF-kB), which is a protein complex involved in regulating inflammatory and immune responses, particularly cancer-related inflammation[33]
- suppresses advanced glycation end products (AGEs), which are glycotoxins found in cancer tissue and linked to oxidative stress and inflammation[34]
- promotes normal cellular replication and apoptosis (cell death), which prevents uncontrolled proliferation of cancer cells[35]
- targets cancer cells, leaving healthy tissues unaffected[36]
- enhances tumor cell sensitivity to drugs[37]
- inhibits metastasis (cancer cell migration) through numerous mechanisms[38]

Spice Up Meals with Turmeric

Although turmeric is generally a staple ingredient in curry powder, some people like to add a little extra of this spice when preparing curries.

And turmeric doesn't have to be used only in curries. Add turmeric to egg salad to give it an even bolder yellow color. Mix brown rice with raisins and cashews and season with turmeric, cumin, and coriander. This spice is delicious on sautéed apples, and healthy steamed cauliflower and/or green beans and onions. Or, for a creamy, flavor-rich, low-calorie dip, try mixing some turmeric and dried onion with a little omega-3-rich mayonnaise, salt, and pepper. Serve with raw cauliflower, celery, bell pepper, and broccoli florets. Turmeric is a great spice to complement recipes that feature lentils. Give salad dressings an orange-yellow hue by adding some turmeric powder to them. For an especially delicious way to add more turmeric to your healthy way of eating, cut cauliflower florets in half and healthy sauté with a generous spoonful of turmeric for 5 minutes. Remove from the heat and toss with olive oil, salt, and pepper to taste.

Saffron

Saffron is a golden yellow spice with a floral taste that is used to add color and zest to a variety of dishes such as bouillabaisse and paella. But this fragrant spice has been used medicinally for centuries to stimulate appetite, treat headaches and depression, and control indigestion. For quite some time, however, researchers have also implicated saffron and its carotenoid component crocin as a phytotherapeutic treatment option for cancer.[39] In one study, scientists examined the effects of saffron in rats with liver cancer and reported that the spice wielded a strong chemopreventive effect by promoting cell death and blocking growth in cancer cells.[40] Crocetin, another constituent of saffron, also inhibits cancer by promoting cell death, blocking replication, and triggering antioxidative activity.[41]

Gene Therapy Fact:
Spice Up Your Genome

I tell my patients to eat an array of plant-based foods that have been shown to combat cancer-causing genes. Here are some anticancer herbs you can incorporate into your meals:

- allspice
- anise
- basil
- caraway
- cardamom
- celery
- chili pepper
- rosemary
- saffron
- tumeric

Rosemary

Rosemary helps protect against breast tumors and is a powerful activator of detoxification enzymes. A member of the mint family Lamiaceae and usually found in warmer climates close to the sea, rosemary can grow to five feet tall and remain in the same place for up to thirty years if handled well. A study showed that rats fed rosemary before ingesting breast cancer–inducing toxins developed 75 percent fewer breast tumors than untreated controls.[42] Similar to green tea, rosemary has also been found to increase the concentration of chemotherapeutic drugs in breast cancer cells. Carnosol, a principal component of rosemary, has ecogenetic effects including increasing the production of enzymes that detoxify carcinogens, promoting cancer cell death and protecting against inflammation. One of the biggest promoters of colon cancer is activating protein 1 (AP-1), and this protein is blocked by the rosmarinic acid in rosemary (as well as by the isoliquiritigenin in licorice and by CLA).[43]

Gene Therapy Fact: Toxins

The buildup of toxins in the body has been linked to problems such as cognitive deficits, depression, fatigue, headaches, allergies, and asthma, and chronic pain via deleterious gene effects, or "toxicogenomics." Toxins enter the body through various conduits: the skin, the nose, and the mouth. The foods you eat and the beverages you drink bring in the majority of toxins into your body. So eating detoxifying foods is the best way to fight years of toxic buildup. Eat clean foods. And that means not conveniently packaged and processed foods—canned vegetables, soft drinks, and prepackaged meals are not clean foods. Conversely, this shouldn't imply that preparations need to be tedious and time-consuming or that purchasing food has to be expensive. That's why I tell my patients to eat clean and colorful foods daily, such as fruits and vegetables.

Beans, Fruits, and Vegetables

These food groups are very high in fiber, which has been shown to reduce the risk of various diseases, especially colon cancer. One major study conducted by the European Prospective Investigation into Cancer (EPIC) evaluated the connection between diet and cancer risk and reported that high dietary consumption of fiber reduces the risk for colon cancer significantly.[44] The study followed more than 519,000 European participants spanning ten countries for four and a half years, during which time 1,065 participants were diagnosed with colon cancer. Individuals whose fiber consumption was in the top 20 percent (35 grams daily) had a 40 percent lower risk for developing the disease than participants who consumed an average of 15 grams daily.

Gene Therapy Fact: Go Organic

Researchers compiled data from fifty studies to compare conventionally produced versus organically grown fruits and vegetables. The results showed that organic foods have a higher nutritional value 40 percent of the time whereas standard food production has a higher nutritional value only 15 percent of the time. The bottom line is that organic produce contains fewer carcinogens, has a better protein quality, and has 20 percent more vitamin C than conventionally grown produce that has been sprayed with fungicides, herbicides, pesticides, and chemical-based fertilizers. The twelve fruits and vegetables most likely to have pesticide residues are apples, bell peppers, celery, cherries, imported grapes, pears, potatoes, strawberries, nectarines, peaches, red raspberries, and spinach. I recommend that my patients buy organic for these whenever possible.

Gene Therapy Fact: Avoid Overcooking

A common question is whether to cook vegetables or eat them raw. While you might think that raw vegetables would better maintain their nutritive integrity, that's not necessarily the case. Italian researchers reported that cooking your vegetables helps to render some of the nutrients more bioavailable.[45] For instance, steaming broccoli helps to increase the amount of available glucosinolates, which are plant compounds with cancer-preventive effects. But be sure to steam—not boil. Boiling glucosinolate-rich vegetables like broccoli saps their anticancer effectiveness by 77 percent.[46]

Lupeol

Lupeol is a phytonutrient that helps to prevent metastasis, shrinking tumors faster than conventional medications, and it can help patients maintain weight during treatments such as chemotherapy.[47] Lupeol is found in mangoes, cabbages, green peppers, olives, and grapes. In addition to its anticancer properties, it has anti-inflammatory and antimicrobial effects, and has even been shown to lower cholesterol.[48]

Ajoene

According to the National Cancer Institute, the sulfur components in garlic and other members of the allium family, such as onions and leeks, possess anticancer properties, and research has linked garlic consumption to a reduced risk of certain cancers, including colorectal cancer. Ajoene is one such organosulfur compound in garlic that has shown promise as a cancer treatment. Specifically, ajoene has been shown to slow tumor growth through mitochondrial-dependent apoptosis.[49] The allyl mercaptan in garlic is an HDAC inhibitor that can restore the function of p21, a tumor suppressor gene, thus inhibiting cancer cell growth.

The chemical makeup of garlic is complex, and the quality of garlic depends on how it is grown, whether it is fresh or manufactured in the form of oil, flakes, or powder, or whether it is a supplement. Peeling fresh garlic releases a compound known as alliinase; after peeling garlic, wait at least fifteen minutes before cooking to preserve its cancer-fighting benefits.

Gene Therapy Fact: Nature's Gene Medicines

One exciting class of anticancer drugs is the histone deacetylase inhibitors (HDAC inhibitors). These drugs work on overactive HDAC, which promotes cancerous change by silencing the tumor suppressor genes. A number of food-based nutrients are also HDAC inhibitors: indole-3, carbinol, and sulforaphane found in cruciferous vegetables as well as in alliums like garlic, chives, and onions. Butyrate, produced by the breakdown of dietary fiber in the gut, is a powerful HDAC inhibitor. This is partly why cruciferous, allium, and fiber-rich vegetables are associated with lower cancer risk.

Lycopene

A study conducted at the Karmanos Cancer Center showed that, when administered preoperatively to men with prostate cancer, lycopene helped to decrease the aggressiveness and size of the tumor. A high intake of lycopene from cooked tomato products has also been associated with lower colon cancer risk, especially in smokers.[50] Most pink and red fruits and vegetables contain lycopene, and sweet potatoes are another excellent source. Pomegranates contain a lycopene-related chemical called punicalagin, which was shown in a 2011 study[51] of men with recurrent prostate cancer to stop the rise of prostate-specific antigen (PSA), which is a biomarker for a protein produced by the prostate gland that, at high levels, is associated with prostate cancer progression.

Gene Therapy Fact: Mom's Cruciferous Cure

When your mother told you to eat your broccoli, she definitely had good reason: cruciferous vegetables are a potent food group containing a vast array of toxin-fighting nutrients, and many studies have shown them to protect against a number of cancers, such as breast, colon, prostate, and ovarian. In fact, the consumption of cruciferous vegetables has been shown to reduce the risk of cancer by up to 54 percent.[52] They also help to maximize the body's detoxification centers in order to prevent toxic buildup and DNA damage.[53] There is a wide range of cruciferous vegetables for you to explore:

- arugula
- black and brown mustard greens
- bok choy
- broccoli
- broccoli rabe
- brussels sprouts
- cabbage
- cauliflower
- collard greens
- horseradish
- Japanese radishes

- kale
- parsnips
- radishes
- rutabaga
- turnips

Gene Therapy Fact: Phyto Gene Defense

In my practice I treat many patients with a mixed cocktail of vitamin E tocotrienols, lycopene, and selenium, which helps keep dormant tumors hibernating for good.

The combination of lycopene, selenium, and full-spectrum vitamin E (all eight forms found in nature, in rice bran oil, rather than a single form found in most supplements) has been shown to be stronger cancer prevention than any of these nutrients alone. What exactly do these micronutrients do on an ecogenetic level? Researchers who administered this trio to mice that had spontaneously developed prostate cancer observed that, together, they activated an inhibitor of angiogenesis to promote tumor dormancy in the early phases of the disease.[54]

Quercetin

Found in grapes, onions, apples, berries, and red wine, quercetin is another one of nature's gene therapy wonders. It inhibits tyrosine kinase, one of the major enzymes associated with cancer. It also helps to activate tumor suppressor genes p53 and p21, which shut off during cancer.[55]

Persin

Not only do avocados contain a good type of fat with anti-inflammatory properties, but their leaves have been shown to inhibit the growth of breast cancer cells. Persin, a plant toxin in the leaves, has been identified as the agent responsible for necrosis and cell death in lactating livestock with mammary cancers.[56] A further study has shown persin to have multiple inhibitory effects on genes known to cause breast cancer. Laboratory studies using human breast cancer cells[57] also demonstrated that persin worked through specific pathways and targeted cell cyclic phases in order to synergistically enhance the cytotoxic effects of breast cancer drug tamoxifen[58] in human breast cancer cells.

Sulforaphane
Sulforaphane, found in broccoli, bok choy, brussels sprouts, and other cruciferous vegetables, has important cancer-fighting properties. It enhances the removal of carcinogens from the body and promotes the activation of tumor suppressor genes. In one study involving more than 1,300 prostate cancer patients, researchers reported that a decreased risk of aggressive forms of prostate cancer was associated with greater consumption of cruciferous vegetables such as broccoli and cauliflower.[59] Sulforaphane has also been shown to reduce the amount of *Helicobacter pylori*, a bacterium that causes stomach cancers.[60] Plus, naturally occurring sulforaphane has been shown to be as effective in cancer prevention as HDAC inhibitor drugs.[61] For your fill of this natural cancer-fighting compound, eat broccoli sprouts, which contain fifty times more sulforaphane than broccoli.

Gene Therapy Fact: Broccoli Beats Peas

Broccoli seems to have profound ecogenetic implications for prostate cancer prevention. In one study, men at risk for developing prostate cancer were given broccoli or peas in addition to their normal diet for over a year. By examining tissue samples obtained before, during, and after the trial, researchers found that gene expression associated with a lower risk for prostate cancer was highly associated with men who ate a broccoli-rich diet. Even more interesting was that men who possessed the gene glutathione S-transferase (GSTM1), which has a role in detoxification, enjoyed even greater chemopreventive effects.[62]

Genistein
Genistein, a compound found in soybeans and soy-based foods, is effective against lung and prostate cancer. Specifically, it can restore the function of cancer-inhibiting genes p16, p65, and p70, leading to reduced risk of developing lung cancer.[63] The average PSA level in men taking genestein as a supplement decreased by 7.1 compared to a 4.1 increase in those taking placebo.[64]

Gene Therapy Fact:
Bee Propolis and Cancer

I suggest 500 milligrams daily of bee propolis (a material used to repair holes in hives), which has been shown to have immune-modulating, antimicrobial, and anti-inflammatory effects.[65] It also reduces the growth of many cancers including colon, prostate, and kidney. It has also been found to be effective in reducing mouth sores associated with chemotherapy and radiation.

Vitamins

You need a well-balanced diet in order to prevent cancer, and if you aren't getting enough nutrients from your whole food intake, you may need to supplement your diet with vitamins and minerals. Vitamins play an important role in maintaining your health through boosting immunity, preventing free radical damage to cells, and upregulating the expression of genes involved in preventing cancer. The following vitamins have been shown to be effective in cancer prevention.

Vitamin B6

One study reported that vitamin B6 prevented human pancreatic cancer cell growth.[66] Although the levels cited in the study were relatively high amounts, the high doses did not appear to lead to side effects; however, further studies are still needed to determine proper dosing levels for pancreatic cancer prevention. In a review of studies conducted in the United States, Europe, and Asia, researchers found that taking vitamin B6 supplements increased blood levels of pyridoxal phosphate (PLP), which decreases the risk of colorectal cancer.[67]

Vitamin C

A daily intake of 200 milligrams of vitamin C has been shown to prevent and reduce various chronic diseases, including cancer.[68] Grapefruit packs a powerful punch because it provides you with all the vitamin C you need, and it contains a plentiful number of phytonutrients that help your body fight cancer. It is especially useful to fight prostate cancer, since it contains naringenin, a citrus flavonoid that repairs damaged DNA in prostatic cancer cells.

Vitamin D

One study showed that women at high risk for developing melanoma—the most severe form of skin cancer—can cut their risk by about half by taking vitamin D and calcium supplements.[69] These same substances could also reduce the melanoma risk for women previously diagnosed with nonmelonomic forms of cancer, such as basal cell carcinoma.

Vitamin E

In a comparison between bladder cancer patients and a healthy control group, researchers found that those who had the highest average intake of vitamin E had a decreased risk—by 34 percent—of developing bladder cancer; they also demonstrated a reduction in the development of bladder cancer cells in those with higher vitamin E intake.[70] In another study, researchers administered doses of a type of vitamin E called tocomin to mice and concluded that the mice that received the vitamin E had significantly lower occurrences of prostate cancer. The findings also concluded that a mixed type of vitamin E prevented prostatic tumors from developing further into high-grade forms.[71]

Vitamin K

A lesser-known but important anticancer nutrient is this fat-soluble vitamin, which serves many physiologic functions, such as aiding in the process of blood clotting and assisting brain and immune function. There are two types of vitamin K: K1 and K2. You are probably more familiar with vitamin K1, which is a dietary form found in leafy green vegetables, such as spinach, broccoli, and lettuce. Vitamin K2 also comes from dietary sources, but it is primarily produced by bacteria in your gut and it occurs as a smaller percentage of the vitamin K in your body. Vitamin K2 works by restoring the cancer cell's ability to die. In a process called apoptosis, normal cells die when they become old in order to make room for new cells; cancer cells lose this ability and continue to divide uncontrollably. Nutrients like K2 that help cancer cells regain the ability to die normally are called "pro-apoptic" nutrients. In one study, the consumption of foods with vitamin K2—especially cheese—helps to reduce cancer risk by 14 percent. Cancer mortality was also reduced by 28 percent.[72]

Targeted Supplements

Targeted Ecogenetic Juice for Cancer

The following juice recipe is for those who are concerned about cancer. But don't feel as though you have to drink this specific juice every day. Shake things up! I've included several juicing recipes at the end of each disease-specific chapter. The ecogenetic juices listed are general recipes that focus on using wholesome ingredients and organically grown produce that have beneficial effects on many body systems. So you don't have to worry about sticking to any specific drink. My patients usually drink one or two ecogenetic juices daily. Mix up the juices you drink to broaden your intake of bioactive nutrients on a weekly basis. If you have a specific health concern, increase your intake of that recommended ecogenetic drink.

> 2 celery stalks
> 1 beet
> 1 apple
> ¼ cup broccoli
> 1 cucumber, peeled
> ½ cup coconut water
> ¼ cup watercress
> 1 tablespoon coconut milk powder
> ⅓ teaspoon ground turmeric

> Juice the celery, beet, apple, broccoli, and cucumber. Blend with the other ingredients for 50 to 60 seconds on medium power. Drink and enjoy.

Targeted Ecogenetic Supplements for Cancer

The supplements listed below are recommendations for cancer prevention and treatment. Don't get overwhelmed and feel that you have to take every supplement listed. Remember: everyone is unique. The supplement list is in no particular order. I recommend them all equally to my patients because each one has anticancer benefits. Many of my patients start off by taking one supplement to determine how well they are tolerating it. Then they add other supplements as needed. When taking supplements, the focus should be to maintain good health. Don't worry about whether you should be taking five, ten, or fifteen supplements. That is not the intent of the supplement list. Do what you can. And take your time in figuring out what works for you: good health isn't a destination; it's a lifelong practice. And supplements are a small part of attaining a healthy lifestyle. Supplements are meant to be an addition to not a replacement for eating a healthy diet, getting adequate sleep, and improving your level of physical activity.

The supplements below are among the most important ones I give to many of my patients. Because every person is different, certain supplements may be more important than others for a given individual.

- Artichoke extract—320 milligrams, once daily
- D-limonene—1,000 milligrams, once daily
- Magnolia extract—200 milligrams, once daily
- DIM (Di-indole methane, a form of indole-3-carbinol)—100 milligrams, twice daily
- Maitake D-fraction—twenty drops daily
- Shiitake extract—500 milligrams, twice daily
- Chaga mushroom extract—500 milligrams, once daily
- Oil of oregano (phytocap)—500 milligrams, once daily
- Vitamin D3—1000 IU, once daily
- Skullcap (*Scutellaria lateriflora* extract)—400 milligrams, once daily
- Blackseed capsule (black cumin seed oil)—500 milligrams, twice daily
- Bee propolis—500 milligrams, once daily

Chapter 5

Diabetes

DIABETES IS ONLY THE SEVENTH LEADING CAUSE OF DEATH IN THE UNITED STATES, but fully 50 percent more people die of diabetes today than they did in 1987.[1] According to the National Diabetes Foundation, more than 8 percent of the entire population, counting children and adults, has an active form of the disease. If you add those with "prediabetes" to the list, the number skyrockets, to more than one hundred million cases, or around one-third of all Americans. By contrast, only about twelve million have ever had a cancer diagnosis (though this figure cannot account for all the creeping cases that have not yet been detected).

Targeted Nutrients for Diabetes at a Glance

Nutritional Ecogenetics	Dietary Sources
juicing	aloe, blueberry, and grape juice
carbohydrates	whole grains (e.g., rye bread, steel-cut oats), broccoli
fats	omega-3 fatty acids
proteins	walnuts, watermelon seed powder
ecogenetic nutrients and supplements	aloe vera, cinnamon, *Gymnema sylvestre* extract, green coffee bean extract, resveratrol

Diabetes doesn't always kill, but it leads the list for causing nonmortal but terribly debilitating conditions such as blindness, amputation, kidney failure, and nerve damage. Heart disease and stroke are also made much likelier by the corrosion of blood vessels that is caused by diabetes.

Despite its enormous prevalence, diabetes is often viewed as a disease of the poor, or of the old, or of the constitutionally infirm. But, as we will see, this is the opposite of the truth. Diabetes is a very real possibility for anyone, particularly for anyone living the way most people live in the United States and in the rest of the developed world. While the risk factors for diabetes may seem to be lurking in every drink, snack, or even fruit, remember that it is never too late to bring back balance. Achieving the ecogenetic balance for diabetes will result in a thinner, healthier you as well.

There are two main forms of the disease, type 1 and type 2. Type 1 diabetes—what used to be called "juvenile diabetes"—is an autoimmune disease. The patient's immune system attacks the special cells in the pancreas (pancreatic beta cells) that produce insulin and allow the body to clear glucose from the bloodstream. Type 2 diabetes, on the other hand, is predominantly a lifestyle and environmental disease. The patient develops insulin resistance over time—often over a very long time—and only in the last stages of acquiring the disease, perhaps as much as thirty or more years later, loses pancreatic function. Over 90 percent of cases are type 2, and that is the form I will consider in this chapter.

Fundamentally, diabetes is a disruption of the body's glucose metabolism. Glucose processing, because it is a primary source of energy for all the body's activities, is naturally a highly managed operation. When you eat a meal, the stomach and intestines break it down into substances that can be transferred into the bloodstream and transported to the cells. Glucose is derived from carbohydrates; when you eat a carbohydrate-rich meal, your blood glucose concentration quickly spikes. The body tries to keep the level in a fairly narrow band, so it must devise a way to "clear" the excess. The way it does this is through cooperation between the cells that sense the rising sugar levels and those that sense the signal to take up and store glucose in the safe recesses of their interiors.

The first part of this system is controlled by the pancreas, which senses the elevation of glucose and then releases the hormone insulin to help abate the flood. The second part involves those cells that receive insulin's signal—the muscle, liver, and fat cells that will ultimately store the energy for future use. Just as the pancreas senses the rising glucose, so these storage cells sense the rising insulin. And in a beautifully symmetrical fashion, as the pancreas releases insulin, the storage cells, in a kind of mirroring, take up the glucose. Sense and release; sense and absorb. The flow is even and regular.

But this harmony can indeed break down. What precisely goes wrong? What are the environments that lead to such a dysfunction?

Success Story

A native Long Islander, Linda is a married thirty-six-year-old stay-at-home mother to a five-year-old boy and a seven-year-old girl. She is an active member of the PTA at her children's school; she coordinates bake sales and arranges book drives to help raise money. She also coaches her daughter's soccer team. At five feet five and 125 pounds, Linda has never gained much weight or worked out vigorously to maintain her slender frame. Even after the birth of her children she was able to shed most of the baby weight. Jokingly, Linda's friends would often say she has the "celebrity post-baby bod gene."

"I was blessed with a fast metabolism, so I could eat anything and not gain weight," Linda said. Before she came to see me, she was in the habit of enjoying breakfast at a local café twice a week and loved to order sugary caffeinated drinks like mochas. Linda often relied on frozen family-size meals like lasagna for dinner.

Over the course of a year, however, Linda reported, "I just couldn't get out of bed most mornings. I was just so tired." She struggled to coach soccer and to participate in her other activities. Most mornings she would get the kids to school barely on time. Her fatigue became crippling; her mother offered to move in to help her with the kids and the household duties. "I'm a doer so it was extremely difficult to ask for help from my friends, family, and neighbors, but I just couldn't do it myself anymore."

When Linda came to see me, her most pressing concern was that she might have developed cancer. She expressed this concern because her aunt had had breast cancer. And during the time

Linda was in college, her mother, a smoker for twenty-five years, had been diagnosed with lung cancer. Linda admitted she'd also smoked cigarettes in high school and college. "But when my mother was diagnosed, it was a no-brainer—I didn't want to get cancer too!" Fortunately, the tests I performed revealed that Linda was cancer-free; however, her blood sugar levels were high. Even though she was thin and athletic looking, she was on the verge of developing type 2 diabetes. She was also vitamin D deficient. Studies show that lower levels of vitamin D are linked to prediabetes among adults.

A self-proclaimed "sugar addict," Linda confessed that she rarely ate fruits or vegetables. To help her improve her diet, I instructed her to cut her sugar intake and get rid of the processed foods. I also introduced her to ecogenetically healthy foods such as green coffee bean extracts (unroasted coffee beans) that have been shown to suppress spikes and after-meal blood sugar surges, and to turmeric, which has been shown to reduce and regulate blood glucose levels. Linda's diet switched from fast food and sugary treats to eating plenty of:

- resveratrol-rich fruits such as red grapes, mulberries, and blueberries
- onion and garlic added to meals because they have proven antidiabetic effects
- vegetables and legumes (especially fenugreek), which all help to keep blood sugar levels under control
- supplements to support glucose control such as *Gymnema sylvestre* extract, berberine, and carnitine

"I feel as though I've gotten my life back," she now says. "The simple things I used to do like carpool or coach my daughter's soccer team became so difficult. Now I savor those moments because I couldn't even get out of bed to make breakfast a few months ago."

The Environments of Diabetes

Inflammation

Glucose entering the stream, insulin entering the stream in response; muscle, liver, and fat cells responding in turn to insulin, and in turn absorbing glucose—the ebb and flow rhythm of the regulation is simple and self-tuning. But as we know, it regularly breaks down. And it tends to break down in a particular sequence, starting on the insulin-sensing, glucose-absorbing side. From this early and very common (and very often undetected) state of insulin resistance, the progression is typically to prediabetes, in which the glucose-sensing, insulin-releasing side begins to struggle, and finally to full-blown type 2 diabetic disease, where both sides are deeply impaired.

Traditionally, diabetes has been thought to result from eating certain kinds of food or from inheriting a certain range of genes. But in just the past few years research has shown that it is predominantly a result of chronic inflammation. This does not mean that nutrition is unrelated to diabetes—on the contrary, your eating patterns are very deeply involved in your diabetes risks. But what you put in your mouth—this piece of bread or that soda or even that candy bar—is not a direct determinant of becoming sick in this way. Rather, the much more significant source of risk is the inflammation that invades the glucose-absorbing cells and keeps them from doing their proper work.

This can be a difficult concept to grasp. It seems natural to think that diabetes, as the disease of sugar regulation, would be somehow closely related to the actual sugars we dump into our bloodstreams. But flooding your bloodstream with sugar from food is *not*, all by itself, going to render your cells insulin resistant. A healthy glucose regulation system can handle that sort of challenge, certainly over shorter time frames.

Chronic high sugar intake is very unhealthy in many ways, and it will also eventually contribute to burning out parts of the regulation system if they are truly overtaxed for extended periods. But it is important to understand the crucial difference between the sugar you eat and your cells' ability to process and store that sugar. Sugar flowing through your blood and washing up on the shores of fat, liver, and muscle cells cannot break the ability of those cells to absorb that sugar.

Gene Therapy Fact: Diabetes Screening

Diabetes has been underreported worldwide due to the antiquated definition of the disease. The most accurate test for measuring blood glucose levels is an oral glucose tolerance test, which detects dangerous postmeal sugar spikes and other glycemic irregularities. Also the hemoglobin A1C is an indication of glucose levels over a longer time period. Your best protection from diabetes is to prevent chronically high blood glucose levels and after-meal sugar surges.

What Insulin Resistance Means

So if sugar is not the culprit in this sugar disease, what is? To get at that, let's step back for a minute and ask a more fundamental question: what exactly do we mean when we talk about "insulin sensing" and "glucose absorption"? It's obvious that the cells somehow get the signal to take in the glucose that's flowing in the bloodstream. But how are those signals actually delivered and received?

Inflammatory Markers

Inflammatory Mediator	Normal Production	Excess Production
Tumor necrosis factor alpha (TNF-alpha)	Important for proper immune response	Excessive amounts can contribute to tumor formation, poor heart pumping, blood clots
Nuclear factor–kappa B (NF-kB)	Required for initiation of inflammatory response	Activated by damaged cells to turn on four hundred–plus genes that promote inflammation
Eicosanoids	Include many mediators pro- and anti-inflammation; release substances in close proximity to the site of inflammation	Prostaglandin E2 and leukotriene B4 are main inflammatory eicosanoids
Interleukins	Play a role in both pro- and anti-inflammatory reactions	Interleukins 10 (G13 allele), 22, 23 have been found to cause inflammation in arteries, lung, skin, and brain

Inflammatory Mediator	Normal Production	Excess Production
C-reactive protein (CRP)	Released immediately by the liver during inflammatory response	Elevated levels are associated with inflammation and predict future risk of coronary artery disease and diabetes

In normal functioning, insulin is received by insulin receptors (IR) on the surface of fat, muscle, and liver cells. The receptors then pass the signal along a chain of further signaling agents within the cells, including the insulin receptor substrates (IRS). This receiving chain, when it is complete, then gives the signal for a second sequence to initiate the process of importing glucose through the cell membrane into the cell's interior. Only then does glucose uptake in fact occur.[2] The initial connection starts the ball rolling, but the *whole chain* of reception has to proceed in order for glucose to be absorbed. It's obvious that the receptors have to be in place, but *so do* the substrates to the receptors. If there's no insulin or no insulin receptor, then there's no glucose uptake; but *also* if there's no insulin receptor substrates, there's no glucose uptake. It takes two to tango, and two or three or four to get sugar into the cells.

Gene Therapy Fact: Metformin and Cancer

Studies are exploring the possible chemopreventive and chemotherapeutic effects of metformin, an antidiabetic drug. Metformin, synthesized from lilac, which has been used in European folk medicine to treat diabetes. A study in the *Journal of Clinical Oncology*[3] evaluated women with very large breast cancers who were not good surgical candidates for either lumpectomy or mastectomy; the women who were taking metformin had a threefold increase in pathologic complete remission rate—meaning that breast tissue samples revealed no microscopic traces of cancer. Metformin is a powerful activator of genes involved in tumor suppression. If you're concerned about metformin's side effects, you don't have to be. Metformin has a good safety profile; its most common side effect is gastrointestinal problems, which can be readily avoided by gradually increasing the drug's dose.

It's important to control blood glucose levels, because diabetes (type 2 in particular) and cancer have similar risk factors—being overweight or obese, having a sedentary lifestyle, eating unhealthily, smoking, consuming excessive alcohol. A collaborative report released by the American Cancer Society and the American Diabetes Association found that people with type 2 diabetes had a higher risk for developing cancer.[4]

Certain studies have shown that metformin may possess anticancer properties.[5] An observational study evaluating the health records of men with diabetes and prostate cancer found that those who were being treated with metformin had a significantly lower risk of death.[6] Many studies have been conducted to investigate the potential promise of metformin as an adjuvant treatment among diabetics with cancer. Furthermore, metformin has shown promise as a cancer-preventive drug in diabetics. It has also been shown to reduce the risk of recurrence among cancer survivors.

This is precisely where inflammation enters the picture, thanks to cytokines, signaling proteins that trigger the reaction. They also gunk up the insulin-receiving process by dysregulating the downstream components of the insulin receptors, notably those insulin receptor substrates. They react and bind with the IRS, which crowds out insulin and insulin receptors from being able to make their own connections. The insulin is still there, waiting outside the cell to be welcomed in, but the cells are already spoken for.

This is what is meant by insulin resistance. It is not that the cells can't "sense" insulin—it's that they have already taken up with other molecules to form a chemical bond. Resistance in this case really means "otherwise engaged."

The Role of Fat

Broken sugar metabolism is not so much a function of sugar but of inflammation. This still leaves the question of where the inflammation comes from. And the answer, based on what we have learned in previous chapters, is fairly predictable.

The dominant source of the inflammation that leads to insulin resistance—

to insulin receptor substrates being tied up with cytokines—is *fat*. As we have seen, fat is now known to be a far more complex and physiologically interesting tissue than previously thought. It is in continuous contact with the rest of the body via its release of hormone-like substances such as leptin, the keystone appetite molecule. But fat sends many other such agents circulating through the blood, including two extremely potent inflammatory molecules: tumor necrosis factor alpha (TNF-alpha) and interleukin-6 (IL-6). The fat cells, and the macrophages that cluster within fat tissue, release these inflammatory agents in proportion to their presence in the body: the more fat tissue, the greater the inflammatory signaling. When fat tissue is abundant, inflammation becomes an almost constant feature of the whole system. This is what is meant by chronic inflammation. Many of the substances that lead the charge against infection, and marshal the troops for acute and necessary high-speed inflammatory responses, are the same ones that, in lower intensities but over much longer periods, steadily bathe the tissues in inflaming fluids.[7]

Gene Therapy Fact: Coconut Oil

Half of coconut oil's content is composed of lauric acid, a compound that contains strong anti-inflammatory properties. In one study, McGill University researchers examined the effects cooking with coconut oil had on the health of people with thyroid disease.[8] Thyroid disease affects various aspects of your health, including energy, metabolism, and weight, and here using coconut oil can help by improving your symptoms. For instance, the researchers reported that people who switched to coconut oil experienced weight loss of about twelve to thirty-six pounds a year. Since coconut oil can be used to make energy within the mitochondria, which is the powerhouse for cellular energy, cooking and preparing meals with it can help to bolster your metabolism and energy.

It is these molecules—above all TNF-alpha and Il-6—that run rampant through the cells and disrupt insulin signal receiving. They do this mainly by triggering secondary cascades of reactions that then bind up IRS, but also by overexpressing proinflammatory genes in the host cells, which then further exacerbate the secondary scavengers.[9] If the cytokines are the Cat in the Hat who brings disaster into the house, these secondaries are Thing 1 and Thing 2 who do the actual damage. IRS is changed and diverted and suppressed, inflammation feeds forward more inflammation, with the result that insulin cannot get its signal all the way through. From the inside out, the cell is being rendered insulin resistant.

So the insulin resistance that ends in the muscle or liver cell's nucleus and IRS *begins* in the body's fat tissue. Diabetes is in the first instance a disease of inflammation, not of sugar consumption, but that inflammation starts when you eat more sugar than you need, which tilts your energy balance *out* of balance and you grow fatter.

In the Engine Rooms of the Cells

Even if fat and muscle cells are being deafened by cascades of inflammatory noise, the pancreas can usually still crank up the volume of insulin so that at least *some* of its signal gets through.

But eventually, as insulin resistance and prediabetes develop into active diabetic disease, the pancreas loses this ability. It too becomes deaf to the warnings, and just as fat and muscle are insensitive to insulin, so the pancreas no longer responds to glucose. And now insulin is being neither released nor sensed, and glucose is being neither sensed nor absorbed. That two-sided breakdown of the balance is the functional definition of diabetes.

To see how this further escalation of the crisis happens, we need to enter the environment of the mitochondria, the little power plants of the cells. The ultimate fate of glucose in the body is to be processed and burned for energy in mitochondrial fires. You eat for energy to power the body. That energy may be stored for use later (in fat, muscle, and the liver) or burned up immediately. But sooner or later it will go to the mitochondria for processing. How that processing misfires is at the heart of diabetic disability.

The Marvelous Machine

The amazing thing about the mitochondria is not that they sometimes fail but just how wonderfully efficient they are when they are working. As glucose and fatty acids enter the cell, they are broken down and then funneled into the mitochondrial matrix, which is like a long assembly line folded in on itself. Here the molecular products are processed and reprocessed in order to generate ATP, the form of energy that the cell can use for its own work.

The last stage of this processing is the electron transfer cycle, a truly remarkable engineering feat that operates within the cells of most living things. In the cycle, the mitochondria push their raw materials through a series of chemical exchanges. At each stage, an electron is "donated" forward to the next stage, and the energy acquired by severing these electrons is used to "pump" protons into the mitochondria's inner membrane. By segregating protons in this inner space, the mitochondria are actually turning themselves into low-voltage batteries. As the cycle is repeated, and more protons are dumped into the holding area, the positive charge builds up and the potential energy increases.

The process is indeed like a battery charging or like a dam holding back a reservoir of water. The higher the water level, the more energy that can be produced by releasing it in a controlled fashion. When you open the gates, the water runs through, it turns the blades of a turbine or waterwheel, and usable energy is generated. This is exactly what happens in the mitochondria. As the stored-up reservoir of electrical current runs out through the membrane's spillway, proton by proton, it physically rotates a propeller-shaped protein and thus generates a single ATP molecule. It is just like a tiny turbine, spinning with the force of its tiny chemical flow.

This cycle is going on all the time. Cells need energy to do their work, and this pumping and rotating machine is how they produce it. So what can go wrong with this marvelous machine? The primary cause of trouble in the case of diabetes is when *too much* energy is being pushed through the transfer stations. The machine pumps faster and faster, the propeller spins too quickly, and things begin to break down.

You can easily imagine why this might be a special difficulty for a body that is already insulin resistant. The mitochondria are constantly processing energy, but they can be overheated by chronic energy excess, and energy excess is precisely what occurs under conditions of hyperglycemia. Glucose is the mitochondria's raw form of fuel—it is the coal being shoveled into the furnace of the steam engine. When fat and muscle fail to soak up glucose in the blood, the sugars eventually flood into many of the other cells of the body. This uncontrolled energy flow begins to overwork the mitochondrial engines. The flux, or flow rate, of glucose into the mitochondria increases; as glucose is processed, the electrical current in the energy reservoir increases; more and more protons are collected; the machine pumps faster and faster; the potential energy level rises; and finally a point of maximum overload is reached.

The Rise of Superoxide

The overload doesn't lead to an explosion, but the energy machine starts to leak. When the stream of glucose down the ATP conversion ramp runs too fast, the mitochondrial machine can pump no more protons into the reservoir and the flow starts to back up. The electrons, instead of being promoted down the chain, get rerouted into a side channel, where they ultimately combine with free-floating oxygen molecules. And just like a crack in the dam or a radiation leak from a power plant, you have a new problem on top of the old one: in this case, one oxygen plus one electron, which equals *superoxide*.

A Bad, Bad Actor

Superoxide is a nasty molecule that is the precursor for most of the damaging free radicals that you may have heard about. Free radicals cause DNA strand breaks, they trigger a whole range of harmful gene expressions, they indiscriminately react with and degrade many substances in the body, and overall they speed the process of DNA and cellular degeneration that constitutes aging.

Superoxide is also the single trigger for most of the pathways that result in diabetic tissue damage: nerve damage, retinal damage, and, importantly, blood vessel damage, which often leads to heart disease.[10] Superoxide is truly a bad actor throughout the body.

This is reason enough to do everything you can to avoid insulin resistance and hyperglycemia. You are literally poisoning yourself with the effluent from industrial-strength glucose processing. But one further effect I want to focus on here is superoxide's role in dysregulating pancreatic cells. For the pancreatic cells are the ones that we should be turning to for help with this problem. In the face of high levels of blood sugar, they should be adjusting by ramping up insulin secretion. And they often do this. But sometimes—and increasingly, with the development of full-blown diabetes—they don't. And the reason they don't has to do with a peculiar feedback loop between superoxide production and insulin secretion. It turns out that the condition that these special cells mean to be correcting—hyperglycemia—is the very one, via overproduction of superoxide, that often keeps them from being able to perform that lifesaving function.

The Final Straw: Glucose Insensitivity

The last environment of diabetes that we need to target is the most specific. It is the moment when the pancreatic beta cell opens its outer membrane to release an insulin molecule into the bloodstream. If that single act happens in proper coordination with the cell's glucose sensing, if rising levels of glucose outside the cell correspond to increased secretion of insulin from within the cell, then diabetes can still be averted. A rough balance of sugar ingestion and sugar storage can still be maintained, even against the relative sluggishness of muscle and fat cells on the uptake.

But once the pancreas fails in that balancing act, diabetes has arrived. Nothing is left to forestall the ravages of sugar on the most vulnerable parts of the body—those that cannot shield themselves at all from the flood of glucose, including, as I mentioned, the eyes, the nerves, and above all the blood vessels, which connect, feed, and irrigate all the other parts.

Among those damages, as a kind of intermediary step that both proceeds from superoxide and exacerbates its effects, is one of the major varieties of pancreatic impairment. When the mitochondria are pumping like mad—collecting protons up to the overload point and then leaking off electrons like steam from an overheated boiler to form superoxide—when this redline is reached, the cell has to hit the safety valve. It cannot tolerate a gross accumulation of superoxide, which is simply too toxic to contain in large amounts. The safety switch is called an uncoupling protein, and it does just what it sounds like: it uncouples or delinks the electron transfer stations from the inner energy reservoir and collapses the voltage gradient between them. All the protons flow out of the reservoir as heat rather than as a charged stream pushing a turbine. As the reservoir empties, the pressure relaxes, and the electrons stop leaking off into superoxide.[11]

This is a basic survival mechanism within the mitochondria, against the excess of its own effects, and although it does not prevent superoxide buildup in all tissues (not all cells have the same kind or amount of uncoupling proteins), it does serve as a frontline antioxidant defense from free radical damage. But the situation in pancreatic cells is, significantly, more complicated. There, hitting the safety valve has a serious side effect: the blunting of insulin secretion. Here's how it works.

Insulin secretion from the pancreas is a complex affair that depends on the production of ATP, the molecule essential for energy transfer in the cell. When the concentration of ATP is high, insulin is released; when the concentration is low, the doors remain closed. Thus the whole energy production operation is *itself* a crucial link between two glucose-related systems: between, on the one hand, the cell's processing of glucose for its own energy and, on the other, the pancreas's special sensitivity to sugar levels on the outside. Effectively, processing glucose through the electron transfer cycle into ATP *is* the pancreas's mode of "sensing" the rising levels of glucose in the blood. Glucose levels rise in the bloodstream; the rising tide reaches the doors of the pancreatic cells; glucose diffuses into the cell, where it is ushered into the mitochondria and converted into ATP; and this end product—the gathering pool of ATP within the cell—*is* the signal that, back out there at the start of the sequence, a mob of glucose is agitating. Given *that* signal, the command is ultimately pronounced to release insulin—the drawbridge is lowered, the portcullis raised, and the knights ride out to do battle with the hordes.

But what if the signal never comes? What if, as indeed they are, these two primary pancreatic purposes—generating energy safely on the inside, and responding to dangerously high levels of energetic fuel on the outside—are in a deep conflict of interest?[12] That is what happens when the mitochondrion, in a self-defensive move intended to stave off free radical depredations, pulls the plug on ATP generation, seals the superoxide leak, and thereby saves its own DNA. But in the process, it shuts its eyes and ears to the floodwaters threatening to drown the city. It is this defensive walling itself off from the flow of glucose that makes the pancreas finally glucose insensitive. The chief glucose supervisor has been forced to go blind to its charge.

This leaves us, at the end, with a paradoxical reversal of the beautiful harmony that we observed at the start. Where the sensing-releasing-absorbing cycle was finely tuned at both ends, now we have only blindness, deafness, and insensitivity. The beautifully self-supporting system has become a self-unraveling one, as in the final undoing the pancreas not only fails to moderate glucose levels but, by saving itself from superoxide, also ensures that those levels will keep rising. The end result: you have diabetes.

The Ecogenetic Way

Diabetes is the disturbance of the beautiful harmony in the body's normal system of glucose regulation. The two sides sense and release, then sense and absorb in a mutually reinforcing way. It's almost like a wave motion tray, or the movement of the tides in the oceans—the gentle rocking of the flow back and forth is the effect of good order. But the balance that keeps itself going can become unbalanced and throw itself out of rhythm and off the tracks. We call the main features of this dysregulation "insulin resistance" and "glucose insensitivity," and it sometimes seems as though they are discrete events that simply disorder cells "out there somewhere" on the spot. But the reality is that these conditions are neither mysterious nor intuitive—they involve separate catastrophes in the deep interior of the cells, catastrophes that originate far from the cellular centers where the damage happens. The ultimate paradox of diabetes is that the cells' ways of interpreting signals coming in from outside is fouled by the very energetic processes they are attempting to assist.

Targeting these interior environments—the insulin receptor chains in muscle and fat cells, the mitochondria in the pancreas—means taking steps to protect those all-important signaling relays.

Know Your Diabetic Ancestor

Surviving famine and surviving disease were the two crucial requirements for our genetic ancestors. If the body routinely failed to handle such crises, it would mean the early death of those individuals and an evolutionary dead end for their suboptimal physiological makeups. So it would make sense for these all-important processes—energy management and infection fighting—over the course of hundreds of thousands of years, to converge on a kind of symbiosis. Thus when these systems are at a good balance point, each tends to reinforce the other's stability. You might *want* fat to be able to send out inflammatory signals if you're threatened by infection. And you might *want* those signals to short-circuit insulin's tissue building or anabolic activity (another of its wide-ranging effects). That way, when you need to direct all your resources toward fighting off pathogens, and inflammation needs to be high, insulin will be checked from using energy to gather more energy reserves and to synthesize new tissues. In that case, it's more important to survive the immediate threat than to pack away food for the future.

But when the systems get out of balance, the opposite happens: they tend to interfere with each other, and dysfunction in one can create dysfunction in the other. This is the case in our contemporary nutritional environment. In fact diabetes and obesity are so clearly related that they are sometimes referred to as "diabesity." Being able to store fat easily against future famine is not especially helpful when you have more food than you need all the time. Now the excess of energy becomes a source of immune responses that foil the regular processing of energy. In fact, it is not far-fetched to think of type 2 diabetes as a kind of environmentally triggered autoimmune disease. The body's immune system, sounding the inflammatory alarm, eats away at its metabolic foundation.

I call this hypothesis "the diabetic ancestor," because retrospectively we can see how those ancient entanglements have led to our being tripped up today. These are in a sense the most basic "environments" of diabetes: our ancestral physiology and our contemporary nutritional abundance. The mismatch between these environments is the "diabetic present" that we find ourselves suffering in now.

This is still a big conceptual challenge for many people. The idea that we have been set up by our evolution to be susceptible to insulin-signaling mixups in the current environment—and that this is true for *all* of us—can be hard to grasp. Many of us still think of diabetes as a peculiarly distant kind of condition. Even people who can imagine that they might one day develop active cancer or heart disease often have trouble thinking of themselves as potentially diabetic.

But we need to shake off this misconception. If cancer is the disease of life processes proceeding unchecked, then diabetes is the disease of modern life and the modern nutritional environment.

Like cancer, diabetes is a permanent risk for every person in the developed world. You can be prediabetic without knowing it; you can gradually develop insulin resistance; you can be increasingly or decreasingly insulin resistant; your pancreatic cells can be more or less glucose sensitive; your mitochondria can be more or less dysfunctional. All of these are states of the disease that are changeable over time, and most of us are moving up and down the scales of risk and healthy functioning in each of these categories all our lives.

This reality needs to become part of the health and sickness perspective that informs our ordinary lives. We need to be able to articulate our behaviors *to ourselves* in terms that take account of our real diabetic susceptibilities. Why not eat a lot of junk food? Because (in addition to all the other detriments) *it is prodiabetic.* Why not sit at the desk all day and enjoy watching TV on the couch at night and take the escalator upstairs to work? *Because lack of exercise is pro-diabetic.*

Fight Inflammation (Again)

All of the advice from previous chapters about curtailing inflammation pertains doubly here. Fat is the primary source of full-body inflammation, so it is crucial to add weight management to the list of inflammation-fighting techniques. It does no good—and in the case of diabetes is directly counterproductive—to eat only healthful foods but to eat so many of them that you destroy your energy balance. But one of the virtues of eating as I recommend is that it is naturally portion controlling—or rather, naturally filling and satisfying. Sugar may not cause diabetes, but added sugar in commercial foods is surely the single biggest collateral cause for Americans' overeating. Unlike vegetables and whole grains and potatoes, or berries and teas and good chocolate, sugar is inherently unfilling. That is precisely why it is added to so many foods in easily processed forms like high-fructose corn syrup: it increases the amount we feel we need to eat, and so increases sales.

Fish oil supplements, olive oil, all the brightly colored fruits and vegetables (especially broccoli and the cruciferous vegetables), turmeric—these and other foods I discuss later are your staples in the battle against systemic inflammation.

Get Out of Bed and Move!

We've seen that fat is not a passive bystander in the body's operations, but a powerful organ in its own right that releases a wide range of hormone-like substances. Scientists have begun to realize that the same is true for our muscles—they have the basic function of allowing us to move our bodies, but they also participate in the hormonal balance of the whole system. Muscles, fit or unfit, are not just sitting there—they are either producing or not producing a range of signaling molecules that help to regulate genetic and epigenetic conditions, including ones that stimulate inflammation.

In one study of the effects of bed rest on muscle inflammation, participants were kept on a particularly tight leash: "All subjects were admitted to the Steno Diabetes Center for ten days and were not permitted to deviate from a half-recumbent position during this period. Toilet visits, limited to a total of fifteen minutes per day, were allowed. Study subjects were allowed to use a laptop computer, watch television, and read in the bed."[13] The results of the study and others like it are telling. The participants experienced many of the same effects, induced by many of the same agents, that have been recorded in the cells of subjects exposed to inflammation stemming from fat. Of particular note was the tendency of bed rest to deactivate genes that are associated with anti-inflammation properties, and, conversely, the potency of physical activity as a promoter of those same genes. Both TNF-alpha and Il-6, those headliner fire-breathing inflammatories, were strongly correlated with sedentariness and activity—aroused by the one, soothed by the other.[14] Muscle *can be* an active anti-inflammatory agent; exercising calls forth the positive expression of genes that send calming signals to the rest of the body. But in order to perform actively for your benefit, the muscles have to be *active*. Under conditions resembling much of modern daily life (i.e., bed rest), muscle mass wastes away, fat tissue accumulates, and genes not only don't help but pile on to the inflammatory burden.

This is why conceiving of exercise as a supplement to health rather than (or in addition to) as a purely competitive endeavor is so important. Why do many football players, wonderfully lean and powerful during their playing days, accumulate, once they retire, huge new fat masses and all the associated health problems, especially diabetes and prediabetes? Partly it is because they no longer exercise regularly, on a daily basis. And why do they no longer exercise? Because for these professional athletes, exercise has always been synonymous with world-class competitive performance. Why exercise after you retire if you are retiring precisely because you can no longer compete at the level where "exercise" is meaningful to you?

But this is a terribly misguided view for health. What health requires is low-level but consistent exertion. If your goal is to keep your genes firing in good order, there is no need to run marathons, no need to lift five-hundred-pound weights, no need to rip your abs or optimize your workout for VO2 max return. Walk for twenty minutes a day, take the stairs in one planned spot as part of your morning routine, join a low-stress exercise class, find a workout buddy.

It's the costs of inactivity you really need to keep in mind. If you don't move your body on a regular basis, if you live a semirecumbent life of TV watching and desk jockeying, your genes are slowly falling asleep. And the longer you let your genes go soft, the more effort it takes, over longer periods, to get your genome back up to baseline. Exercise—again, not strenuous, world-class performance, but moderate, daily physical activity—is like water. It is that fundamental to human health. Its absence is deadly. If you don't drink water, you die pretty quickly (around a week). If you don't exercise, you die more slowly, but you're still *dying*.

Hit the Emergency Brake on Body Fat

Diabetes is epidemic in the modern developed world not because people have suddenly lost their willpower, or because tastes for foods have dramatically changed, or because the human genome has begun to express itself in some new way. The rise in insulin resistance, prediabetes, and diabetes itself is directly due to a nutritional excess unprecedented in human history.

Not every obese person will become diabetic, and not all diabetics are obese, but the correlation is very high, for all the reasons outlined above. Obesity simply is a chronic energy imbalance in which the excess is stored as more and more fat tissue. And fat, as we now know, can no longer be ignored as a passive rider on an otherwise dynamically interactive body. Fat is a *participant* in that dynamic; it is deeply involved in the most intimate workings of our cells. And fat is the unignorable evidence of the diabetic ancestor's presence within us—his setting us up to overstimulate our energy systems and thus trigger an inflammatory backlash. But we can also take the confluence of energy and emergency pathways as an evolutionary hint. Too much nutrition is indeed too much of a good thing. Expanding fat stores are *dangerous*—and a sign to start hitting the brakes.

The Ecogenetic Way: Diabetes Summary

Here's a quick review of the essential steps you can take to improve your diabetes environments:

- **Know your diabetic ancestor.**
  - *We are evolutionarily predisposed to develop diabetes in the modern nutritional world. This makes diabetes, and its constituent disorders of obesity and metabolic syndrome, uniquely specific to modern life.*
  - Everyone *is vulnerable because everyone has inherited essentially the same genetic and physiological legacy. This makes adopting a preventive attitude the most important first step in maintaining healthy glucose metabolism.*
  - *Take account of diabetes—it is emphatically* not *only a disease of certain kinds of other people.*
- **Fight inflammation (again).**
  - *Diabetes is profoundly a disease of inflammation. Thus quieting systemic sources of inflammation is a first response.*
  - *Reduce weight if you are too heavy—excess fat is inherently inflammatory and will weaken and age you prematurely.*
  - *Eat the wide range of foods that have anti-inflammatory properties.*
  - *Consider taking fish oil supplements.*
  - *Use olive oil.*

- **Get out of bed and move!**
  - *Exercise is not simply good for you. Not exercising is actively and powerfully bad for you. Sedentariness overexpresses genes in the muscles that do many of the same corrosive things as fat-derived inflammation. And sedentariness and obesity together are a wicked inflammatory cocktail.*
  - *But there is no need to do more than you can. Exercising for health, as opposed to extreme performance, is much more effective when done regularly at low intensities.*
  - *Walk, carry light weights, join a gym with a friend.*
  - *However small, be sure to start to do something. It's the inactive person who can least afford to remain inactive.*
- **Hit the emergency brake on body fat.**
  - *Losing weight, or maintaining it at a healthy level, is one of the surest ways to reduce your diabetes risk. Especially if you are not yet diabetic or insulin resistant (or don't know that you are), keep tabs on your shape. Gaining weight is already a warning sign that your diabetic ancestor is living on in you. Fat tissue is ground zero for insulin resistance—shrink its size and you shrink the risk. Every other part of your body will thank you.*

Targeted Nutrition for Diabetes

The Glycemic Index

The difference between simple and complex carbohydrates is an important concept for managing sugar metabolism. With a few exceptions, complex carbs mainly slow down the absorption of sugar in the blood, which is measured by a value known as the glycemic index (GI). The glycemic index for carbohydrates ranges from 1 to 100 (1 is the slowest absorption, 100 is the fastest absorption). Pure glucose has a glycemic index of 100; carbohydrate-rich foods such as honey and puffed rice are close behind (though honey is a simple carb that is also healthful). The table below from the American Diabetes Association provides a GI overview of certain carbohydrates.

Glycemic Index	Foods
■ ≤ 55 (low)	■ 100 percent stone-ground whole wheat or pumpernickel bread ■ Oatmeal (rolled or steel cut), oat bran, muesli ■ Pasta, converted rice, barley, bulgur ■ Sweet potatoes, corn, yams, lima/butter beans, peas, legumes, lentils ■ Most fruits, nonstarchy vegetables, carrots
■ 56–69 (medium)	■ Whole wheat, rye, and pita bread ■ Quick oats ■ Brown, wild, or basmati rice; couscous
■ ≥ 70 (high)	■ White bread or bagel ■ Corn flakes, puffed rice, bran flakes, instant oatmeal ■ Short-grain white rice, rice pasta, macaroni and cheese from mix ■ All white potatoes, pumpkins ■ Pretzels, rice cakes, popcorn, saltine crackers ■ Melons, pineapple

Use this table loosely, because the glycemic index of food isn't fixed. In fact, various factors influence the GI of food, such as whether or not it has been cooked or processed. Other factors that affect the glycemic index of food:

- **Starch type:** Barley is broken down and absorbed more slowly than potato starch.
- **Fiber:** Foods with more fiber tend to have a lower GI.
- **Ripeness:** Fruit that is riper contains higher concentrations of sugar, which raises the GI.
- **Amount of acid or fat:** The more acid or fat a food contains, the lower the GI.

Gene Therapy Fact: Good Carbs/Bad Carbs

Try to take all the factors into consideration, but don't skip out on a nutritious form of carbohydrate just because it has a higher glycemic index. Likewise, lower GI does not automatically equate to high nutrition. It's more important that you use this information to help evaluate, rather than dictate, what you eat.

Foods for Glycemic Control

Category	Food Sources	Why?
Omega-3 fatty acids	Salmon, rainbow trout, mackerel, sardines (eat two or more times weekly); omega-3 fatty acid supplements	Reduce the risk of cardiovascular complications (lower triglycerides and blood pressure); groups who eat a diet high in fish have lower rates of heart disease and diabetes (e.g., the Japanese)
Vitamins C and E	Vitamin C: brussels sprouts, broccoli, strawberries, oranges Vitamin E: almonds, sunflower seeds, mustard/turnip greens	Both are antioxidants that lower the risk of cardiovascular disease
Minerals	Chromium: onions, tomatoes, bran cereals Magnesium: black beans, cashew nuts, sesame seeds, soybeans, spinach	Chromium: supplements improve glucose utilization Magnesium: levels are depleted in diabetics; studies show supplementation improves insulin sensitivity and glycemic control

Nutrient-Depleted Carbs

Both simple and complex carbohydrates can be further categorized as refined or unrefined sugars. Refined sugars aren't great dietary choices because they are mainly processed foods that are devoid of any nutrients and fiber. Snacks and packaged foods may seem convenient, but these processed foods are major players involved in our growing waistlines as well as conditions like diabetes.

Gene Therapy Fact: Refined's Not Fine!

Important nutrients, vitamins, and minerals are removed from refined carbs. When wheat is converted into white flour, the process removes large amounts of vitamins and minerals. How much? *A Revolution in Health Through Nutritional Biochemistry*[15] illustrates how essential vitamins and minerals are removed from food during food manufacturing. For example, over 80 percent of vitamin E and magnesium are lost from wheat when it's processed. Interestingly, vitamin E and magnesium are also depleted in people diagnosed with diabetes. Coincidence? No, not at all. In fact, studies show[16] that vitamin E and magnesium not only improve glycemic control, but also keep in check "memory" associated with diabetes-like cardiovascular problems. Chromium and zinc are also important minerals removed from refined carbohydrates, and these metals are necessary for digesting and metabolizing carbohydrates.

The biochemical process of converting carbohydrates into energy is quite complex. To put it simply, the conversion of sugar into energy requires oxygen, minerals, vitamins, and trace elements. Many carbohydrate-rich foods contain these compounds, which is one good reason to eat sufficient amounts of good carbs. But just because you're consuming carbohydrates in your diet doesn't mean you're getting adequate amounts of these substances. In fact, most carbohydrate-rich products that you buy at the grocery store have been stripped of many of these nutrients. What you are left with in the processed shell is mostly sugar in the form of glucose.

Gene Therapy Fact: A Kernel of Truth

Unless you have a digestive condition such as celiac disease, you should not decide to eat gluten-free food because you think it's healthier to do so. Instead, you're actually increasing your sugar intake. How could this be, right? Gluten-free is supposed to be healthier. Well, that's not entirely true. Gluten is a sticky protein in grains like wheat, barley, oats, rye, and spelt. It is found in almost all processed foods like cereals, bagels, bread, and other baked goods. For those looking to eat healthier and lose a couple of pounds, buying gluten-free alternatives to your favorite dietary indulgences such as cake and cookies isn't any better, because it's all still processed food that contains loads of other processed starches such as rice flour, corn, and cassava starch.[17] Starchy foods increase blood glucose levels and put insulin into overdrive, a process that leads to insulin resistance, in which cells lose their sensitivity to the hormone and fail to absorb glucose. Also, a lot of the necessary vitamins and minerals you need are eliminated from gluten-free food. So even if you do have celiac disease, it's important for you to speak with a nutritionist to ensure that you are eating a balanced, nutritious diet.

Even worse, because many of these processed foods are nutritionally denuded, they actually function as "nutrient leeches" when you eat them. When the body doesn't get what it needs from food, it uses its internal stores to make up the difference. Given a continuously empty diet, the body will continue to supply its needs from its own stores, ultimately becoming nutrient deficient. And indeed, that is the condition of a remarkably high number of people who subsist on mostly processed food, including many who are in the process of becoming diabetic.

Gene Therapy Fact: Whole Grains: Not Entirely Wholesome

All whole grains contain compounds (e.g., lectins and phytates) that our bodies aren't capable of breaking down. Lectins, for example, can damage the intestinal lining and be absorbed across the gut and wind up in the bloodstream. They can also bind to insulin receptors, and the more lectins bound to insulin receptors mean there are fewer available receptor sites for insulin to bind to, thus minimizing sugar uptake into cells. That means blood sugar levels rise—resulting in type 2 diabetes! Still whole grains and whole grain flours are a better choice than white and refined grains and flours.

Many healthy whole grains exist for you to choose from, such as amaranth, bulgur, flaxseed, millet, quinoa, and steel-cut oats. When shopping for whole-grain breads, you should be aware that some brands add coloring so that their breads appear the desired unprocessed color of brown. Make sure the first ingredient on the back of the label says *"whole wheat flour."* That way, you ensure that you're eating the intact grain that has important nutrients, such as B vitamins, minerals, and fiber. Processed grains lack the healthy outer and inner layers and leave the carb-rich middle layer intact, which is why eating too many refined grains causes obesity and diabetes.

Gene Therapy Fact: The Best Sugar Substitute

Coconut crystals, made from the sap of the coconut tree, are the best sweetener you can use. This sweetener has the consistency of sugar but a much lower glycemic index, meaning it requires less insulin to metabolize. It is rich in vitamin C, amino acids, and B vitamins. Unlike table sugar, which is usually subjected to high heat and contains 90 percent sucrose, coconut crystals contain inulin, which is a fiber that slows glucose absorption, which explains why it has a lower glycemic index than regular sugar.[18] It is also richer in short chain fatty acids that enhance healthy gut bacteria. They are a sweet probiotic nutrient that fosters intestinal health. I recommend Coconut Secret brand (www.coconutsecret.com), which is free of pesticides and uses no chemicals in the extraction process.

Antioxidants

Carnitine
Carnitine is an antioxidant that is also involved in converting fat into energy. Research shows that carnitine levels are depleted under conditions of insulin resistance. An animal study showed that oral carnitine supplements may lead

to increased glucose uptake.[19] I suggest that my patients take carnitine supplements to regulate blood glucose and to effectively convert fats into energy.

Acety-L-Carnitine

L-carnitine is an amino acid involved in fat metabolism that has been shown to have an impact on the management of blood glucose levels and hypertension. In one study, researchers provided a twice daily dose of L-carnitine to patients with prediabetes over 24 weeks. The results revealed that a twice daily dose of acetyl-L-carnitine yielded a reduction in blood glucose levels, and ameliorated insulin resistance and hypertension.[20] Adiponectin, a fat cell derived hormone that improves glucose utilization, also increased.[21]

Herbs and Legumes

Gymnema sylvestre

Gymnema sylvestre extract, which comes from a plant native to India, has been shown to boost insulin activity and C-peptide to lower the levels of blood glucose. A study showed that taking a sixty-day supplement of the plant extract resulted in substantial improvements in glycemic control.[22]

Fenugreek

Fenugreek, a pungent and bitter legume found widely in the Middle East and Asia, is high in protein, fiber, and iron. It also has antioxidant, anti-inflammatory, and chemopreventive properties. Various animal and clinical studies have shown that it also serves an antidiabetic function.[23] One study reported that including 25 to 100 grams of fenugreek in your daily diet is effective at controlling diabetes.[24]

Garlic

Garlic has antioxidative, anti-inflammatory, and antidiabetic properties. In animal studies, garlic induced the secretion of insulin, thereby reducing blood glucose levels.[25] Another study reported that raw, rather than cooked, garlic significantly reduces the levels of blood glucose.[26] Onions, in the same allium family of vegetables as garlic, also demonstrate antidiabetic effects.[27]

Gene Therapy Fact: What Exactly Is Yucca?

Yucca (*Yucca schdigera*) is a flowering plant growing throughout the deserts, canyons, and chaparrals of the Southwestern U.S. and Mexico. It has long been a source of food and natural medicinals among Native Americans. It is rich in anti-inflammatory and anti-oxidant polyphenols, such as resveratrol and stilbenes. After feeding Yucca extracts for 3 weeks to diabetic rats, researchers found that glucose levels improved and cholesterol and triglycerides levels declined.[28]

Turmeric

Turmeric, which gives Indian curry dishes and American yellow mustards their yellow color, is effective for fighting diabetes. One study reported that the combination of turmeric and garlic reduced blood sugar levels and HbA1c as well as improved lipid levels.[29] Another study showed that turmeric may help to prevent or treat type 2 diabetes by activating proteins called PPAR-gamma, which are located in adipose cells and reduce insulin resistance.[30] Turmerin, an antioxidant component found in turmeric, has been shown to block the activity of diabetes-related enzymes.[31] And yet another study reported that nine months of treating prediabetic people with curcumin—the active component of turmeric—lowered the risk for developing type 2 diabetes and enhanced the performance of pancreatic beta cells.[32] If Indian cuisine is not for your palate, then try adding yellow mustard to your meals. You can sneak the zesty condiment into your sandwiches, burgers, and meats.

Gene Therapy Fact: Hurry for Curry

Since most Americans do not eat curry daily, a curcumin supplement is useful. Meriva-SR (made by Thorne) is a slow-release form that many of my patients find quite palatable.

Curcumin is a major gene therapy nutrient with myriad healthful benefits. I mention it over and over again in this book because it has such widespread effectiveness. But be aware that turmeric needs to be aged properly in order to work best. Most growers harvest it when it turns its signature yellow color. But that is too early—the herb still needs time for its phytonutrients, curcuminoids, and sesquiterpenoids to reach their maximum concentrations. To ensure you're getting curcumin supplements that are harvested *after* they've matured, look for pharmaceutical-grade brands that put supplements through testing to produce high-quality products. While curcumin supplements are healthful, I prefer turmeric supplements because you get the full range of other natural compounds found in the spice, not just curcumin alone.

Aloe

Aloe is widely known to help maintain youthful skin, yet it has many other potential therapeutic benefits, including treating type 2 diabetes. In one study, five compounds called phytosterols were extracted from aloe vera gel to assess their effect on controlling elevated glucose levels. When researchers administered these phytosterols to diabetic mice for twenty-eight days, they observed reductions in the mice's fasting blood glucose (FBG) ranging from 28 percent to 64 percent.[33] Many of my patients don't like aloe's bitter taste, which is why I suggest that they add a teaspoon of aloe gel to juice.

Neem

Neem is a colossal evergreen tree that grows in India, where it is commonly referred to as the "miracle" tree because of its versatility as a medicinal plant. Its Sanskrit name, *arishta* ("reliever of sickness"), is apt because virtually every part of the tree has been shown to treat conditions such as diabetes, arthritis, and gastric ulcers. Several compounds extracted from neem leaves, seeds, and bark have demonstrated hypoglycemic, anti-inflammatory, antimicrobial, and immunomodulatory functions.[34] Neem has also been shown to increase the utilization of glucose by blocking the effect of epinephrine (the fight-or-flight hormone, which increases blood glucose levels) on glucose metabolism.[35] Researchers also reported a marked decrease in blood sugar levels in diabetic rabbits that were administered a neem leaf extract and seed oil, and the hypoglycemic effect was comparable to glyburide, a pharmaceutical drug used to treat type 2 diabetes.[36]

Holy Basil

Holy basil, or tulsi, is a salutiferous plant with ecogenetic properties that guard against diabetes. This aromatic herb is abundantly found in India, where it is used to manage stress and is grown around Hindu temples since it is considered to be a sacred plant. The plant is widely used in Ayurvedic medicine to treat conditions such as the common cold, heart disease, tuberculosis, and diabetes. As an antidiabetic agent, tulsi has been shown to stimulate the release of insulin from beta cells, which helps to reduce blood glucose levels in the body.[37] Another study showed that tulsi decreases levels of both glucose and cortisol (a stress hormone that raises glucose levels and can contribute to diabetes).[38]

Bay Leaves

Bay leaves, which come from the Mediterranean evergreen *Laurus nobilis*, possess antidiabetic properties and are also a good source of vitamin A, vitamin C, and folic acid. As an antidiabetic agent, the pungent leaves regulate insulin to help control glucose levels. Certain compounds in bay leaves affect gene expression and blood sugar levels, and offset sugar spikes. In one clinical study, type 2 diabetics who took varying doses of ground bay leaves had significantly lower blood glucose levels than those who'd received a placebo.[39]

Gene Therapy Fact: The Radical Reishi Mushroom

While reishi mushrooms have been known in the West for only a few decades, they've been widely used in Asia for thousands of years for their varied medicinal effects: in liver disorders, cardiovascular disease, autoimmune diseases, arthritis, and much more. Six species of the reishi mushroom—red, black, blue, white, yellow, and purple—have been extensively studied. Of these, the red and the black reishi mushroom are known to have the most health-boosting effects.[40] In particular, the red reishi mushroom (*Ganoderma lucidum*) is the most commonly used in treating diabetes, especially in Chinese medicine. Bioactive compounds found in the mushroom also work at preventing the formation of new fat cells, which is important since diabetes and obesity are so closely linked.[41]

And reishi helps to keep cholesterol levels down—good news

not only for obesity and diabetes but for cardiovascular diseases as well. The mushroom also inhibits alpha-glucosidase, which is an important enzyme needed to convert starches into sugars.[42] By blocking this enzyme, reishi curbs rapid increases in blood glucose levels after meals—a problem in diabetes that worsens with age. Finally, the consumption of reishi extracts has been shown to slow the disruptive effects of advanced glycation end products (AGEs), molecules that promote advanced aging.[43]

Coffee and Tea

Green coffee bean extract, which contains the polyphenol chlorogenic acid, is a potent ecogenetic nutrient. Chlorogenic acid exerts an antidiabetic effect on glucose-6-phosphatase (G6P), an enzyme involved in blood glucose control. As we saw earlier, green coffee beans are those that haven't been roasted, leaving them with just a faint aroma and bitter taste. Researchers have reported that:

- Chlorogenic acid from green coffee beans reduced blood sugar levels after meals by 32 percent.[44]
- In a Japanese study, blood sugar levels dropped 43 percent in mice that were fed green coffee bean extract.[45]
- The consumption of coffee is associated with a reduced risk of type 2 diabetes,[46] and chlorogenic acid is responsible for these antidiabetic effects by lowering blood sugar.[47]

Black tea also regulates the absorption of sugars obtained from a meal. Researchers have reported that the enzyme alpha-glucosidase, which is responsible for the absorption of sugar from the gut, is dramatically inhibited by black tea.[48] Black tea is more effective than white tea, and white tea more so than oolong.[49] Considering that many new diabetes drugs, such as acarbose, are aimed at inhibiting alpha-glucosidase, a tea bag is an easily accessible, cost-effective way to be on the cutting edge.[50]

The compounds in green tea have numerous salubrious effects as well, including the regulation of blood sugar.[51] EGCG, a potent catechin in green tea, regulates blood glucose levels through several mechanisms: its insulin-like effects improve glucose absorption;[52] it blocks gluconeogenesis,[53] a process in which the liver makes glucose; it limits the amount of sugar that is absorbed from the gut;[54] and it reduces amylase production, an enzyme that converts starch into sugar.

Minerals and Vitamins

Calcium, chromium, magnesium, potassium, and zinc are only some of the minerals that play an important role in carbohydrate metabolism.

- A study followed fifty-two overweight insulin-resistant nondiabetics who had normal magnesium levels. The researchers reported improvements in insulin sensitivity, blood glucose control, and even blood pressure in the magnesium-supplemented group.[55]
- In a meta-analysis of seven large studies that included close to 290,000 people, researchers found that participants who increased their daily intake of magnesium by 100 milligrams experienced a 15 percent drop in developing diabetes.[56]
- A study evaluating Chinese women demonstrated the protective effects of calcium and magnesium against the development of type 2 diabetes.[57]
- High levels of potassium correlated to a lower risk for the development of diabetes, and people with the lowest potassium levels had a 64 percent greater risk than people with high levels.[58]
- Researchers investigating the effects of selenium on dysglycemia (the whole range of glucose-related conditions) reported lower risks of abnormal blood glucose levels.[59]

Vitamins have also been shown to have benefits:

- Researchers compared personalized dietary regimens—a low-calorie diet versus an antioxidant-enriched diet—and reported that antioxidants such as vitamins C and E improved insulin sensitivity in patients with metabolic syndrome. They also enhanced the effects of metformin.[60]
- Vitamins K1 and K2 have both been shown to lower diabetes risk in men and women.[61]
- A 2011 study demonstrated that vitamin D may play an important role in improving insulin secretion and insulin sensitivity among those with the highest risk for developing diabetes.[62]

- Vitamin D deficiencies have been linked to myriad health complications, such as osteoporosis, fractures, and cardiovascular disease. Vitamin D supplementation improves many of these conditions, including lowering diabetes risk.[63]
- Another study established an inverse relationship between vitamin D and hemoglobin A1C, the marker for prolonged elevated blood sugar. In individuals with low levels of vitamin D there was an increase in A1C, whereas in those with high dietary supplementation there was a corresponding decrease.[64]

Grapes

Grapes, like red wine, contain resveratrol, a potent polyphenol that has demonstrated many beneficial effects on diabetes. Closely related to resveratrol is pterostilbene, also present in grapes and also very effective in diabetes treatment and prevention. (You can also munch on a handful of blueberries for a decent dose of this polyphenol.) Among their benefits:

- Research has shown that pterostilbene, a resveratrol-like compound, has been found to up-regulate the gene that codes for PPAR alpha, which leads to decreased triglycerides and LDL, and supports healthy glucose levels.[65]
- A study on mice demonstrated that a powdered blend of green, red, and black grapes led to a remarkable reduction in the risk of developing metabolic syndrome.[66]
- In another study, participants with type 2 diabetes who were given daily doses of 10 milligrams of resveratrol experienced lower insulin resistance.
- Scientists have now synthesized a resveratrol-like compound that improves insulin sensitivity in diabetic mice. The major difference between this man-made version and the naturally occurring one is that the synthetic version is a thousand times stronger.[67]

Many scientists believe that resveratrol's effects may be attributed to antioxidant activity that inhibits oxidative stress associated with insulin resistance. Another hypothesis is that resveratrol has a specific intracellular insulin-dependent protein that is responsible for the uptake of glucose into cells.[68]

As for the related pterostilbene, various animal studies also show that this polyphenol helps to:[69]

- regenerate pancreatic cells that produce insulin
- inhibit high blood sugar levels and block insulin resistance
- regulate weight, blood sugar, and inflammation in people diagnosed with type 2 diabetes
- decrease bad fats (e.g., triglycerides, LDLs, and VLDLs) in people with diet-related hyperlipidemia
- reverse age-related cognitive decline[70]

In addition to its presence in grapes, pterostilbene is also derived from *Pterocarpus marsupium*, a tree indigenous to India and Sri Lanka. Pterostilbene extracts from the tree's bark and heartwood have been used in Ayurvedic medicine in the treatment of diabetes.

Gene Therapy Fact: Wine vs. Beer

While wine has many demonstrated health benefits when consumed in moderation (lowering cardiovascular risk, inhibiting cancer cell growth, promoting longevity), oenophiles aren't the only beneficiaries of the amazing health benefits found in a fermented beverage. A study shows that people diagnosed with diabetes and certain cancers who drink beer experience health improvements.[71] Researchers are focusing on humulone, the derivative of hops that gives beer its specific flavor, as the source of the benefit. Humulone is inhibitory against cancer, helps induce sleep, and builds stronger bones. It can also be taken in supplement form, as hops extract (310 milligrams, at bedtime).

Gene Therapy Fact: Apple Cider Vinegar

Another fermented food product shown to have healthful benefits is vinegar, particularly apple cider vinegar. This vinegar is produced from fermented apples, a process that involves bacteria and yeast breaking down sugar (glucose) in apples until it becomes alcohol; the continued fermentation of alcohol will eventually yield vinegar. Vinegar is acidic because of acetic acid, but it is made up of other beneficial components, such as vitamins and amino acids. In the United States, the medicinal beginnings of this vinegar started in the 1950s with the publication of D. C. Jarvis's health book *Folk Medicine: A Vermont Doctor's Guide to Good Health*. Since then, various claims have been made about the health benefits of apple cider vinegar, not all of which are backed up by science. But when it comes to diabetes, some studies have demonstrated its health benefits. For instance, a study looking at type 2 diabetics reported that two tablespoons of apple cider vinegar taken before bed helped to lower blood glucose levels after meals by 20%,[72] and lowered hemoglobin A1c levels.[73]

Targeted Supplements

Targeted Ecogenetic Juice for Diabetes

The following juice recipe is for those who are concerned about diabetes. But don't feel as though you have to drink this specific juice every day. Shake things up! I've included several juicing recipes after the disease-specific chapters' section. The ecogenetic juices listed are general recipes that focus on using wholesome ingredients and organically grown produce that have beneficial effects on many body systems. So you don't have to worry about sticking to any specific drink. My patients usually drink one or two ecogenetic juices daily. Mix up the juices you drink to broaden your intake of bioactive nutrients on a weekly basis. If you have a specific health concern, increase your intake of that recommended ecogenetic drink.

  ¼ cup blueberries
  1 tablespoon spirulina powder
  15 drops ChlorOxygen (chlorophyll)
  1 tablespoon raw cacao powder
  1 teaspoon bee pollen
  ¼ cup brewed green tea
  1 teaspoon magnesium powder (by Calm)
  1 teaspoon aloe vera juice, whole leaf

  Blend all ingredients until smooth. Drink and enjoy.

Targeted Ecogenetic Supplements for Diabetes

The supplements listed below are recommended for achieving and maintaining healthy blood glucose levels. Don't get overwhelmed and feel that you have to take every supplement listed. Remember: everyone is unique. The supplement list is in no particular order. I recommend them all equally to my patients because each one has benefits in the prevention and management of diabetes. Many of my patients start off by taking one supplement to determine how well they are tolerating it. Then they add other supplements as needed. When taking supplements, the focus should be to maintain good health. Don't worry about whether you should be taking 5, 10, or 15 supplements. That is not the intent of the supplement list. Do what you can. And take your time in figuring out what works for you: good health isn't a destination; it's a lifelong practice. And supplements are a small part of attaining a healthy lifestyle. Supplements are meant to be an addition to not a replacement for eating a healthy diet, getting adequate sleep, and improving your level of physical activity.

The supplements below are among the most important ones I give to many of my patients. Because every person is different, certain supplements may be more important than others for a given individual.

- Alpha lipoic acid—300 milligrams, twice daily
- Apple pectin—500 milligrams, twice daily
- Cinnamon extract—500 milligrams, twice daily
- Chromium—250 milligrams, twice daily
- Garcinia—1,000 milligrams, once daily
- Cayenne fruit capsules—450 milligrams, twice daily
- Saffron—100 milligrams, once daily
- Astaxanthin—4 milligrams, once daily
- Banaba extract—450 milligrams, once daily
- Cordyceps—400 milligrams, once daily
- Fenugreek seed extract—500 milligrams, once daily
- Bitter melon (momordica)—500 milligrams, once daily
- Green coffee bean extract—500 milligrams, once daily

Chapter 6

Aging

THROUGHOUT THIS BOOK I've made the point that various disease processes can rumble along beneath the surface for years, whether or not they ever become symptomatic. But no matter how well we manage to avoid specific disease entities, the one impairment we are all subject to is aging. Aging is simply the process that takes us toward death—and that, you can be assured, is the end for all of us. However, even if you have developed age spots, wrinkles, thinning hair, and stiff joints . . . well, by now you may have guessed . . . it is never too late to bring back balance. There are ecogenetic factors and imbalances that accelerate aging. You can restore balance and change your gene expression to delay and even reverse the process.

Which is why the anti-aging business is enormous and projected to keep growing fast. This is true even on the purely cosmetic end of the spectrum, where over $33.3 billion was spent on cosmetics and beauty products in 2010. As baby boomers age, they are determined to stay *looking* forever young. But the outsized emphasis on superficial things belies an important truth. Who cares how you look if all the time you *feel* terrible—tired, weak, bloated, inflamed? The real point is to feel better, and to feel better *longer*—over the course of more years, over more of the course of a full lifetime.

Gray hair and wrinkles show us what aging looks like on the outside. But what's going on *inside*? I'll go into the details of those interior environments in just a moment, but first I want to link the *idea* of aging to the kinds of ideas of disease we have examined in previous chapters.

You may have noticed a pattern in which we start by identifying the true sources of disease and then move into the best access points or "environments" for affecting those sources. Time and again, we have found that the moral of the story is not to avoid disease but to *slow* disease processes. And this is the approach we want to take for the aging process as well.

Aging is akin to the cellular changes in cancer or the blood vessel changes in cardiovascular disease—part of the total context of what being human entails. Gray hair and wrinkles will get us all eventually, but wouldn't it be nice if underneath we could remain as alert and spry and responsive as we were in our prime? And that is the spirit in which I would like to address the causes of aging, with the goal not being to vanquish it, but simply to live longer *better*.

The Environments of Aging

Cells divide throughout our lives. The longer the span of time, the greater the number of divisions. The more divisions, the more chances for something to go wrong, especially when you consider the inevitable wear and tear.

When your cells divide in order to create new cells for any given tissue, they split right down the middle. The most crucial part of the cell to be divided and copied is the nucleus and its precious cargo—the long strands of DNA wound up in their spools along the forty-six chromosomes. Chromosomes *are* DNA—they are great strings of bunched-up genetic code.

At the tip of each end of each chromosome is a section called a telomere (after the Greek for "end part"). This tip does not carry genetic instructions but is designed merely to protect the active and useful genes during the process of cell division and copying. During division and copying, the long, long DNA strands are first severed down the middle of their double helix bond. Copier proteins follow along behind the cut line to reproduce a new left strand for the right side, and a new right strand for the left side. Once the process is complete, two identical, whole DNA double strands—two identical chromosomes—exist side by side. The cell does this forty-six times, drags the two groups of chromosomes to opposite ends of the nucleus, then divides itself in half.

The tricky part of this process is when the cutting-and-copying team reaches the *ends* of the chromosome. Because of the way the divided strands are oriented, there is not room in front of one strand for the cutting and copying to get far enough ahead of the spot it wants to paste its copy back onto. It's a bit like painting yourself into a corner. In the case of the DNA, if the cutting and copying simply stopped when it ran out of room, it would effectively snip off that little bit of unreplicated end every time the cell divided, as if cutting off the unpainted corners. This would result in continual loss of vital genetic information, and over time would lead to just what you might expect: DNA damage, mutations, cancer, and possibly the death of the cell.

This is the dilemma that the telomeres are designed to solve. By being made of DNA but storing no genetic information, telomeres are a kind of sacrificial dummy material that offers itself up for damage in place of the actual gene-bearing ends of the chromosomes.

But over time, telomeres get worn down, and even though it's their function to sacrifice themselves and get shorter and shorter with each cell division, this process reaches a limit. After around fifty divisions and reductions, the telomeres are short enough that the cell may no longer divide without endangering its DNA. At that point the cell stops dividing and goes into a state called senescence. The cell may simply lie dormant at a very low level of functioning or it may die. But it can no longer renew itself, nor carry out the work required for the organism of which it is a part.

As we age, we accumulate more and more cells with shorter telomeres. Our body cannot restore its lost functioning by replicating new cells. Gradually the process of self-restoration slows; the cells become senescent and so do we. We age as our cells age.

Ironically, one of the things that makes a cancer cell cancerous is that it is immune to this process of senescence. Because of a substance called telomerase, a cancer cell has the ability to regrow its telomeres, which gives tumors an unlimited ability to replicate and grow.

Mitochondria and ROS

A second major "theory of aging" is that the mitochondria, the cells' energy-producing centers, suffer incremental damage and gradually lose efficiency. This may result in lower energy levels throughout the body (a real problem for older people), but the more immediate cause of trouble is the side effects of that inefficiency. As they become less precise at transforming glucose and fatty acids into ATP, the mitochondria spill off increasing levels of noxious free radicals.

Free radicals are molecules that have lost an electron. Typically, atoms like to have their electrons paired up in twosomes—this is a stable configuration in which the atom or molecule is well set, or "satisfied," electromagnetically. For stable molecules, there is no impulse either to shed or to acquire an additional electron in order to even out the set. Such molecules are not seeking to react with other molecules in order to steal their electrons.

In contrast, a free radical is a *highly* reactive molecule—it is constantly on the prowl for that one extra electron that can fill its empty slot. To find that missing piece, it will happily crash into neighboring molecules and rip off their electrons. If the victim molecule is then transformed into an electron-missing reactor, it too has become a free radical, and it too will go spinning off to steal its neighbors' electrons. These chain reactions can go careening through the tissues with alarming speed and violence. At the end, when the last radical in the line crashes into a substance that does not immediately radicalize in turn, the reaction has stopped but the damage has often been done. That final target, while it may not become a free radical itself, does suffer the loss in its proper atomic shape. It can no longer function in the proper way, and the result may be any manner of local dysfunction. If the dysfunction occurs in fats or proteins, the result might be wrinkles. If it occurs in DNA, the result may be strand breaks and further cascades of malfunctions originating from inaccurate gene expressions, including cancer.

As we saw in the chapter on diabetes, it is the sped-up process of energy production that generates the most and the most toxic free radicals. Superoxide is the primary villain here. As the keystone free radical, it serves as the gateway or progenitor for most of the most damaging free radicals, those that involve oxygen, called reactive oxygen species (ROS). These degrade DNA, wreck proteins, and even punch holes in the lipoprotein capsules that transport cholesterol through the bloodstream. Some superoxide is generated from sources outside the body, such as cigarette smoke and ultraviolet radiation. But by far the largest proportion of ROS is produced internally, from the normal process of energy burning in the mitochondria.

It is the random, small-scale change in well-ordered systems that is at the heart of the free radical problem. In its overall effect, free radical damage is not unlike the course of cancer in its mutations. Both begin with small, often repairable errors. But gradually, more and more damage is done—in DNA sequences for cancer, in atomic structures for free radicals. A long, slow accumulation of such damage ensues, until eventually we begin to see and feel more manifest, systemic dysfunction. In the case of genetic coding, we call that dysfunction "cancer." In the case of free radical damage, we call it "aging."

A whole host of diseases and health problems has been associated with ROS and specifically with superoxide and its adjuncts. These include heart disease, diabetes, cancer, Alzheimer's, and the many smaller deteriorations of aging in general. For example, it was recently discovered that graying hair in middle-aged people is due to a buildup of hydrogen peroxide in the hair follicles. Hydrogen peroxide is an especially reactive ROS that is a direct descendant of superoxide in the mitochondria. As we age, the mitochondria spring more and more leaks, more and more superoxide tends to get generated, more of this is converted to hydrogen peroxide, and more of the wear-and-tear breakdowns of an aging body show up—such as gray hair.

AGEs

One promising place to look for the sources of aging is a particular kind of molecule known as advanced glycation end products (AGEs). These are the result of unregulated bonds between sugar and DNA, proteins, and fats. When these irregular bonds are made, the tissues that the sugar bonds to are rendered stiff and rigid. They become less flexible and, depending on their function, may be deeply disordered. If AGEs attach to the collagen proteins of the skin, for example, the skin loses its natural suppleness, its ability to bend and stretch and bounce back into place. This AGE-induced flaccidity is what often forms wrinkles. If AGEs attach to the collagen in the blood vessels, the same general thing happens, but now with more dire effects: the wonderfully expandable blood tubes harden; they respond less flexibly to the variable blood flow; and, being brittle, they are more prone to cracking, which may lead to infiltration by LDLs, heart disease, and stroke.

Where Do AGEs Come From?

The major sources of AGEs are the foods we eat and free radicals produced in the body. In foods, AGEs are what we normally call "browning": the crust that forms when sugars react with fats or proteins in the absence of an enzyme (like water). These kinds of AGEs are primarily in animal products—due to the curing, pasteurizing, and storing processes, uncooked meats already harbor substantial numbers of AGEs, which cooking then increases. Dry heat is the main culprit in the home—cooking in this way increases AGEs in foods from ten- to a hundredfold over their uncooked levels. For example, bacon fried without oil has over ten times as many AGEs as bacon microwaved.

Gene Therapy Fact: Avoid Acrylamides

Acrylamide is a carcinogen created when high-starch foods are baked, toasted, or roasted, like those crunchy chips you may consume as snacks or with lunch. Cigarette smoking also generates large amounts of acrylamide. In 2007 Dutch researchers noted that high dietary intake of acrylamide could raise the risk of endometrial cancer by 29 percent and the risk of ovarian cancer by 78 percent.[1] Even more disconcerting was a 2008 Danish study that measured blood levels of acrylamide in women with and without breast cancer. The study found that women with the highest levels of acrylamide were twice as likely to develop breast cancer as women with the lowest levels.[2]

But even beyond the obvious animal sources, AGEs due to heat processing and added ingredients are all over the place. Crackers, cookies, cakes—all the crispy, crunchy snacks that you eat a bag at a time—are quite high in AGEs because of their excessive heat processing, which is used to extend shelf-life and how that process reacts with the added butters, oils, and sugars. When we talk about the dangers of "processed" foods, this is what we mean—food stripped of its nutrients, cooked and packaged to make it look good, and pumped full of tasty additives that prematurely age your body. In general, vegetables, fruits, whole grains, and other whole food carbohydrates are significantly lower in AGE content.

The second main source of AGEs takes us back into the mitochondria. Diabetics are especially warned not to eat excessive AGEs, because they produce so many AGEs themselves. This is the result of those reactions we traced in the previous chapter—particularly the superoxide backup during hyperglycemia-induced glucose processing.

AGE production in diabetes is another example of how the falling lines of biological dominoes lead both forward and backward into all sorts of unexpected places. When the fast-pumping mitochondria leak off electrons that then go on to form superoxide, they trigger several different chain reactions. The first is the scenario we saw in the previous chapter: as superoxide builds up in the pancreatic beta cells, the cell hits the safety valve and depressurizes the energy gradient across its inner membrane. The stored protons come rushing out, ATP production goes down, and superoxide levels stop rising. But the cost of this detoxifying procedure is quite high. Since ATP production declines, the cell "senses" less glucose, it therefore releases less insulin, and thus actually exacerbates the condition—hyperglycemia—it is supposed to remedy.

But there are a number of other reactions triggered by superoxide that are equally damaging. Because superoxide and its products can be so dangerous to the DNA as their levels rise, the nucleus sends out defenders to prevent and repair the damage—in this case a DNA repair enzyme called PARP. It's like the police sending out patrol cars to keep hooligans from vandalizing your property. But, as is often the case, there are hidden consequences of taking this protective action. In order to do its work, PARP needs to modify other substances, some of which could be doing important work of their own elsewhere.

And indeed, GAPDH is just such a protein that normally interacts with a range of other metabolites involved in glucose processing. When it is unavailable to do this interacting work due to being tied up with PARP, GAPDH goes missing at the other site, and those other metabolites begin to pile up. And one of the effects of that unattended overexpression is—you guessed it—*AGE formation*.

The Ecogenetic Way

All disease is pro-aging because it increases your chances of dying. Thus the best thing we can do to prevent or slow aging is to prevent or slow those major diseases that are the greatest risks to our lives. If we are tilting ourselves systematically away from disease and toward good functioning, we are already living in the most "anti-aging" way possible.

But when we talk about "aging," we're also talking about the nonlethal deteriorations in many bodily functions that seem to pile up with each passing year. Gray hair, wrinkles, loss of muscle mass—we don't die from these developments (at least not right away!), but they are an inherent part of the process of decline.

If we ask what actually causes these surface effects, we lead ourselves back into the substantial interior of the body's environments—back into the nucleus and back into the mitochondria. These are the scenes of basic and powerful operations that shape our lives in fundamental ways. The telomeres cap not only the chromosomes, but also the normal life span of each cell. When *we* gray, or begin to lose our hearing, or have trouble remembering names, it's in part because our *cells* are aging. When we gun the mitochondrial engines by flooding them with glucose, we release superoxide poisons, which go zipping through many tissues in the body, wreaking havoc and disordering everything in their path. Superoxide corrodes the tissues, but it also calls forth opposing, protective reactions that lead indirectly to further problems upstream. AGEs are one prominent source of "above the dam" trouble. AGEs are well named: just like the free radicals that steal electrons from neighboring molecules, AGEs are highly reactive, binding themselves indiscriminately to the proteins and fats they attack. And just like an aging person, AGE-bound tissues become rigid, brittle, and prone to breakdown.

Shrinking telomeres, free radical overproduction, AGE proliferation—the causes of gray hair and sagging skin go much deeper than their cosmetic effects. Targeting aging in the superficial sense may mean buying into the latest cure-in-a-bottle. But targeting aging for real means thinking seriously about the environments in which life itself is being played out. Protect and nurture those environments, and they will help you grow long and well. Neglect them, and your life becomes shorter and more brittle. And if, by taking care of your *insides*, you happen to look better on the outside too, then that's a pleasant side benefit you can enjoy as well!

The best thing you can do to slow down your aging process is to slow down the disease processes that are already going on in you and that are by far the greatest threats to your life. If you take the steps to target cancer, heart disease, obesity, and diabetes, you are giving yourself the best chance for a good, long life.

Get Out the Mop and Bucket

Floods of glucose are really bad for your engine. They burn out the motor and corrode the gaskets. We are all susceptible, in our snack-filled modern world, to living in a messy glucose state. Too much high-fructose corn syrup, too many heat-irradiated luncheon meats—too much food in general—gunk up the works. But this means that we need to become better and more vigilant mechanics. We need to keep things clean, run the machine within safe limits, and make sure the insulin levels are topped off. And if things get really messy, we need to roll up our sleeves, get out the mop and bucket, and be better *janitors* for our mitochondria.

Above all, we need to reduce inflammation to prevent neurodegenerative diseases such as Alzheimer's. This means reducing fat mass, keeping the energy balance *in* balance, and eating a range of anti-inflammatory foods. Polyphenolic substances contained in foods such as grapes have been shown to have anti-inflammatory and antioxidant effects that protect brain health. One study showed that concord grape juice helps to reduce dementia and improve cognition in older adults.[3] Another showed that concord grape juice supplementation improves memory function in older adults with mild cognitive impairment.[4]

Help your body to help you—move, exercise, activate those inflammation-suppressing genes in the muscles. This is how you keep the rhythm flowing and the engine room clean.

And because of the intimate links between glucose regulation and free radical production, these are also the best ways to control superoxide—not to mention AGE—levels. By targeting the precursor condition of inflammation that leads inexorably to insulin insensitivity, hyperglycemia, and runaway glucose processing, you give yourself a huge preemptive antioxidant defense. If you don't give glucose a chance to overrun your cells, you can stop superoxide before it starts.

Get Out of the High-AGE Pool

The AGEs you produce in your body come mostly from superoxide-mediated breakdowns in upstream glucose processing. There is a long chain of linked events whose branching contingencies it may sound difficult to address. But in fact the linkages make things easier; acting in *one* place, your action ripples along lines of connection and has widely ramifying effects. You can stop inflammation to stop superoxide. And stopping superoxide will stop the devastations of free radicals and AGEs.

If you choose your actions well, you can kill three or four birds with one stone. Eat more healthful, more naturally satiating foods → cut down on calories and energy imbalance → reduce fat mass → reduce inflammation → defend and restore insulin sensitivity → avoid hyperglycemia → avoid redlining the mitochondria → reduce superoxide production → reduce AGE production. That's a pretty long line! But the magic of ecogenetics is that we can regard each step as an *environment* of the next one. Keep backing up, and before long you've reached a point where you can intervene to make a decisive difference in the *whole* complex of linkages.

But there are many other reasons to eat in a nutritionally targeted way. In the case of AGEs, there are also exogenous sources, and these are predominantly from what you put in your mouth. The deep end of the high-AGE pool is filled with meats, fats, proteins, cheeses, fish, and eggs. Butter, cream cheese, and mayonnaise are all high-AGE foods, as are nuts and oils (though the smaller typical serving size limits total exposure). McDonald's French fries are very high, as are many fast-food sandwiches. The typical cracker, such as Fritos or Goldfish or even plain oyster crackers, has from fifteen to thirty times more AGEs than an equivalent slice of Wonder Bread. A butter croissant from Starbucks might have ten times as many as a bagel.

In general, carbohydrates are low in AGEs—15, 20, or 100 AGEs per serving rather than 5,000 or 6,000 for some scorched meats. So this is the shallow end, where you want to spend most of your time. Fruits, vegetables, and whole grains are all very low in AGEs, owing to their low fat and protein contents, to their comparatively higher water contents, and also to their typically being eaten at lower temperatures than meats. But even carbohydrates have enough protein and fat in them to drive AGE levels up when they are cooked high and dry. Broiled tofu has seven times the AGEs of raw tofu.

Here are some additional findings from the latest survey:[5]

- An apple has about 13 AGEs per serving; a baked apple has around 45.
- Raw eggplant has about half the AGEs of grilled eggplant.
- Grilled broccoli and carrots have nearly twenty times the AGEs of raw, though both forms are still quite low in absolute terms.
- Packaged cocoa mixed with nonfat milk has over thirty times the AGEs of nonfat milk alone microwaved for two minutes.
- A fast-food cheeseburger, fried fish sandwich, or fried chicken nuggets will each set you back 5,000 to 6,000 AGEs.
- Pizza or a toasted open-faced sandwich with melted cheese both have over 5,000 AGEs.
- Veggie burgers and Boca Burgers are both low-AGE foods.
- Mustard has virtually no AGEs, and ketchup has tiny amounts.
- Most liquids are very low: coffee is around 10, tea around 5 AGEs. But coffee sitting on a hot plate for an hour more than triples its AGE count.

Two main rules can guide you when estimating and trying to reduce AGEs in foods you eat and prepare. First is that the *type* of food determines much of its AGE potential. High-fat, high-protein foods are full of the kinds of molecular substances that can be, or may already have been, converted into AGEs.

The second and even more important principle is that the *method* of preparing foods has a tremendous influence on their AGE levels. High heat is inherently AGE producing. And dry heat—food heated in the absence of water or even oil—is the most AGE producing of all. Poached chicken contains about one-fourth the AGEs of roasted chicken. Salmon broiled with olive oil contains almost three times the AGEs of salmon steamed for ten minutes.

Another crucial point is that *processing* makes an enormous difference, even before the food enters your home. Crackers, cookies, snacks—these stand out among carbs as unusually high-AGE foods. In part this is due to added fats and sugars, but it also reflects the methods of producing such items. Foods that come in boxes or wrapped in plastic, and are intended to sit on store shelves for weeks, are typically prepared or "sterilized" with high-heat processing. This makes them safer from decay and contamination, but it also sets in motion the glycating process, which can continue for a very long time, even when the foods are returned to a cooler environment. Simply sitting there on the shelf, a box of crackers may be slowly glycating its way to more and more AGEs.

Gene Therapy Fact: Fast Food, Early Grave

One study looking at Chinese people living in Singapore showed that those who ate fast food only once a week raised their risk of dying from a heart attack by 20 percent. The risk jumped by 80 percent among those in the study who consumed fast food more than four times a week.[6]

My advice? Eat more whole foods. Eat more fruits, vegetables, spices and herbs, and whole grains. Drink water, tea, and coffee. Eat some foods raw. When you cook food, go "low and slow"—there's no need to blast every meal under a broiler or in a sauté pan. Treat your food gently, and it will treat you the same way.

The Ecogenetic Way: Aging Summary

Here's a quick review of the essential steps you can take to improve your aging environments:

- **Don't die.**
  - *I admit this is a hyperbolic way of putting it, but it's still true. The best way to slow aging is to slow the diseases that are the biggest risks to your life. You haven't aged too far if you're not dead. Staying alive is the first principle of anti-aging.*
- **Reread, rehearse, repeat.**
  - *The best way to stay alive better and longer is to follow the advice from the previous chapters. All the worst risks are addressed there; if you're tilting your disease environments in your favor, you're way ahead in the aging game.*
- **Get out the mop and bucket.**
  - *Glucose and fatty acids spilling into cells is the chief cause of superoxide and free radical production.*
  - *You can help your body mop up glucose spills by keeping it in good, anti-inflammatory shape. Keep your fat and muscle cells responsive to insulin by keeping inflammation out of the house.*
  - *Reverse engineer your free radical defenses. Diabetes causes massive aging, so do the things you would do to prevent diabetes.*
  - *Reduce fat mass.*
  - *Move your body daily to keep expressing the muscles' anti-inflammatory genes.*
  - *Include anti-inflammatory foods in your daily diet.*
- **Get out of the high-AGE pool.**
  - *AGEs are like sugar-glazed free radicals that stick to their targets and make them weak and brittle. AGEs come mainly from effects following superoxide production. Stop superoxide (see above), and you mostly stop AGEs.*
  - *High-fat and high-protein foods, especially animal products, have high AGE potential—and often are already full of AGEs, even when uncooked.*
  - *High-heat cooking multiplies AGEs in food. Dry-heat cooking is the worst. Browning is a sure sign that sugars are fusing to fats and proteins in an AGE-accelerating way.*

- *The processing in processed foods includes high-heat preparations that trigger AGE formation. Eating processed foods is inherently aging.*
- *Eat more vegetables, fruits, and whole grains. Eat more whole foods. Eat some food raw. Cook food gently—low and slow.*

Targeted Nutrition for Aging

General Anti-Aging

Researchers in Canada conducted an animal study that demonstrated the potential effectiveness of nutritional supplements on aging.[7] The researchers targeted five central sources of the ravages we associate with old age:

- inflammation
- insulin resistance
- membrane integrity
- mitochondrial dysfunction
- oxidative stress

A thirty-ingredient nutrient cocktail was developed to target these five mechanisms, and relying on many of the ingredients I have already discussed throughout this book: B vitamins, vitamin C, vitamin D, acetyl-L-carnitine, garlic, beta-carotene, and coenzyme Q10. In the study, the nutrient cocktail improved cognition and mobility in mice as well as expanded their life span by approximately 28 percent. While clinical trials are still warranted to determine the efficacy of this cocktail in humans, the initial results of this targeted therapy are very promising. Other researchers have confirmed these findings, and I believe that supplementing humans with a similarly effective cocktail could add nine years of life and enhanced activity and cognition to the average eighty-year-old person.[8]

Here are other promising ingredients:

Phloridzin

Phloridzin is a potent polyphenol found in the skin of apples that slows three types of aging processes: oxidative stress, inflammation, and glycation. One study reported that phloridzin extended the life span of yeast cell cultures 2.3 generations. Specifically, scientists found that the polyphenolic substance increased yeast cells' resistance to oxidative stress from free radicals. Eating this ecogenetically powerful food will help prevent the development of various age-related conditions, such as cancer, diabetes, and cardiovascular disease. A good anti-aging dose would be 300 to 600 milligrams daily.

Reishi

Sometimes called the "mushroom of immortality," reishi is a potent-tasting fungus with many bioactive compounds shown to slow down factors associated with unhealthy aging. It can also help in the fight against pathological conditions that lead to advanced aging, such as cancer, diabetes, autoimmune diseases, Alzheimer's, and Parkinson's. A good anti-aging dose is 200 to 300 mg daily.

Olive Oil

A staple in the Mediterranean diet, olive oil has been shown to have antioxidant effects on free radicals and to have protective effects against diseases such as cancer.[9] One study showed that olive oil may increase the average life span by 13.4 years. By evaluating dietary information for more than forty thousand people, researchers determined that those whose olive oil intake was in the top 25 percent had a 44 percent lower risk of dying from heart disease and a 26 percent lower risk of dying from any other cause.[10] Olive oil decreases the expression of proinflammatory genes in humans and partially explains why there is a reduced risk of cardiovascular disease, dementia, and cancer among people living in Mediterranean countries.[11] Olive oil is sensitive to heat, though, which changes the beneficial compounds in it—so it is best to use it on salads or in dips rather than in cooking.

Yucca

Yucca, the flowering plant discussed earlier in the diabetes chapter, contains steroidal saponins, which possess antimicrobial activity by blocking gut microbes that contribute to arthritic joints. One study showed that arthritic patients who took yucca tablets (a powdered form of the yucca plant) experienced reduced pain and swelling.[12] Different mechanisms have been proposed to explain its anti-inflammatory effects. Overall, the beneficial effects of yucca's active compounds—its polyphenols and steroidal saponins—make it an excellent choice in preventing and treating arthritis.

Boswellia

Boswellia, an Ayurvedic herb with profound anti-inflammatory activity, has been used for both arthritis and joint stiffness. It also blocks the activation of cancer-promoting genes caused by tumor necrosis factor alpha (TNF-alpha) and nuclear factor–kappa B (NF-kB), which are two of the most powerful activators of cancer. Two large randomized studies have shown boswellia improves joint function, pain, and stiffness in knee osteoarthritis.[13] Boswellia has also been reported to decrease symptoms of asthma[14] by improving lung function, and inflammatory bowel disease[15] by decreasing inflammation of the gut. I recommend 300 to 400 mg daily.

Methionine-Containing Nutrients

Methyl sulfonyl methane (MSM), a sulfur-containing organic compound that is found in a variety of fruits, vegetables, and grains, has been shown to improve joint function and to help maintain normal joint cartilage, as joints require sulfur and cysteine for healthy functioning.

CoQ10

Research has shown that coenzyme 10, or CoQ10, can add up to nine years to your life expectancy by tuning up the efficiency of the mitochondria's energy production and by protecting against oxidative stress. Lab studies have shown that animals supplemented with CoQ10 had an 11.7 percent increase in mean life span and a 24 percent increase in maximum life span.[16]

Although our bodies produce CoQ10, its levels rapidly decrease with increasing age and are found to be low in patients with chronic diseases. Because of the role of oxidative stress in creating wrinkles and altered pigmentation, the topical application of CoQ10 has been reported to improve the appearance of aging skin.[17] My patients take 100 to 200 mg daily.

Pumpkin

With age, a loss in muscle and sphincter tone can lead to weakened bladder control. Studies have shown that pumpkin seed extract, along with soy isoflavones, can improve the function of an overactive bladder, a problem affecting approximately 16 percent of men and women. The pumpkin seed prevents the symptoms of urgency and frequency. One study reported that administering pumpkin seed and soybean germ extract over a six-week period significantly reduced the number of daytime and nighttime urinations.[18] Another study showed that using the combined extract improved sleep because participants experienced less nighttime urinary frequency.[19]

Pumpkin seed extract has also improved urinary symptoms in men suffering from benign prostatic hyperplasia or an enlarged prostate.[20] In one study, older adult men who received pumpkin seed extract for three months experienced a 40 percent improvement in urinary flow and a 30 percent reduction in urinary frequency compared with those in the placebo group. I usually recommend 250 to 500 mg daily.

Lutein

Lutein is the carotenoid that gives the yellow or orange pigment to fruits and vegetables such as carrots, corn, sweet potatoes, squash, mangoes, zucchini, and tomatoes. Lutein is also found in dark leafy green vegetables like spinach, romaine lettuce, kale, collard greens, and bok choy. But surprisingly, the best source of lutein appears to be egg yolk.

Lutein has been shown to protect against the development of two age-associated eye disorders: cataracts and macular degeneration. It is also protective against atherosclerosis. Researchers reported that individuals with the highest consumption of lutein at baseline did not have any additional arterial plaque buildup at the end of an eighteen-month study, whereas arterial clogging had worsened among participants with the lowest amounts of lutein.[21] Surgically removed sections of human arteries further demonstrated the efficacy of lutein against plaque formation in blood vessels. The resected arterial tissues were treated with lutein and found to attract fewer white blood cells, which are involved in the development of diseased arteries.

Some of its other benefits:

- Lutein plays an important role in slowing down the effects of an aging brain. In one lab study, rats that were fed spinach (as well as blueberries and strawberries) showed signs of reversed age-related deficits in brain and behavioral aging.[22]
- The consumption of 6 to 10 milligrams of lutein daily has been shown to provide antioxidants that reduce oxidative damage to the skin.[23]
- Researchers have reported that the consumption of lutein may improve lung tissue, a particularly important finding because of its implications for smokers.[24]
- A Dutch study in patients with rheumatoid arthritis showed that arthritic symptoms of the knee decreased among people with the highest consumption of lutein.[25]
- Lutein has been shown to increase apoptosis, impair DNA repair, and inhibit angiogenesis in cancer.[26]

While a growing number of studies have established lutein's anti-aging properties, the verdict is not yet in on the best approach to consumption. Are the same effects found in supplement form as dietarily? How much lutein do you need to prevent or treat health problems? Some experts recommend 4 to 6 milligrams daily. But a typical Asian diet, which is considered to be high in lutein, provides only about 2 milligrams daily. The USDA suggests adding one egg and a cup of spinach to a salad to reach your daily recommended amount of lutein. Although egg yolk is a great source of lutein, you should limit your intake if you have high cholesterol. Focus instead on eating fruits and vegetables that are high in lutein.

Brain Health

A study showed that feeding old rats a combination of mitochondrial metabolites, acetyl-L-carnitine (ALC), and lipoic acid helped to improve the animals' ambulatory activity and cognitive function. A review of twenty-one double-blind clinical trials in which ALC was used to treat mild cognitive impairment and mild Alzheimer's disease also showed improved mitochondrial function.[27]

A study has reported that men who drink tea regularly (three cups per day or more) experience a five-year increase in life span when compared with men who drink little tea (a quarter cup or less of tea per day). The results were attributed to increased length in the telomeres of the tea-consuming men.[28] In addition, a large Japanese study found that a higher consumption of green tea is associated with a lower incidence of cognitive impairment in humans.[29]

A combination of vitamin C and vitamin E has been shown to be a protective antioxidant against cognitive decline among older adults. Elder participants in a five-year Canadian study who combined vitamins C and E were less likely to experience significant cognitive decline.[30] Another study, at Johns Hopkins, found similar results and also showed that this combination provided protection against Alzheimer's disease.[31]

Swedish researchers showed that high levels of all eight forms of vitamin E correlated to a dramatic reduction in the risk of Alzheimer's disease for people over eighty.[32]

Vitamin D appears to have protective properties against Parkinson's disease. In a Finnish study, participants with lower levels of vitamin D in their blood were three times as likely to develop Parkinson's disease.[33]

Grape-derived polyphenols may provide protection against Alzheimer's disease, as shown in a study that administered grapeseed extract to mice with neurotoxins in their brain similar to those found in Alzheimer's disease. This neurotoxic protein was substantially reduced in the brains of these mice.[34]

Green tea has neuroprotective effects when used in combination with L-theanine, a protein similar to glutamate. L-theanine readily enters the brain to stop brain cell death after a stroke or transient ischemic attack by blocking the effects and formation of glutamate. One study showed that elderly participants with normal cognition or mild cognitive deficits who were administered L-theanine and green tea experienced significantly lower cognitive dysfunction than those in a placebo group.[35]

Studies have demonstrated the protective effects of EGCG, an antioxidant found in green tea, in making the amyloid plaque protein involved in Alzheimer's disease more soluble by using its enzyme alpha-secretase. Unfortunately, an enormous amount of EGCG would be needed in humans to have this effect. One study has demonstrated that when EGCG is combined with fish oil, the activity of green tea's antioxidant is enhanced compared with using either fish oil or EGCG alone.[36]

In another study, Alzheimer's patients who received a nutritive cocktail of choline (vitamin B), DHA (an omega-3 fatty acid), and uridine (an amino acid) showed a significant increase in the number of dendrites in their brains, which meant increased synaptic transmission between nerve cells. These participants had a 40 percent increase in delayed verbal recall compared with those untreated.[37]

Low levels of vitamin B6 are associated with an increased risk for developing Parkinson's disease. One study showed that people taking a daily supplement of vitamin B6 had a 54 percent drop in their risk of developing the disease.[38]

A study showed that older adults who took a supplement of the omega-3 fatty acid DHA demonstrated an improvement in age-related cognitive decline, showing significant improvements in episodic memory, learning faculties, and verbal memory.[39]

Vitamin B3 supplements are important because they aid in cellular repair. Normally, injured or old cells undergo apoptosis or cell death to make room for new cells. Unfortunately, not all cells have the same ability to produce new cells. Nerve cells, unlike skin cells, have a limited ability in replacing cells that die. In particular, NAD+, which is a precursor to B3, declines when nerve tissue is damaged.

But a group of scientists has reported that nicotinamide riboside, a compound readily found in milk, replenishes NAD+, which is important because B3 promotes cell repair after nerve injury.[40]

Rhodiola is a root from an arctic plant that helps the body manage stress. Research has shown that rhodiola decreases anxiety, depression, and fatigue. It has also been shown to improve cognitive decline in humans, as well as support memory and brain function in animals.

In conjunction with rhodiola, I recommend three additional herbs: *eleutherococcus, huperzia,* and *schisandra.* The main active ingredient in *huperzia,* which comes from Chinese club moss, is *huperzine H*, a neuroprotective compound that increases acetylcholine. It also protects the brain from formation of amyloid, which is a plaquelike substance that causes memory loss and cognitive decline. And studies have shown that *huperzine H* reverses memory loss and agitation in people who are diagnosed with senile dementia.

Bone Health

Hesperidin, a phytochemical classified as a bioflavonoid, is an antioxidant, anti-inflammatory, anticarcinogenic, vasoprotective, cholesterol-lowering agent. It is found mainly in citrus fruits, with the highest concentration within the white parts and pulp of the skin. Hesperidin has been shown to strengthen bones,[41] as well as lower total cholesterol levels and triglycerides.[42, 43] Moreover, the phytochemical was found to exhibit the same mechanism of action as statins, which are cholesterol-lowering drugs. Incorporating dietary sources of hesperidin can improve both bone health and lipid levels, two adverse changes that occur in postmenopausal women.

Among its many healthful effects, curcumin has been shown to improve arthritis symptoms. In one study on patients suffering from osteoarthritis of the knee, participants who received a daily curcumin supplement reported a 58 percent decrease in pain and discomfort, and demonstrated more stamina, when they were observed walking on a treadmill.[44]

Not surprisingly, bone health improves with exercise. One study found that bone health increases in postmenopausal women who perform tai chi, and also in those who take a supplement of green tea antioxidants.[45]

Vitamin C may play an important role in minimizing the risk of fractures in older adults. One major study showed that men and women with a high vitamin C intake (whether from food or supplements) had much lower risk for fractures than those who took little vitamin C.[46]

The combination of vitamin D and calcium reduces the risk of fractures as well. A meta-analysis of 137 studies assessing the efficacy of vitamin D supplementation on fracture risk found that the combination of vitamin D and calcium supplements reduced the risk for fracture more than vitamin D alone.[47] Because there aren't any available ways to measure the production of vitamin D in the body from exposure to sunlight, the adequate amount of vitamin D from dietary sources remains unclear. In addition, other researchers found that, over a three-year period, calcium and vitamin D supplements lowered the risk of mortality.[48]

Research shows that girls with low levels of vitamin D, especially those who participate in high-impact physical activity (such as gymnastics), are more likely to have stress fractures.[49] Because bone strength in young girls is linked to bone health later in life, it is especially important for them to consume foods that are high in vitamin D, such as yogurt and milk (the daily recommended amount of vitamin D is 600 IU).

Skin Health

Goji berries, a potent source of antioxidants, are loaded with vitamin C, important for collagen synthesis, and vitamin E, which helps prevent dryness and wrinkles. Goji berries have been shown to boost antioxidant activity by 57 percent,[50] and to reduce free radical formation by 82 percent.[51] These berries contain bioactive components that help to maintain a healthy, youthful appearance of skin by blocking collagen-destroying enzymes.[52]

Phyllanthus emblica, or Indian gooseberry, has antioxidant and anti-inflammatory properties.[53] Think of it as edible SPF—it has been shown to protect against harmful effects of UV rays, especially damage to collagen, which makes the skin vulnerable to fine lines, age spots, skin discoloration, and wrinkles. One study, looking at the effects of Indian gooseberry on human skin exposed to UV radiation, showed that the berries blocked the formation of matrix metalloproteinase, an enzyme that destroys collagen in UV-damaged skin.[54] Indian gooseberry has also been shown to boost collagen synthesis,[55] prevent collagenase (a collagen-destroying enzyme) activity,[56] and promote skin repair.[57]

Pycnogenol, a natural extract from pine tree bark, can help improve elasticity and minimize collagen loss and to help maintain youthful, healthy, supple skin. Pycnogenol contains bioactive compounds such as procyanidins and bioflavonoids, which target the processes in the body that cause skin to age prematurely. Many of these processes cause tissue damage, such as oxidative stress, inflammation, and DNA damage, even in other parts of the body. When these processes begin to take their toll, your skin bears the first visible signs of premature aging. Studies exploring the health effects of Pycnogenol have demonstrated that it inhibits mechanisms that promote premature aging. In one clinical trial, supplementing participants with 25 to 75 milligrams of Pycnogenol daily was protective against UV light exposure. Pycnogenol also aids in improving skin elasticity and smoothness, as shown in a controlled double-blind study.[58]

Targeted Supplements

Targeted Ecogenetic Juice for Aging

The following juice recipe is for those who are concerned about aging. But don't feel as though you have to drink this specific juice every day. Shake things up! I've included several juicing recipes after the disease-specific chapters' section. The ecogenetic juices listed are general recipes that focus on using wholesome ingredients and organically grown produce that have beneficial effects on many body systems. So you don't have to worry about sticking to any specific drink. My patients usually drink one or two ecogenetic juices daily. Mix up the juices you drink to broaden your intake of bioactive nutrients on a weekly basis. If you have a specific health concern, increase your intake of that recommended ecogenetic drink.

> ½ cup Knudsen organic tomato juice
> ¼ cup cilantro leaves and delicate stems
> 1 tablespoon spirulina powder
> juice from 1 lime
> 1 tablespoon honey
> 1 teaspoon royal jelly
> 1 teaspoon Barlean's Omega Swirl
> 1 teaspoon ground ginger

> Blend all ingredients for 15 to 20 seconds on low. Drink and enjoy.

Targeted Ecogenetic Supplements for Aging

The supplements listed below are recommended for aging well. Don't get overwhelmed and feel that you have to take every supplement listed. Remember: everyone is unique. The supplement list is in no particular order. I recommend them all equally to my patients because each one has benefits that prevent or reverse premature aging. Many of my patients start off by taking one supplement to determine how well they are tolerating it. Then they add other supplements as needed. When taking supplements, the focus should be to maintain good health. Don't worry about whether you should be taking five, ten, or fifteen supplements. That is not the intent of the supplement list. Do what you can. And take your time in figuring out what works for you: good health isn't a destination; it's a lifelong practice. And supplements are a small part of attaining a healthy lifestyle. Supplements are meant to be an addition to not a replacement for eating a healthy diet, getting adequate sleep, and improving your level of physical activity.

The supplements below are among the most important ones I give to many of my patients. Because every person is different, certain supplements may be more important than others for a given individual.

- Boswellia—300-400 milligrams, once daily
- Yucca extract—500 milligrams, once daily
- MSM—1,000 milligrams, once daily
- Calendula extract—500 milligrams, once daily
- Krill oil—500 milligrams, once daily
- Ashwagandha root—500 milligrams, once daily
- Holy basil leaf extract—500 milligrams, once daily
- Phosphatidylserine—250 milligrams, once daily
- Moducare C (plant sterols)—20 mg, once daily
- PQQ—20 milligrams, once daily
- Biotin—5 milligrams, twice daily
- Bamboo extract—300 milligrams, twice daily
- *Bacopa monnieri* extract—500 milligrams, twice daily
- Triple Bee Complex by Y.S. Eco Bee Farms (royal jelly 200 mg, bee pollen 600 mg, bee propolis 200 mg)—twice daily
- N-acetylcysteine (NAC, a precursor of glutathione)—600 milligrams, once daily
- Gingko—120 milligrams, once daily
- Inositol—750 milligrams, twice daily
- Glycerophosphocholine (GPC)—300 milligrams, once daily
- Rhodiola—100 milligrams, twice daily

Part II

Implementing the Plan

Chapter 7

The Gene Therapy Questionnaire

IN THE FIRST PART OF THIS BOOK, I provided you with the scientific underpinnings that make the ecogenetic approach make sense and that allow you to make better choices about the foods and beverages you bring into your epigenetic environment.

In this second part, I want to offer more practical advice that brings the science down to the level of day-to-day nutrition and meal planning, first offering a guide to supplements and then a series of meal plans and recipes to demonstrate that nutrigenetics is not only healthful but delicious as well.

Supplements are not regulated by the U.S. Food and Drug Administration, they are not required to undergo rigorous clinical trials before being marketed to the public, and in most cases they are easily obtainable without a prescription, which means that your safety and assurance of value lies in being an informed and cautious consumer. Some commentators are skeptical of supplements altogether. But dismissing supplements out of hand is like saying one should avoid fastening one's seatbelt because it's uncomfortable. The fact is, certain supplements are often a necessity so you can be sure that you are getting either some or all of many specific nutrients required for optimal health.

Here are some tips to consider before you start using any supplements:

- Always discuss your plan for supplemental nutrition with your physician before beginning any new regimen.
- Check the FDA Web site. Although the agency does not regulate supplements, its Web site does carry a list of recalled drugs, including supplements. There are many other reliable Web sites backed by medical and government organizations that can provide helpful information.
- Follow your gut. Does the advertisement for a supplement sound too good to be true? It probably is. If the manufacturer is making claims that are mind-boggling or boasting extremely rapid results, you should steer clear.
- Look for the following seals or symbols: United States Pharmacopeia (USP), NSF International.
- Know where your supplement was manufactured; the label should include contact information as well as a list of all the ingredients.
- Be sure to identify the serving size provided for each nutrient (you don't want to consume an excessive amount of any one nutrient).
- The rising cost of prescription drugs is evident, but resist the urge to shop around for a supplemental alternative to a prescription drug your physician has prescribed—especially outside the United States, since the regulatory standards are quite different in many other countries.

When I see any new patient, I go through a consultation that lasts two and a half hours. Much of that time is spent going over the questionnaire I ask new patients to fill out to give me a picture of their overall condition and medical history. This helps me enormously in trying to determine the regimen of supplements that might be best for them.

I've provided that questionnaire just below, each question correlated with specific recommendations for supplemental nutrition.

The Gene Therapy Nutrition and Supplements Questionnaire

1. Do you have a first-degree family member, such as a parent or sibling, with cancer?

There are genetic predispositions to cancer such as the BRCA1 mutation, which predisposes one to breast, ovarian, and pancreatic cancer, and the MSH mutation, which predisposes one to colon cancer. Both of these genes are responsible for DNA repair. However, a 2000 study showed that women born before 1940 with the BRCA1 mutation had a far lower risk of developing either breast or ovarian cancer than women born after 1940, suggesting that exposure to numerous environmental toxins causes a deleterious gene-environment interaction.

Top Five Anticancer Supplements

- Di-indole methane (DIM)—100 milligrams, twice daily (Brand recommendation: Source Naturals). Found in broccoli, brussels sprouts, cauliflower, and cabbage, this compound induces an enzyme that promotes healthy estrogen metabolism in women and inhibits prostate cancer cell proliferation in men.
- Magnolia—200 milligrams, once daily (NutriCology). This herb has been found to inhibit skin, breast, prostate, and pancreatic cancer growth by promoting apoptosis, inhibiting abnormal angiogenesis, and decreasing the body's production of inflammatory mediators. It contains the nutrients honokiol and manganol.
- Artichoke extract—320 milligrams, once daily (Integrative Therapeutics). This substance contains rutin, quercetin, and gallic acid, which promote tumor cell death and inhibit tumor cell proliferation.
- Chaga mushroom extract—500 milligrams, twice daily (Host Defense). This mushroom, which grows in cold climates on birch tree bark, has been found to stimulate the part of the immune system that protects against cancer and has direct inhibitory effects against a variety of cancers, such as breast, prostate, and skin.
- Black cumin seed oil—500 milligrams, twice daily (Amazing Herbs). Also known as blackseed, this herb has profound anti-inflammatory activity but also promotes the ability of cancer cells to undergo apoptosis. It has been found to inhibit pancreatic, breast, and liver cancer cell growth.

Top Ten Foods to Inhibit Cancer
In the recipe section you will find preparation suggestions for these cancer-preventive foods:

- Olive oil
- Ginger

- Garlic
- Cruciferous vegetables—cauliflower, cabbage, brussels sprouts, and broccoli
- Rosemary
- Beets
- Walnuts
- Carrots
- Cooked tomatoes
- Blueberries

2. Is your weight appropriate for your height, or are you more than 10 percent above your ideal body weight for your height?

Studies have shown that being within 10 percent of your ideal body weight is essential for reducing your risk of heart disease, cancer, and diabetes. Being overweight promotes inflammation, which leads to premature aging and degenerative diseases, such as arthritis, macular degeneration, and dementia.

Top Five Supplements for Weight Loss

- Guggul—650 milligrams, twice daily (Now Nutrition). Found in an Indian tree bark, guggul contains a gum resin filled with compounds known as guggulsterones. Numerous studies have shown use of this extract to result in improved cholesterol and triglyceride profiles. It has also been shown to improve metabolic rate and the body's efficiency in burning calories.
- Glucomannan—665-milligram capsules, two before meals (Nature's Way). This is a sugar made from the corm of the konjac plant, which is used in traditional Japanese cooking as a food thickener. A bulky fiber, it expands in the digestive tract, creating a sense of fullness and reducing the absorption of carbs and cholesterol. It has been associated with lower cholesterol and blood sugar in people with type 2 diabetes. To avoid constipation, it is important to drink at least 8 ounces of water with every gram of glucomannan, and it is taken before meals.
- Forskohlii root—385 milligrams, twice daily (Solaray). A member of the mint family, this plant grows on the mountain slopes of Thailand, India, and Nepal. Studies have shown that it increases the rate of fat

burning and decreases inflammatory compounds associated with heart disease and weight gain.

- Conjugated linoleic acid (CLA)—750 milligrams, twice daily (Jarrow Formulas). This is an omega-9 fatty acid that naturally occurs in organic dairy products and beef. Studies have shown that CLA helps the body burn more fat and control appetite. It has also been found to lower triglycerides.
- Resveratrol—100 milligrams, once daily (Jarrow Formulas). Found in the skin of red grapes and red wine, this compound blocks inflammatory mediators associated with weight gain. It also inhibits the growth of new fat cells by interfering with their ability to form new blood vessels and decreasing their growth rate.

Top Ten Foods for Weight Loss
In the recipe section you will find preparation suggestions for these weight-busting foods:

- Grapefruit
- Wheatgrass
- Romaine lettuce
- Celery
- Flounder
- Curry powder
- Yogurt
- Aloe vera
- Miso soup
- Asparagus

3. Do you live in a part of the country with a latitude that has limited sun exposure between November and April of each year (north of Reno, Nevada; Kansas City, Missouri; or Cincinnati, Ohio)?

Studies have shown that people living closer to the equator have higher 25-hydroxy vitamin D levels, which is related to the body's production of vitamin D3. People with normal levels of 25-hydroxy vitamin D have lower incidence of cancer. People who reside where sun exposure is limited for six months per year cannot form adequate amounts of this vitamin, and there is a marked variation in how people absorb D3. Most people require supplementation with 1,000 or 2,000 units per day. I happen to be a very poor absorber of D3 and require 50,000 units per week to keep my levels in the mid normal range. This is not a supplement to guess the dosage with, though. Too much can damage the kidneys and create problems with your calcium. Therefore, it is essential that you work with your physician to follow your levels regularly and find the correct dose for you.

4. Do you have difficulty falling asleep or staying asleep?

Sleep is critically important for the immune function as well as healthy glucose utilization. Sleep deprivation has also been linked to heart disease and obesity.

Top Five Supplements for Sleep

- Melatonin—3 to 6 milligrams, at bedtime (Pure Encapsulations). This hormone made by the pineal gland in the brain regulates sleep and wake cycles. Its levels often drop with age and some adults make little or none. Small amounts are found in grains, fruits, and vegetables, but a supplement with this dose is useful for many people.
- 4-amino-3-phenylbutyric acid—300 milligrams, at bedtime (Biotics). This substance is related to a neurotransmitter in the brain responsible for drowsiness, and it is an excellent sleep aid. It was synthesized by Russian scientists for use by cosmonauts to help them sleep without impairing their cognitive or physical performance the next day.
- Passion flower extract—350 milligrams, at bedtime (NOW Foods). Native to the southern United States, this plant contains numerous nutrients important to central nervous system activity, such as quercetin, glycosides, and phytosterols. It's excellent for relieving anxiety and stress, allowing deeper, more restful sleep.
- Lemon balm—400 milligrams, at bedtime (Solaray). This herb is a member of the mint family and has been used since the middle ages to promote sleep. Studies have shown that essential oils within lemon balm leaves contain terpines, which account for its relaxing effects.
- Magnolia—200 milligrams, at bedtime (NutriCology). The bark from this tree has been used in Chinese medicine for hundreds of years to treat anxiety and insomnia. Its nutrients have been found to increase neurotransmitters in the brain responsible for relaxation, sleep, and mood.

Top Ten Foods for Sleep

In the recipe section you will find preparation suggestions for these restful, sleep-assisting foods:

- Chickpeas—a good source of tryptophan, an amino acid necessary for the synthesis of melatonin and other essential neurotransmitters related to sleep
- Shrimp—another excellent source of tryptophan
- Almonds—rich in magnesium, required for neurologic function related to sleep
- Romaine lettuce—containing lactucarium, which has sedative effects on the brain
- Halibut—high in vitamin B6, which is required for production of melatonin and serotonin, both necessary for healthy sleep
- Pistachio nuts—also high in vitamin B6
- Cherries, especially the tart variety—naturally boost levels of melatonin
- Chamomile tea—associated with an increase of glycine, an amino acid that acts directly as a sedative, as well as an increase in neurotransmitters associated with relaxation
- Honey—a low-glycemic sugar that slightly raises insulin levels, thereby allowing tryptophan to function more effectively in producing sleep
- Kale, spinach, and mustard greens—very rich in calcium, needed by the brain, along with tryptophan, to manufacture melatonin

5. Are you on any medication or chemotherapy?

Chemotherapy

Chemotherapy drugs often cause depletion of antioxidant vitamins. This is due to their prooxidant effects caused by the destruction of cancer cells, which in turn releases inflammatory mediators, resulting in the growth of more resistant cancer cells. Other medications can interfere with the absorption of vitamins such as B12 and folic acid, as well as vitamins A, D, and K. Nearly half of all American adults take a prescription medication, and there are several classes of drugs that may be associated with nutritional deficiencies.

As an oncologist, I prescribe chemotherapy frequently. The evaluation necessary to help a patient on chemotherapy—induced nutritional deficiencies as well as the host of other side effects caused by chemotherapy drugs that can be alleviated with nutritional interventions—is beyond the scope of this book. I suggest, however, that you seek out advice from your oncologist and have him or her work in conjunction with an integrative oncologist.

Hormone Replacement Therapy

Hormone replacement therapy has been associated with deficiencies of folic acid, magnesium, and vitamins B6 and B12. For patients on these medications, I recommend the following:

- P5P50 (the active form of vitamin B6)—50 milligrams, once daily
- Vitamin B12—500 micrograms under the tongue, once daily
- Magnesium glycenate—240 milligrams, once daily
- Folic acid—400 micrograms, once daily
- Riboflavin—50 milligrams, once daily
- Zinc—25 milligrams, once daily

Psychotropic Drugs

Lithium carbonate, used to treat bipolar disorder, depletes vitamin B8 (inositol) and folic acid. I recommend patients take folic acid (400 micrograms, once daily) and inositol (750 milligrams, twice daily) if they are taking this medication.

Antidepressant medications require an adequate supply of precursors of neurotransmitters such as serotonin and dopamine. I recommend that my patients who take these medications include in their diet the following foods, which contain nutrients necessary for neurotransmitters:

- Foods rich in omega-3 fatty acids—deep coldwater fish like salmon, haddock, and cod, as well as flaxseed and pumpkin seed
- Eggs—a protein-rich food that provides amino acids necessary for the production of dopamine, a key neurotransmitter
- Chicken and turkey—contain tryptophan and proteins necessary for norepinephrine and dopamine, and are good sources of CoQ10, required for optimal brain function
- Bananas—excellent sources of tyrosine and potassium, critical for both adequate neurologic function and for serotonin, norepinephrine, and dopamine
- Apples—contain quercetin, important for normal brain function and decreased inflammation
- Cheese—loaded with amino acids required for neurotransmitter synthesis
- Cottage cheese—loaded with vitamin D3, essential for brain function, and provides key proteins necessary for neurotransmitter synthesis

- Beets—contain betaine, an amino acid critical for production of SAM-e, an important part of neurotransmitter synthesis and balance
- Beans—rich in proteins and amino acids required for production of dopamine and norepinephrine
- Wheat germ—a good source of phenylalanine, a key amino acid required as a precursor to the amino acid tyrosine, required to manufacture dopamine
- Watermelon—rich in vitamin B6, necessary for most of the neurotransmitters needed for mood and regulating sleep

High Blood Pressure Medications

There are a variety of medications commonly used to treat hypertension. These include diuretics, ACE inhibitors, beta-blockers, and calcium channel blockers.

Diuretics can decrease magnesium, zinc, potassium, calcium, vitamin B6, and vitamin B1. Talk with your doctor about taking the following daily supplemental regimen:

- Calcium—750 milligrams
- Potassium—100 milligrams
- Vitamin B1—300 milligrams
- P5P50—50 milligrams
- Zinc—25 milligrams
- Magnesium glycenate—240 milligrams

Beta-blockers lower blood pressure by reducing the effects of epinephrine and norepinephrine on blood vessels. These drugs deplete CoQ10, which is necessary for mitochondrial function in the heart and brain. They also reduce production of melatonin. Talk with your doctor about taking CoQ10 (200 to 300 milligrams, once daily) and melatonin (6 milligrams, at bedtime) if you are on this class of drug.

Cholesterol-Lowering Drugs

Statins are the most commonly used medications for lowering cholesterol. These drugs deplete the body of CoQ10. Talk with your doctor about taking CoQ10 (200 to 300 milligrams, once daily) if you are on a statin.

Stomach Ulcer and Acid Reflux Medications
These include antacids, histamine two receptor blockers, and proton pump inhibitors. The aluminum antacids as well as the calcium carbonate–based antacids reduce stomach acid, which is required for nutrient absorption.

Both proton pump inhibitors and H2 blockers decrease the absorption of vitamin B12, folic acid, iron, and zinc. When used for over one year, proton pump inhibitors can cause such marked deficiencies of calcium and vitamin D that the risk of hip fracture doubles. This is because of an impaired ability to build new bone. I recommend my patients who are taking chronic acid-reducing medications supplement with the following daily regimen:

- Vitamin D3—at least 2,000 IU (or more if necessary based on regular lab testing)
- Phosphorus—500 milligrams
- Chromium—500 milligrams
- Zinc—25 milligrams
- Vitamin B12—500 micrograms, taken either intranasally or under the tongue
- Folic acid—400 micrograms
- Red algae–derived calcium—750 milligrams

Anti-Hyperglycemic Medications
Medications to treat hyperglycemia, such as metformin (Glucophage), may interfere with the body's absorption of vitamin B12, folic acid, and CoQ10. I prescribe metformin in many patients to prevent the development of diabetes and cancer. To this I regularly add supplemental vitamin B12 (500 to 1,000 micrograms under the tongue, once daily), folic acid (400 micrograms, once daily), and CoQ10 (200 milligrams, once daily).

6. Do you have a problem with hair thinning or hair loss?

Hair thinning or hair loss can be caused by nutritional deficiencies as well as by underlying medical conditions, such as hypothyroidism, estrogen or testosterone abnormalities, diabetes, or autoimmune disease. Hair is 97 percent protein and it is essential to consume enough protein in your diet in order to replace hairs that are shed naturally each day.

Top Five Healthy Hair Supplements

- Biotin—5,000 micrograms, twice daily (NutriCology)
- Thorne Amino Complex (powder containing eleven amino acids)—1 teaspoon in water, once daily
- Bamboo extract (contains silica)—900 milligrams, twice daily (Chi's Enterprise)
- Methyl sulfonyl methane (MSM)—1,000 milligrams, twice daily (Nature's Way)
- Pantothenic acid—100 milligrams, once daily (Source Naturals)

Top Ten Foods for Healthy Hair

In the recipe section you will find preparation suggestions for these foods:

- Walnuts—contain omega-3 fatty acids, biotin, and tocotrienols
- Salmon—rich in omega-3 fatty acids, amino acids, and vitamin D3, all essential for hair and scalp health
- Shrimp—rich in zinc, important since zinc deficiencies are common as we age and can lead to hair loss and dry scalp and skin
- Eggs—excellent sources of protein, zinc, selenium, and iron
- Kale—an excellent source of folic acid, iron, carotenoids, and vitamin C, all necessary for hair follicle growth and scalp oil synthesis
- Pumpkins and squash—contain a variety of carotenoids that the body uses to make vitamin A, as well as other skin, hair, and scalp protective nutrients
- Lentils—loaded with biotin, zinc, protein, and iron
- Greek yogurt—contains both vitamin B5 and vitamin D3, essential for maintaining healthy hair growth
- Strawberries—rich in vitamin C and resveratrol
- Chicken—not only an excellent source of protein but also contains biotin, zinc, and iron, essential for healthy hair

7. Do you have skin dryness, age spots, or premature wrinkles?

The following supplements are necessary for synthesizing enough collagen and elastic, which are the fibers that support skin structure and help prevent wrinkles and age spots. They also help reduce free radical damage and inflammation caused by sun exposure and pollution.

Top Five Supplements for Skin Health

- Biotin—5,000 micrograms, twice daily (NutriCology)
- PABA—500 milligrams, once daily (Pure Encapsulations)
- Lycopene—10 milligrams, once daily
- Astaxanthin—4 milligrams, once daily
- Moducare (phytosterols from maritime pine)—twice daily

Top Ten Foods for Healthy Skin
In the recipe section you will find preparation suggestions for these foods:

- Plums
- Salmon
- Walnuts
- Brazil nuts
- Green tea
- Water—eight glasses per day
- Spinach
- Peas
- Spinach
- Apricots

8. Are you prone to prostatitis (men) or urinary tract infections (women)?

Prostatitis in men and urinary tract infections in women should be evaluated by a physician. Both cause chronic inflammation, which has been associated with an increased risk of cancer.

Top Five Supplements for Prostate Health

- Saw palmetto—540 milligrams, once daily (Nature's Way)
- Pygeum—50 milligrams, once daily (Solaray)
- Nettle root—250 milligrams, once daily (NOW Foods)
- Turmeric root—500 milligrams, once daily (Thorne)
- Pumpkin seed oil capsules—1,000 milligrams, once daily (Solaray)

Top Ten Foods for Prostate Health
In the recipe section you will find preparation suggestions for these foods:

- Brussels sprouts
- Cilantro
- Linseed oil
- Tofu and miso
- Watercress
- Rosemary
- Dandelion leaves
- Basil leaves
- Thyme
- Blueberries

Top Five Supplements for Urinary Tract Health

- D-mannose—1,000 milligrams, twice daily (Solaray)
- Oil of oregano capsules—460 milligrams, once daily (Gaia Herbs)
- Nettle root extract—250 milligrams, once daily (NOW Foods)
- Marshmallow root extract—480 milligrams, once daily (Solaray)
- VSL probiotic—once daily

Top Ten Foods for Urinary Tract Health
In the recipe section you will find preparation suggestions for these foods:

- Cranberries
- Peaches
- Wheatgrass
- Celery
- Black raspberries

- Parsley
- Greek yogurt with kefir cultures
- Garlic
- Oregano
- Thyme

9. On a normal day do you eat five or more servings of fruits and vegetables? (A serving size is a half cup of nonleafy vegetables—raw or cooked—or one cup of leafy green vegetables. For fruits, it is one medium-size piece of fruit or a half cup of berries.)

I recommend at least six servings of fruits and vegetables daily. However, many people have busy schedules or travel frequently and are unable to cook or eat at healthy restaurants. Juicing is an invaluable way of getting several servings of fruits and vegetables at one time.

Top Five Supplements for Days When You Cannot Have the Recommended Number of Servings of Fruits and Vegetables

- Meriva-SR slow-release turmeric extract—500 milligrams, twice daily (Thorne)
- Kyolic deodorized garlic—600 mg, once daily
- Oil of oregano capsules—460 milligrams, once daily (Gaia Herbs)
- Black raspberry powder—1 teaspoon in water, once daily (Nutri-Fruit)
- Coconut milk powder—1 tablespoon in water, once daily

Top Ten Ecogenetic Fruits and Vegetables
In the recipe section you will find preparation suggestions for these healthy fruits and vegetables:

- Mangoes
- Blueberries
- Black raspberries
- Oranges
- Grapes
- Watercress
- Flaxseed
- Pumpkin
- Romaine lettuce
- Olives

10. Do you consume more than one serving of alcohol per day?
(A serving size is 5 ounces of wine, 12 ounces of beer, or 1 ounce of hard liquor.)

I advise patients to consume no more than one drink per day. If you do consume more than this, it is essential to do everything possible to protect your liver and enhance the detoxification of alcohol, as alcohol increases inflammation and oxidative stress on the body. Patients with underlying liver disease or who are taking certain medications should abstain from alcohol altogether.

Top Five Liver Support Supplements

- Milk thistle—300 milligrams, once daily (NOW Foods)
- EPA/DHA fish oil—1,000 milligrams, once daily (Nordic Naturals)
- OncoPLEX glucoraphanin—100 milligrams, once daily (Xymogen)
- N-acetylcysteine (NAC)—600 milligrams, once daily (Pure Encapsulations)
- Alpha lipoic acid—300 milligrams, twice daily (Jarrow Formulas)

Top Ten Foods for Liver Support
In the recipe section you will find preparation suggestions for these liver-healthy foods:

- Turmeric
- Salmon
- Kale
- Blueberries
- Grapes
- Wheatgrass
- Pumpkin seeds
- Brazil nuts
- Olive oil
- Lentils

11. Do you drink more than two cups of coffee per day?

Consumption of two or more cups of coffee per day has been linked to lower risk of many types of cancer, including liver, colon, prostate, and head and neck. Coffee contains phenols and polyphenols similar to those found in green tea, which work to promote healthy gene expression. Coffee is heavily treated with chemicals as it is grown, so it is best to consume certified organic coffee. If it is labeled organic, at least 95 percent of the coffee beans are required to have been cultivated under organic conditions.

12. On average, do you consume two or more servings of calcium-rich foods per day? (A serving size is one cup of milk or enriched soy or rice milk, one cup of yogurt, two cups of cottage cheese, or three domino-size pieces of hard cheese.)

The conventional wisdom is that all postmenopausal women should be taking calcium supplements in high doses to prevent osteoporosis, and premeno-pausal women should be taking calcium in more modest doses for the same reason. Calcium is a critical mineral for muscles, nerves, bone formation, and hormone and enzyme synthesis. It is important to keep in mind that magnesium and vitamin K2 are equally important for formation of proper, healthy, strong bones. Magnesium is critical for strong bones and for DNA, RNA, and protein synthesis; it also helps to prevent high blood pressure and heart disease. However, most calcium supplements are derived from chalk, limestone, or coral. We do not consume chalk, limestone, or coral in our diets, so our bodies cannot process or use supplements derived from these substances in a healthy way.

Studies involving older adults have shown that synthetic calcium supplements neither consistently improve bone density nor reduce fracture rates in postmenopausal women. Synthetic calcium supplements have also been associated with a significantly increased risk of heart attack and stroke.[1] It is hypothesized that synthetic calcium supplements are deposited in parts of the body where calcium is in fact detrimental, such as arterial walls and breast tissue. This is because calcium obtained from natural sources is more slowly absorbed while synthetic supplements cause an abnormally abrupt elevation in blood levels of calcium.

I often recommend calcium supplements for both men and women with low bone densities or for those who have difficulty getting adequate calcium from their diet. However, I recommend only calcium supplements derived from a natural source of red marine algae known as *Lithothamnion calcareum*. This supplement is more bioavailable and is the only one derived from a naturally occurring whole food. Because of its enhanced bioavailability, lower doses have been found to be effective in improving bone density.[2] It is also rich in other key minerals, like selenium, magnesium, boron, and zinc.

Top Five Supplements for Bone Health
Common dosages range from 1,000 milligrams to 1,300 milligrams daily. Discuss dosage with your physician.

- Natural Calcium (Lifestream)
- Bone Strength Take Care (New Chapter)
- DensiMAX (Flora Force)
- Organic Calcium (North Coast Naturals)
- Green Calcium (Green Nutrition)

Top Ten Foods for Calcium
In the recipe section you will find preparation suggestions for these calcium-rich foods:

- Sardines—3 ounces contains 325 milligrams of calcium
- Salmon—3 ounces raw without bones contains 80 milligrams of calcium; 3 ounces canned with bones contains 190 milligrams of calcium
- Tofu—a half cup contains 435 milligrams of calcium
- Greek yogurt—one serving contains 187 milligrams of calcium; while some of the calcium content is lost in the extensive straining process, I recommend it to my patients and use it in the recipes in this book
- Oatmeal—one bowl (35 grams) contains 100 milligrams of calcium
- Sesame seeds—1 ounce contains 250 milligrams of calcium
- Kale—one cup provides 90 milligrams of calcium
- Soybeans—one cup boiled contains 250 milligrams of calcium
- Dried figs—two dried offer 55 milligrams of calcium and are also rich in iron and magnesium
- Almonds—a quarter cup contains 95 milligrams of calcium

13. Are you a strict vegan (consuming a diet without meat, dairy, eggs, or fish)?

I do not agree that meat, eggs, and all animal fats are uniformly bad. Nor does the data show that people enjoy superior health by avoiding them. Nonetheless, I do have patients who are strict vegans and I tell them that there are several classes of nutrients they must include or supplement with. It is essential that vegans consume enough omega-3 fatty acids, especially since they are not consuming deep coldwater fish. Omega-6 fatty acids are found in most vegetable or seed oils. For Americans the ratio of omega-6s to omega-3s consumed is anywhere from 15:1 to 50:1, but for optimum health should be closer to 3:1. Many omega-6 fatty acids promote the formation of leukotrienes, which promote inflammation and abnormal angiogenesis by affecting gene expression. This in turn leads to conditions such as heart disease, cancer, and obesity. There are beneficial omega-6 fatty acids, like oleic acid, found predominantly in olives, avocados, almonds, pecans, and macadamia nuts, which protect against cancer, heart disease, and obesity. I recommend that patients avoid oils made from canola, corn, and soy, as well as margarine. Extra-virgin olive oil has an omega-6 to omega-3 ratio of 10:1, but is loaded with nutrients that have powerful anticancer effects, such as squalene. The best cooking oils are coconut oil, which contains medium chain fatty acids, and grapeseed oil, because both of these have very high heat coefficients that prevent them from being damaged by cooking. Consuming fats and oils damaged during cooking only puts more free radical stress on the body.

For vegans who do not consume enough foods rich in these nutrients, it is very often necessary to supplement with vitamin B12, vitamin D3, iron, zinc, magnesium, long-chain fatty acids like DHA, calcium, protein, and carotenoids. The most abundant detoxifying enzymes in the body are all dependent on adequate glutathione stores. Glutathione is a peptide made of glycine, glutamine, and cysteine. Taurine is also an extremely important amino acid, critical for heart and neurological function, found in meat and seafood. Vegans need more zinc in their diet than meat eaters, as it is important for brain function, vision, and adequate hormone production. Zinc deficiency can sometimes cause white spots on the fingernails.

Top Five Supplements for Vegans

- Taurine—500 milligrams, once daily (Thorne)
- Methylated B12—500 milligrams, one under the tongue, once daily (Jarrow Formulas)

- DHA Neuromins—100 milligrams, three capsules, twice daily (Solaray)
- Zinc—25 milligrams, once daily (Allergy Research)
- Carnosine—500 milligrams, once daily (Pure Encapsulations)

Top Ten Foods to Include in a Vegan Diet
In the recipe section you will find preparation suggestions for these foods:

- Blueberries—rich in resveratrol and amino acids that form glutathione
- Kale—contains glycine, glutamine, and cysteine, which are precursors for glutathione
- Seaweed—rich in taurine as well as chlorophyll and other antioxidants
- Flaxseeds—contain the omega-3 fatty acid ALA, about 10 percent of which is converted into the omega-3 fatty acid DHA
- Avocados—rich in carnitine, important for heart and muscle function
- Lima beans—very rich in zinc
- Shiitake mushroom—excellent source of zinc and nutrients that stimulate a healthy immune system
- Brussels sprouts—loaded with zinc and nutrients that promote detoxification
- Beets—contain iron, magnesium, and zinc
- Pecans—loaded with zinc and magnesium

14. On average, do you consume two or more 3-ounce servings (about the size of an iPhone) of deep coldwater fish per week, such as salmon, haddock, cod, halibut, or tuna?

Omega-3 fatty acids are critically important. The Mediterranean diet has about a 3:1 ratio of omega-6s to omega-3s. This is what I consider to be optimal. Most omega-6 fatty acids promote inflammation by turning on the genes responsible for the production of inflammatory mediators, whereas omega-3 fatty acids reduce inflammation and promote gene expression that protects against obesity, diabetes, degenerative disease, cancer, heart disease, and autoimmune diseases.

The worst oils that contain only omega-6 and no omega-3 are safflower, sunflower, corn, cottonseed, and peanut oils. Even if you do not cook with these at home, you very likely are consuming them if you eat processed or packaged foods or regularly eat out.

Top Five Supplements for Omega-3 Fatty Acids

- Pro Omega—1,000 milligrams, once daily (Nordic Naturals)
- Krill Oil (EPA 150 milligrams, DHA 60 milligrams, phospholipids 400 milligrams)—one capsule, twice daily (Thorne)
- Neuromins DHA (derived from marine algae)—100 milligrams, three capsules, twice daily (Solaray)
- Cod liver oil—1 teaspoon, once daily
- Vegetarian Omega-3—270 milligrams, twice daily (Nature Made)

Top Ten Foods for Omega-3 Fatty Acids
In the recipe section you will find preparation suggestions for these omega-rich foods:

- Salmon
- Cod
- Basil
- Walnuts
- Flaxseed oil
- Oregano
- Wheat germ oil
- Arugula
- Haddock
- Watercress

15. Are you currently a smoker, or have you been regularly exposed to secondhand smoke or chemicals in the workplace?

We must all do what we can to reduce our exposure to environmental toxins. If you are a smoker, do what you need to do to quit. Try to eat organic as much as possible. Find green alternatives to pesticides and herbicides inside and outside your home. Use only nontoxic green bathroom and kitchen products. Practice "safe tech," which means using a hands-free device when talking on your cell phone, and do not place laptop computers directly on your lap or keep your cell phone close to your body, such as in a pants or shirt pocket.

Top Five Supplements to Boost Detoxification and Minimize DNA Damage from Environmental Toxins

- Broccoli seed extract (sulforaphane)—50 milligrams, once daily (Thorne Crucera-SGS)
- Black cumin seed extract—500 milligrams, twice daily (Amazing Herbs)
- Alpha lipoic acid—300 milligrams, twice daily (Jarrow Formulas)

- Black raspberry powder—1 tablespoon in water, once daily (Nutri-Fruit)
- Rosemary leaf extract—400 milligrams, twice daily (Nature's Way)

Top Ten Foods to Boost Detoxification and Minimize DNA Damage from Environmental Toxins

In the recipe section you will find preparation suggestions for these purifying foods:

- Brussels sprouts
- Basil
- Oregano
- Parsley
- Olives

- Red beans
- Tomatoes
- Oranges
- Pinto beans
- Artichokes

16. Do you get more than one or two colds or upper respiratory tract infections per year?

People who are prone to developing more than two colds per year or frequent bouts of earaches, sinusitis, or bronchitis often have underlying problems with inflammation, structural abnormalities such as bronchiectasis (a condition that weakens the walls of the small airways), or a deviated septum within the sinuses.

Top Five Supplements for Upper Respiratory Health

- Oil of oregano (phytocap)—460 milligrams, once daily (Gaia Herbs). Oregano has been found to have antifungal and antiviral properties.
- Cordyceps—400 milligrams, once daily (Mushroom Science). Cordyceps is a mushroom that improves oxygenation in elderly people with upper respiratory infections or asthma. It has also been found to improve natural killer cell function and number, and to improve cellular energy, stamina, and athletic performance.
- Shiitake extract—300 milligrams, once daily (Mushroom Science). Shiitake mushroom boosts the part of the immune system that fights viruses and lowers inflammation.
- Echinacea—500 milligrams, once daily (Gaia Herbs Echinacea Supreme). Echinacea fights influenza and viral colds by increasing the production of cytokines such as interferon and interleukin, as well as T cell activity.

- Green tea—three cups a day. Green tea has been found to have significant antiviral properties.

Top Five Foods for Upper Respiratory Function and Fighting Infection
In the recipe section you will find preparation suggestions for these immune-boosting foods:

- Ginger—has anti-inflammatory and immune-boosting properties that relieve inflamed bronchial tubes. Make an herbal tea for colds by adding a teaspoon of ground ginger and a teaspoon of turmeric powder to a cup of boiling water, then mix in a teaspoon of honey.
- Garlic—has antibiotic and antiviral properties. For colds or bronchitis, add three peeled and minced garlic cloves to a glass of warm orange juice.
- Turmeric powder—use with ginger in tea, as above.
- Edible camphor—put a half teaspoon in a cup of boiling water and stir, then mix in honey and a quarter teaspoon of paprika.
- Almonds—loaded with essential oils and minerals needed for your immune system.

17. Do you exercise at least thirty minutes or more three times per week?

This is the minimum amount of exercise you should aim for. I recommend to my patients that they exercise for thirty minutes, five times per week. This should be an equal mix of aerobic exercise and weight training. Muscle burns almost three times the number of calories as fat when you are at rest. Exercise affects gene expression important for immune function, carbohydrate metabolism, risk of obesity, cardiovascular function, and even memory.

Top Five Supplements for Getting the Most out of Your Exercise Routine

- Vital Whey—one heaping tablespoon (35 grams whey protein) before exercise (Well Wisdom). For more rapid muscle recovery and strength.
- Daxibe—one packet immediately before and immediately after each workout (Thorne). Provides branched-chain amino acids, essential for repairing and building muscle tissue, of which the most important is the amino acid leucine.

- Carnosine—500 milligrams, once daily (Pure Encapsulations). Important for the mitochondrial function of muscle.
- Perfusia (arginine)—1,000 milligrams (Thorne). The amino acid arginine is converted by the body to nitric oxide, which assists in increasing muscle strength as well as reducing body fat during exercise. Do not take arginine supplements if you have a history of oral herpes simplex or genital herpes as it may increase the chances of an outbreak.
- Green tea—2-3 cups daily. Green tea has been shown to assist in burning more fat during exercise.

Top Ten Foods to Eat Before and After Working Out

In the recipe section you will find preparation suggestions for these restorative foods:

- Grilled chicken—one serving provides lean protein and the necessary carbohydrates that assist in muscle recovery while leaving you feeling full
- Grilled vegetables with olive oil—one serving provides the necessary carbohydrates and amino acids for post-workout recovery
- Greek yogurt—one serving before exercise provides your body with the necessary energy, carbohydrates, proteins, and fatty acids for an optimal workout
- Eggs—provide an excellent source of protein, minerals, and fatty acids
- Avocados—assist in the absorption of fat-soluble vitamins like A, D, E, and K, critical for healthy muscle function and carbohydrate utilization
- Fruit smoothie—any of the fruit smoothies discussed in this book are excellent pre-exercise nutritional boosts
- Mixed vegetable juice—any of the vegetable juice recipes discussed in this book are excellent for post-exercise recovery as they provide your body with the necessary minerals, vitamins, and ecogenetic nutrients required to reach your exercise-related goals
- Salmon—excellent post-exercise meal as it contains amino acids, peptides, and proteins that assist in regulating carbohydrate metabolism, decreasing inflammation, and building muscle
- Sweet potatoes or yams—excellent post-exercise snack as these contain complex carbohydrates to help restore glycogen levels, which are depleted during a vigorous workout

- Pear slices with 1 tablespoon of cashew or almond butter—the synergistic nutrient combination of carbohydrates, minerals, and anti-inflammatory nutrients prevents insulin surges and corresponding drops in blood sugar during exercise to optimize energy levels

18. Have you or a first-degree family member been diagnosed with a cardiovascular disease such as high cholesterol, hypertension, stroke, or heart attack?

If several members of your family have been affected by cardiovascular disease, ask your doctor about testing for Factor V Leiden (FVL) mutation as well as MTHFR mutation, which can lead to elevated homocysteine levels. These mutations cause the arteries to clog at an earlier age.

Top Five Supplements for Heart Disease

- Carnosine—500 milligrams, once daily (Thorne). This powerful amino acid, found primarily in red meat, prevents the glycation of LDL cholesterol, thereby preventing plaque formation on arterial walls. It also helps protect the heart and blood vessels against oxidative stress and has been shown to help protect heart and brain tissue deprived of adequate oxygen.
- Grapeseed extract—300 milligrams, once daily (NutriCology). The phytonutrients found in grapeseed improve circulation and help to lower cholesterol. By decreasing inflammation and inhibiting the stickiness of platelets, they also help protect against the development of plaque formation in the heart's main arteries.
- Sytrinol—150 milligrams, once daily (Next Pharmaceuticals). A formulation of citrus and palm fruit extracts containing flavonols and tocotrienols, which have been shown to increase good cholesterol while lowering bad cholesterol and triglycerides.
- P5P50 (activated pyridoxine, or vitamin B6)—50 milligrams, once daily (Pure Encapsulations). Lowers homocysteine, associated with an increased risk of heart attack and stroke.
- Quercetin—250 milligrams, once daily (Pure Encapsulations). This polyphenolic compound, found in red grapes, apples, and onions, has numerous beneficial effects on the cardiovascular system, including

improved blood pressure, decreased stickiness of platelets, and improved arterial blood flow.

Top Ten Foods to Prevent Heart Disease

In the recipe section you will find preparation suggestions for these heart-healthy foods:

- Watercress
- Goji berries
- Kale
- Pomegranate
- Almonds

- Apples
- Salmon
- Avocados
- Scallions
- Ginger

19. Have you or a first-degree family member been diagnosed with a rheumatologic illness such as rheumatoid arthritis, lupus, or osteoarthritis?

Rheumatologic diseases include autoimmune diseases as well as degenerative diseases involving the joints, skin, or spine, such as osteoarthritis, rheumatoid arthritis, lupus, and mixed connective tissue disease (MCTD). Late effects from Lyme disease can also affect joints and other organs. Inflammation in other organ systems can affect joints, such as in Crohn's disease and colitis.

Top Five Supplements for Joint Health

- Boswellia—600 milligrams, once daily (NOW Foods). An Ayurvedic herb that decreases joint inflammation and blocks inflammatory mediators.
- Chinese skullcap root extract—400 milligrams, twice daily (Oregon's Wild Harvest). Decreases inflammation by blocking inflammatory mediators.
- Gingerroot extract—550 milligrams, once daily (NOW Foods). Contains compounds known as gingerols, which preserve joint function by minimizing oxidative stress.
- Yucca stalk extract—520 milligrams, once daily (Nature's Way)—Contains saponins and yuccaols, anti-inflammatory and antiarthritic compounds.

- Holy basil leaf extract—500 milligrams, twice daily (NOW Foods). Contains anti-inflammatory and antioxidant oils that reduce joint pain and swelling.

Top Ten Foods to Improve and Maintain Joint Function
In the recipe section you will find preparation suggestions for these foods:

- Deep coldwater fish such as salmon and cod—their omega-3 fatty acids help inhibit joint inflammation
- Cruciferous vegetables such as broccoli, cauliflower, and brussels sprouts—their anti-inflammatory properties protect against the development of arthritis
- Greek yogurt and cottage cheese—rich in vitamin D3, which helps maintain strong bones and prevent osteoarthritis and rheumatoid arthritis
- Extra-virgin olive oil—rich in polyphenols, omega-3 fatty acids, and squalene, which have been found to reduce pain and swelling in patients with rheumatoid arthritis
- Ginger—its antioxidant and anti-inflammatory compounds help alleviate arthritis symptoms
- Kidney beans—rich in vitamin C and other compounds that reduce the risk of developing rheumatoid arthritis
- Strawberries—rich in anthocyanins, which help reduce inflammation as well as the corresponding inflammatory blood marker known as C-reactive protein
- Carrots—rich in beta-cryptoxanthins, anti-inflammatory and antioxidant compounds known to protect against arthritis
- Brown rice—a whole grain shown to reduce inflammation and corresponding inflammatory blood markers such as C-reactive protein
- Spinach—contains abundant tocopherols and tocotrienols, which protect joints from proinflammatory molecules

20. Do you have food sensitivities or food allergies to dairy, gluten, nightshade vegetables, or any cosmetic products?

Food sensitivities usually result in symptoms such as nausea, abdominal cramping, or indigestion. They are very often the result of "leaky gut," which is excess intestinal permeability caused by toxins, parasites, bacterial overgrowth, inflammation, and certain nutritional deficiencies. This results in the overab-sorption of certain food molecules, thus creating an inflammatory or even aller-gic response.

A food allergy is the result of one's immune system becoming hyperactive—on either a genetic or an environmental basis—and subsequently forming anti-bodies against certain foods. Symptoms can be as severe as anaphylactic shock, or milder symptoms such as hives, diarrhea, and itching. Food allergies are rarer than food sensitivity and intolerance.

Food intolerance, characterized by abdominal pain, cramps, bloating, or diar-rhea, is the result of an inability to digest certain nutrients, such as gluten or lac-tose. Lactose, a nutrient in most dairy products, is the most common substance to cause food intolerance, affecting about 10 percent of Americans. The bacteria that live in the gut are the largest part of what is known as the microbiome. Just as over-growth of invasive bacteria on the teeth (plaque) eats away at the protective enamel, toxic bacteria in the gut can release proinflammatory molecules and chemicals called lipopolysaccharides, which create chronic inflammation and trigger insulin and leptin resistance, resulting in food intolerance, obesity, and diabetes.

Like human DNA, the microbial DNA in the gut is largely inherited as well. Infants pick up their microbiome as they pass through the birth canal. The micro-biome in the birth canal is composed of healthy bacteria, which is probably why children born in cesarean delivery are more likely to develop food intolerance, aller-gies, asthma, childhood obesity, and diabetes. It is estimated that the total human microbiome consists of a collection of microorganisms that make up 99 percent of the body's total genetic information, outnumbering human cells ten to one. Just as the epigenome allows DNA to be modified, the microbial genome can be influenced by nutritional and environmental factors as well. It is essential for you to enhance the intestinal microbial environment to promote health rather than disease.

Top Five Supplements for Food and Chemical Sensitivities

- Probiotics—at least one-billion colony-forming units per gram, once daily (Natren Healthy Trinity or VSL). These beneficial bacteria main-tain proper pH, produce essential nutrients and enzymes within the intestines, and prevent colonization by harmful yeast and bacteria. Choose coated capsules to protect the probiotics from stomach acids. Best if taken on an empty stomach.
- Prebiotic fiber supplement—1 tablespoon in water, once daily (Meta-genics UltraClear Sustain). Containing oligofructose and inulin, which

promote digestive health, gut symbiosis, and nutrient absorption. These work primarily in the small intestine.

- Saccharomyces Boulardii (5 billion colony-forming units per gram) MOS 200 milligrams—once daily (Jarrow Formulas). Contains an important probiotic yeast that survives passage through stomach acid, plus an important oligosaccharide. Take one capsule daily with water either with food or on an empty stomach.
- Artichoke extract—320 milligrams, three times daily (Integrative Therapeutics). An excellent source of prebiotic fiber.
- Super Enzymes—one pill fifteen minutes before meals (NOW Foods). A mixture of plant-based digestive enzymes for healthy digestion.

Top Ten Foods for Preventing Food and Chemical Sensitivities
In the recipe section you will find preparation suggestions for these foods:

- Greek yogurt with kefir cultures
- Leeks
- Sprouted whole grain bread
- Raw asparagus
- Bananas
- Apples
- Brown rice
- Winter squash
- Sweet potatoes
- Garlic

21. Do you frequently eat when you are not hungry or have recently consumed a meal? Do you eat out of boredom or anxiety?

If so, you may be eating too much white sugar or white flour, which is causing your glucose to drop about two hours after eating a meal and thereby leading to hypoglycemia. This also may be a sign of emotional eating. The key to both of these is to replace white sugar and white flour with healthy alternatives that will leave you feeling full.

Top Five Supplements to Combat Binge and Emotional Eating

- Glucomannan—665 milligrams, three capsules before meals (Nature's Way). This fiber expands in the stomach, making you feel more full.
- White kidney bean extract—1,000 milligrams, one before meals (Nature's Way). Blocks the enzyme that assists in the absorption of carbohydrates.
- Whey protein—20 grams (1 tablespoon) in water three times daily (Well Wisdom Vital Whey). Regular consumption of protein assists in satiety.

- Maitake mushroom elixir—twenty drops, twice daily (Grifron). Contains beta-glucans, which exhibit fiberlike activity, lowering cholesterol, assisting in carbohydrate metabolism, and promoting weight loss.
- Mango seed fiber—900 milligrams, once daily (Natural Health Labs). Leads to lower cholesterol and makes you feel more full.

Top Ten Foods to Control Binge Eating and Emotional Eating
In the recipe section you will find preparation suggestions for these satiating foods:

- Sweet potatoes or yams—lower in calories than white potatoes and have a high water content and carotenoids, which help control blood sugar
- Oatmeal—contains both soluble and insoluble fiber, which assist in staying full longer; a half-cup serving is only 150 calories
- Grapefruit—largely made up of water and contains a moderate amount of fiber; eating three slices about five minutes before each meal results in more balanced insulin secretion and better portion control
- Celery—rich in fiber and plant-based digestive enzymes; eating three celery stalks immediately after a meal assists with digestion and also leaves you feeling full longer
- Almonds—one of the best diet foods, as their rich protein, fiber, and fatty acid ratio helps inhibit hunger
- Canned salmon—a high-protein, low-carb food rich in omega-3 fatty acids that will leave you more satisfied
- Apples—a great source of soluble and insoluble fiber and have a high water content, keeping hunger at bay
- Chickpeas—assist in the release of the hormone cholecystokinin, which signals to the brain that you are full
- Popcorn—has a higher fiber content than many packaged snacks and is low in calories, but consume only air popped with no butter added (avoid microwave popcorn)
- Greek yogurt—an excellent source of protein, carbs, and water, in a ratio that leaves you feeling full longer

22. Do you feel fatigued either upon waking up or in the afternoon?

Fatigue has many causes, including anemia, vitamin deficiencies, hormone imbalances, infectious diseases, and not getting enough sleep. It should always be evaluated by a physician. However, many people find that they are fatigued with apparently no underlying medical cause. In that case, I work with my patients to determine whether they are exposed to foods or chemicals that are causing sensitivity or intolerance. I also look for heavy metal toxicity. There are many ecogenetic nutrients that our bodies require and that most of us do not consume in adequate amounts for optimal energy levels.

Top Five Supplements for Optimal Energy and Peak Performance

- PQQ (pyrroloquinoline)—20 milligrams, once daily (Quality of Life). A critical vitamin for function of the mitochondria, the energy centers of every cell in the body.
- Royal jelly—500 milligrams, once daily (Y.S. Eco Bee Farms). A food from bees loaded with micronutrients for cellular energy. Consumed only by the queen bee in the hive, she lives forty times longer than the other bees due to the epigenetic effects of this substance.
- Bee pollen—500 milligrams, once daily (Y.S. Eco Bee Farms). Contains twenty-two amino acids and hundreds of micronutrients, including minerals, vitamins, enzymes, amino acids, and fiber. It also contains various energy-supplying nutrients (50 percent of bee pollen protein consists of free amino acids that can be used to directly produce proteins).
- Spirulina—500 milligrams, twice daily (Nature's Way). A single-celled alga rich in protein, chlorophyll, vitamin B12, and energy-enhancing minerals.
- Ashwagandha—450 milligrams, once daily (NOW Foods). Used in India since ancient times, it improves mitochondrial health, supports neurologic and adrenal function, and has anti-inflammatory effects.

Top Ten Foods for Combating Fatigue
In the recipe section you will find preparation suggestions for these energizing foods:

- Wheatgrass juice
- Pumpkin seeds
- Greek yogurt with kefir cultures
- Steel-cut oatmeal
- Cashews
- Dark chocolate
- Green tea
- Watermelon
- Red bell peppers
- Ginger

23. Has your doctor checked the following labs within the past year?

The following are basic lab tests that I use for evaluating new patients. They are by no means complete, nor are they meant to be used for self-diagnosis or treatment.

Throughout this book I have provided you with a road map to take control of your genetic destiny. However, your physician needs to be your partner for health and wellness. Discuss what you have learned in this book, and show him or her that there is ample scientific data for this approach. The following labs, in conjunction with this questionnaire, should begin to customize your gene therapy lifestyle.

I do not believe you must necessarily find a new physician to have these blood tests or to incorporate the knowledge found in these pages. It is important that *you* become an advocate for your health. Remember, it's never too late to bring back balance, and your doctor should be your partner in this quest.

Men and Women
- Lipid profile: total cholesterol, LDL, HDL, triglycerides
- Metabolic profile: glucose, liver function tests such as AST, ALT, LDH, alkaline phosphatase, GGT, and bilirubin
- Kidney function tests such as BUN, creatinine, and uric acid
- Fasting blood glucose and hemoglobin A1C
- Blood minerals such as calcium, magnesium, phosphorus, sodium, selenium, and zinc
- Vitamin levels such as 25-hydroxy vitamin D, vitamin B12, folate, CoQ10
- Heavy metal toxicity such as mercury, arsenic, and lead
- Food allergy panel
- Inflammatory markers such as C-reactive protein and sedimentation rate
- Cardiac markers such as high-sensitivity C-reactive protein, homocysteine
- Screening for infectious disease markers such as hepatitis A, B, and C, Lyme disease, and HPV (oral for men and women, and cervical as well for women)
- Immune function such as immunoglobulin levels plus natural killer cell number and activity

- Complete blood count including red blood cell count, white blood cell count with differential of lymphocytes, monocytes, neutrophils, basophils, eosinophils, and platelet count
- Hormone levels such as free and total testosterone, DHEA, estradiol, TSH, T4, T3, fasting insulin, insulin-like growth factor 1 (IGF-1)
- Detoxifying enzyme levels such as GST, CYP2D6

Men Over 45
- Prostate-specific antigen (PSA)

Women Over 45
- Progesterone
- CA-125

Chapter 8

Sample Meal Plans

DURING MY CHILDHOOD YEARS, I spent a lot of time learning how to cook from my mother. I assisted her with kitchen tasks such as chopping, mixing, and blending. Since then my passion for food and healthy meals has evolved into a union that grinds in science, marinates with medicine, and tosses in nutrious, flavorful ingredients.

This part of the book includes many recipes to help you begin your transition toward eating better. These recipes, however, are not disease-specific. My recipes are meant to provide you with the framework to achieve robust health. By consistently eating foods that contain bioactive compounds and applying the rule of one-thirds, you will develop sound dietary habits: the driving force behind good health.

Don't worry, however. *The Gene Therapy Diet* isn't a rigid, uncompromising regimen. Because a 220-pound man doesn't require the same amount of calories as a 100-pound woman, serving sizes will vary. Furthermore, it is perfectly fine (and expected) if you splurge from time to time. So don't feel bad if you're at a birthday party—go on and have a slice of cake. It won't throw off all the work you've done. Just make sure you're not overindulging, since you now understand how processed foods affect your health. The main point of this meal plan is to develop habits that are wholesome. Many patients who follow my meal plans report that their caloric intake has improved and that they are not overeating or craving processed, sugar-filled foods anymore. As a result, they feel more energized during the day, sleep better at night, and feel and look great.

To help jumpstart your Gene Therapy Diet, I've provided a four-week guide for healthy meals. Many of the meals included below refer to the recipes provided in the next chapter. The recipe section includes more recipes if you want to swap it for something besides what I listed in the guide. Before you try these recipes, review the tips below, which will help make your trip to the grocery store easier.

Shopping Guidelines

Cookware: Perfluorooctanoic acid (PFOA) is a compound used to make the nonstick coating of Teflon pans; PFOA has been linked to cancer in birds, but it hasn't been found to cause cancer in humans. With that said, however, I do not use Teflon pans because under high heat they release fumes that cause flulike symptoms called "polymer fume fever." Use stainless steel or cast iron cookware, which is virtually nonstick once well seasoned.

Dairy: I strongly recommend organic dairy products, which are epigenetically superior to conventional. Buy organic milk, yogurt, butter, and cheese when you can. For milk and yogurt, always choose low-fat.

Herbs and Spices: Because conventional spices and herbs undergo irridation to kill bacteria, contain GMOs, and are treated with harmful chemicals, aim to buy organic herbs and spices. To ensure that your herbs and spices are fresh and nutrient-filled, (1) buy the amount you need from bulk bins, (2) check the store-bought label for an expiration date, and (3) discard if old or unaromatic. There are, however, certain items you should avoid because they are not good for you such as licorice, MSG (monosodium glutamate), rue, and sumac. Be aware of nonnutritious spices: cinnamon, for instance, is sold in two forms—Ceylon and Cassia, the latter, which is inexpensive and more popular in North America, contains high levels of coumarin, a blood thinner known to cause liver damage.

Oils: Extra-virgin (and only extra-virgin) olive oil should be consumed daily if possible. Given that it denatures with heating, it is best to pour olive oil over salads, vegetables, pasta, or grains after they're cooked. Choose coconut oil or expeller-pressed grapeseed oil or ghee butter (it comes in jars) to cook with or grease pans. They are healthier options and the most resistant to heat damage.

Meat: Buy poultry or beef that is 100% grass-fed or organic. The American Grass-Fed Association regulates the labeling of animals that have been grass-fed for their entire lives. (See page 104 for the benefits of grass-fed meat.) Whereas, "organic" labels mean that the animal was fed only organic feed and received no antibiotics or hormones.

Produce: Organic fruits and vegetables are the best options: they haven't been treated with pesticides or are too costly: But don't forgo fruits and vegetables if organic choices aren't readily available and they may be nutritionally superior: instead, take your time to wash nonorganic fruits and vegetables thoroughly and buy the occasional organic item.

Groceries and Pantry Staples

An essential part of creating healthy meals is stocking your pantry and refrigerator with great ingredients. If you do, then everything you eat out of your own kitchen will be epigenetic and promote good health.

Fruits and Vegetables

They're all good, and the more varieties you eat, the better. Make sure to include these.

Apple
Avocado
Banana
Beets
Blackberries

Blueberries
Boysenberries
Broccoli
Broccoli sprouts
Brussels sprouts
Carrots
Cauliflower
Celery
Grapefruit
Herbs such as rosemary, basil, parsley, dill, cilantro
Kiwi
Orange
Papaya
Romaine lettuce
Scallions
Sweet potatoes
Tomatoes
Winter squash

Dairy

Organic butter
Organic Low-fat Greek yogurt
Organic Low-fat milk
Unsweetened almond milk

Grains

We've become accustomed to looking for "whole grain" as an ingredient in packaged processed foods, but the best way to consume whole grain is to cook and eat whole grains! They're all as easy to cook as rice and just as versatile. Try a variety.

Brown rice
Bulgur
Quinoa
Spelt
Steel-cut oats

Beans

Nothing beats the convenience of canned beans, but dried are easy to prepare and tastier. Buy beans either way.

    Chickpeas
    Lentils

Pasta

For dried pasta, look for vegetable-based and whole grain varieties made from buckwheat, brown rice, barley, and spelt, in addition to whole wheat.

Miscellaneous

    apple cider vinegar
    coconut sugar crystals
    rye crisps
    sprouted-grain sandwich bread
    wheat germ

Nuts and Seeds

For the varieties sold that way, raw is best.

    Almonds (with the skin)
    Cashews
    Chestnuts
    Pine nuts
    Pistachios
    Pumpkin seeds
    Sunflower seeds
    Walnuts

Spices

    Black pepper
    Cayenne
    Cinnamon
    Coriander

Cumin
Curry powder
Garlic powder
Ginger
Oregano
Paprika
Saffron
Sage
Sea salt
Turmeric

Cooking Oils

Coconut oil
Extra-virgin olive oil
Grapeseed oil

The following four-week menu consists of breakfast, lunch, and dinner options.

Now that you have your shopping and pantry lists, you can just focus on preparing fresh, tasty, ecogenetically inspired meals. Feel free to substitute ingredients such as nuts, spices, and vegetables to your taste.

Week One

Day 1
Breakfast: Option 1: Rye crisp (three or four) with low-fat cottage cheese and grapefruit
Option 2: Veggie Frittata
Lunch: Organic turkey breast (two or three slices) and low-fat mozzarella cheese sandwich
Dinner: Basil Salmon and Wild Rice

Day 2
Breakfast: Option 1: Scrambled eggs (one or two) on multigrain toast and orange juice
Option 2: Mixed fruit (one cup apples, pears, and peaches) and multigrain cereal
Lunch: Chicken Spinach Salad
Dinner: Cod and Roasted Scallions

Day 3

Breakfast: Option 1: Boiled eggs (one or two), sprouted whole grain bread (one or two slices) with ghee butter

Option 2: Blueberry Banana Cottage Cheese with Almonds

Lunch: Thai Chicken Salad

Dinner: Broiled Flounder with Sautéed Red Peppers and Quinoa

Day 4

Breakfast: Option 1: One cup low-fat plain Greek yogurt and blueberries

Option 2: Breakfast Burrito

Lunch: New England Clam Chowder

Dinner: Herb Roasted Turkey Breast with Mustard Caper Sauce

Day 5

Breakfast: Option 1: Plain oatmeal and apple (sweetened with honey)

Option 2: Nutty Papaya Yogurt

Lunch: Cucumber Curry Ginger Soup

Dinner: Ziti with Zucchini

Day 6

Breakfast: Option 1: Scrambled eggs (one or two) with rye bread (one or two slices)

Option 2: Steel-Cut Oatmeal and Fresh Berries

Lunch: Baked potato with tahini sauce (ground sesame seeds mixed with lemon juice, garlic, and salt)

Dinner: Spiced Roast Chicken with Watercress Salad

Day 7

Breakfast: Option 1: Sliced banana and strawberries in low-fat plain Greek yogurt (½ or 1 cup)

Option 2: Chocolate Super Waffles

Lunch: Salmon Burger

Dinner: Orange Fennel Roast Chicken and Baked Garlic Yucca Fries

Week Two

Day 1

Breakfast: Option 1: One cup low-fat plain Greek yogurt with blueberries (¼ cup or ½ cup) and sprouted whole wheat bread (2 slices) with almond butter

Option 2: Exotic Banana Pancakes

Lunch: Cobb Salad

Dinner: Broiled Snapper with Lime

Day 2

Breakfast: Option 1: Low-fat
plain yogurt (one cup) with
raspberries and crunchy
whole grain cereal

Option 2: Scrambled eggs (one
or two) with rye bread (one or
two slices)

Lunch: Organic turkey breast
(two–three slices) and low-fat
mozzarella cheese sandwich

Dinner: Wine-Braised Lamb
and Vegetables

Day 3

Breakfast: Option 1: Mixed fruit
(one cup apples, pears, and
peaches) and multigrain cereal

Option 2: Cinnamon Peach Pancakes

Lunch: Seitan Veggie Wrap

Dinner: Olive Baked Salmon

Day 4

Breakfast: Option 1: Scrambled
eggs stuffed in a pita bread

Option 2: Almond Butter Waffles

Lunch: Cilantro Kale Soup

Dinner: Orange Fennel Roast
Chicken and Baked Garlic
Yucca Fries

Day 5

Breakfast: Option 1: Rye crisp
(three–four) with low-fat
cottage cheese and a banana

Option 2: Eggless Cinnamon
French Toast

Lunch: Tomato Swiss Melt

Dinner: Manhattan Shrimp Chowder

Day 6

Breakfast: Option 1: Oatmeal
and banana

Option 2: Scrambled eggs (one
or two) on multigrain toast
and orange juice

Lunch: Mango, Spinach, and
Feta Cheese Salad

Dinner: Lemon Dill Halibut with
Garlic Cauliflower Purée

Day 7

Breakfast: Option 1: Cottage cheese
and mini bagel with almond butter

Option 2: Breakfast Burrito

Lunch: Chicken, Apple, and
Watercress Salad

Dinner: Red Snapper with Red
Potatoes and Asparagus

Week Three

Day 1

Breakfast: Option 1: Eggless
Cinnamon French Toast

Option 2: Steel-Cut Oatmeal
and Fresh Berries

Lunch: Vegetable Soup

Dinner: Halibut and Broccoli
over Pasta

Day 2

Breakfast: Option 1: Oatmeal (half cup) with blueberries and cinnamon

Option 2: Nutty Papaya Yogurt

Lunch: Turkey Avocado Wrap

Dinner: Flounder and Endive Nut Salad

Day 3

Breakfast: Option 1: Strawberries and multigrain cereal

Option 2: Scrambled eggs (one or two) on multigrain toast, a banana, and orange juice

Lunch: Kombu Chicken Soup

Dinner: Eggplant and Lentil Stew

Day 4

Breakfast: Option 1: Plain yogurt and figs (three)

Option 2: Almond Butter Waffles

Lunch: Fresh Pea Soup

Dinner: Chicken and Vegetable Casserole

Day 5

Breakfast: Option 1: Low-fat cottage cheese and sliced peaches

Option 2: Cinnamon Peach Pancakes

Lunch: Fresh Asparagus Soup

Dinner: Chicken and Moroccan Brown Rice Pilaf

Day 6

Breakfast: Option 1: Oatmeal with organic maple syrup

Option 2: Scrambled eggs (one or two) with rye bread (one or two slices)

Lunch: Thai Chicken Salad

Dinner: Curried Red Snapper with Asian Pear Cabbage Slaw

Day 7

Breakfast: Option 1: Low-fat Greek yogurt and banana

Option 2: Exotic Banana Pancakes

Lunch: Onion Soup

Dinner: Tangy Barbecue Chicken

Week Four

Day 1

Breakfast: Option 1: Low-fat plain yogurt with banana and coconut

Option 2: Chocolate Super Waffles

Lunch: Almond Caesar Salad with Grilled Chicken

Dinner: Easy Salmon Pesto Pasta

Day 2

Breakfast: Option 1: Acai Berry
Juice

Option 2: Oatmeal and Fresh Berries

Lunch: Winter Squash and
Chickpea Soup

Dinner: Coconut Curry Chicken
and Brown Rice

Day 3

Breakfast: Option 1: Rye bread
and boiled eggs (one or two)

Option 2: Nutty Papaya Yogurt

Lunch: Avocado Kale Smoothie

Dinner: Rigatoni with Pesto
Tomato Sauce

Day 4

Breakfast: Option 1: Steel-
cut oats

Option 2: Breakfast Burrito

Lunch: Kiwi Berry Smoothie

Dinner: Orange Fennel Roast
Chicken and Baked Garlic
Yucca Fries

Day 5

Breakfast: Option 1: Scrambled
eggs (one or two) and
sprouted whole grain bread
(one or two slices)

Option 2: Blueberry Banana
Cottage Cheese with
Almonds

Lunch: Turkey Avocado Wrap

Dinner: Sesame Pork
Tenderloin and Pine Nut
Salad

Day 6

Breakfast: Option 1: Oatmeal,
honey, and blueberries
(¼ cup)

Option 2: Vegetable Frittata

Lunch: Almond Butter
Smoothie

Dinner: Sesame Chicken with
Broccoli and Brown Rice

Day 7

Breakfast: Option 1: Steel-
cut oats

Option 2: Sprouted whole grain
bread (one or two slices) with
almond butter

Lunch: Seitan Veggie Wrap

Dinner: Saffron Chicken with
Sesame Green Beans and
Spelt

Recipes

If you're looking to shake up your eating habits with foods that reignite your health, you can start here. Rooted in the epigenetic fundamentals of reversing genes that make way for diseases, the ingredients and cooking techniques in the recipes that follow aim to reroute your health trajectory toward longevity and wellness. You should recognize that the snacks, shakes, and meals are not GTP-specific but rather are designed for overall wellness. In my practice, I talk to patients at length and request a variety of diagnostic tests and scans. That information allows me to tailor a plan that targets their health problems with foods that are primed to replenish natural antioxidants, boost anti-inflammatory molecules, and pinpoint epigenes. While many of the ingredients in these recipes are clearly aligned with certain health benefits, I have identified recipes that target obesity, heart disease, cancer, diabetes, and aging in the chart on page 293.

These recipes offer only a glimpse into how nutrients can be used to make wholesome, delicious meals. If you have old family recipes or new favorites from a cooking show, look to see which ones are already consistent with my recommendations. Others can be modified to boost their ecogenetic profile. The recipes that follow are not rigid culinary prescriptions for gene therapy. Don't hesitate to diversify your meals and please yourself by substituting certain ingredients for others. For instance, if you've been following a recipe that uses rosemary, try sage; brown rice, quinoa; walnuts, almonds. Swap ingredients for other ones to expand the spectrum of nutrients you eat. And look for ways to make small improvements that will have long-term benefits. Add a second vegetable to every dinner plan. Make a simple vinaigrette to eliminate the corn syrup and other poor quality additives in almost all bottled salad dressings. The key is to enhance wholesomeness by eating a diversity of fruits, vegetables, whole grains, herbs, and spices.

Before you get started, I have three GTP kitchen rules for you: the first rule is to recognize that flavor and nutrition do go together, because better nutrition isn't at the expense of good taste. The second rule is practice makes perfect; work to improve your eating habits each day, but don't beat yourself up—remember that good health is achieved steadily. Finally, the third rule is to have fun and enjoy cooking. Taking pleasure from preparing food and consuming it thoughtfully are great motivators for sticking with a healthy lifestyle. Bon appétit!

Ecogenetic Juices, Smoothies, and Snacks

Basil Tomato Juice
Serves 1

½ cup water
½ cup chopped tomatoes
⅛ teaspoon ground cumin
½ teaspoon ground turmeric
¼ cup chopped red bell pepper
⅛ teaspoon freshly ground pepper
½ cup fresh basil leaves
¼ cup peeled and chopped cucumber
1 ½ teaspoons bee propolis
2 teaspoons grated ginger

Blend all ingredients until smooth.

Coconut Water

Serves 2

1 coconut (coconut water yield varies based on size)
4 cups water
¼ teaspoon salt
honey or organic maple syrup to taste

Coconut water is a refreshing and healthy way to replenish lost electrolytes. Because coconut water is a natural electrolyte replacement drink, it is readily available in stores. You can purchase coconut water or make it yourself.

Use corkscrew to open a hole in the coconut by screwing into one of the three eyes. Drain coconut water into a Mason jar.

Add ½ cup of water to small pot. When it boils, remove from heat. Add honey (or syrup) and salt to hot water and stir until dissolved. Mix remaining water, honey mixture, and coconut water together. Refrigerate and serve when cold. Enjoy!

Blueberry Coconut Juice

Serves 1

½ cup blueberries
2 tablespoons spirulina
2 tablespoons GI Revive powder
2 tablespoons basil, finely chopped
4 tablespoons bee pollen
1 cup coconut water

Blend all ingredients until smooth.

Aloe Juice

Serves 1

2 ounces aloe vera gel (Lily of the Desert)
¼ cup unsweetened almond milk
1 banana, sliced
1 tablespoon ground flaxseeds

Blend all ingredients on low for 15 seconds.

Acai Berry Juice

Serves 2

1 carrot
1 beet
1 tablespoon acai berry powder
½ teaspoon spirulina
½ teaspoon cacao powder
1 tablespoon rice protein powder
½ cup brewed green tea
¼ cup Hunza raisins
¼ cup peeled and chopped cucumber
⅓ cup sunflower seed kernels
½ cup chopped tomato

Juice the beet and carrot. Blend with all other ingredients until smooth.

Black Raspberry Smoothie
Serves 1

¾ cup brewed black tea
1 tablespoon lime juice
1 tablespoon black raspberry powder
1 teaspoon camucamu berry powder
¼ cup noni juice
1 lemon, peeled, deseeded, and chopped
¼ cup goji berries

Blend all ingredients until smooth.

Spiced Apple Smoothie
Serves 1

1 peeled cucumber
2 celery stalks
1 beet
2 apples
¼ cup watercress
1 cup shredded, dried, unsweetened coconut
⅛ teaspoon ground turmeric

Juice cucumber, celery, beet, and apple. Blend with other ingredients until smooth.

Coconut Milk
Serves 1

1 tablespoon coconut milk powder
½ cup shredded, dried, unsweetened coconut
2 cups unsweetened almond milk
1 teaspoon wheat germ

Blend all ingredients at medium speed for 30 seconds. (You can use store-bought coconut milk or use this recipe to make your own.)

Coconut Cream and Almond Smoothie
Serves 2

1 ½ cups coconut water
6 raw, unsalted almonds
¼ cup shredded, dried, unsweetened coconut
1 banana
1 tablespoon organic lecithin powder
1 tablespoon aloe vera gel (Lily of the Desert)
¼ cup low-fat plain yogurt

Blend all ingredients until smooth.

Orange Berry Slushie
Serves 1

¼ cup blueberries or black raspberries
¼ cup mandarin orange segments
½ cup coconut water
4 ice cubes

Blend all ingredients on low until smooth.

Go Green Smoothie
Serves 2

3 celery stalks
1 green apple
¾ cup fresh pineapple juice
½ cup romaine lettuce
1 cup kale
¼ tablespoon parsley
1 teaspoon grated ginger
1 tablespoon vanilla-flavored protein powder

Juice celery, green apple, lettuce, and kale. Blend with other ingredients until smooth.

Tomato Juice
Serves 1

3 medium tomatoes
½ cucumber, peeled
¼ teaspoon salt
1 tablespoon lemon juice
1 celery stalk
parsley to garnish

Juice tomatoes and cucumber. Mix with salt and lemon juice. Serve with celery stick and garnish with parsley.

Apple Ginger Juice
Serves 2

2 apples, peeled and cored
2 cups water
1 teaspoon ground ginger
½ cup fresh lemon juice
1 tablespoon honey
1 tablespoon whey protein powder

Juice apples. Blend with other ingredients until smooth.

Acai Grape Juice
Serves 2

1 small pink grapefruit
1 cup red grapes (seedless)
1 cup green grapes (seedless)
1 tablespoon acai berry powder
1 teaspoon honey

Juice grapefruit and grapes. Blend juice with honey and powder.

ABC Smoothie
Serves 1

2 apples
3 beets
2 carrots
1 tablespoon fresh ginger
1 tablespoon whey protein powder

Juice apples, beets, and carrots. Blend with other ingredients until smooth.

Citrus Juice
Serves 1

2 tangerines
1 orange
½ cup fresh pineapple
1 lime
½ teaspoon ground ginger

Juice tangerines, orange, pineapple, lime. Add ginger and stir.

Fruit Smoothie
Serves 1

1 orange
2 green apples
1 banana
1 cup strawberries
1 pear, peeled and cored
1 tablespoon black raspberry powder

Juice orange and apples. Blend with other ingredients until smooth.

Berrylicious Smoothie
Serves 2

½ cup blackberries
½ cup blueberries
½ cup fresh cranberries
½ cup boysenberries
1 cup strawberries
1 teaspoon coconut crystals
1 tablespoon whey protein powder
1 tablespoon organic lecithin powder
3 ice cubes
½ cup unsweetened almond milk

Blend all ingredients until smooth.

Carrot Kale Wheatgrass Juice
Serves 2

4 large carrots
6 kale leaves
1 cup trimmed wheatgrass
1 green apple
1 fennel bulb
½ teaspoon ground ginger
½ cup orange juice

Juice carrots, kale, wheatgrass, apple, and fennel, and blend with ginger and orange juice.

Pear Coconut Juice

Serves 1

> 2 pears
> 1 tablespoon coconut milk powder
> 1 cup coconut water

Juice pears. Blend with other ingredients until smooth.

Strawberry Cherry Lavender Juice

Serves 2

> 1 cup strawberries
> ½ cup frozen, pitted cherries
> ½ teaspoon fresh organic lavender blossoms, plus lavender sprigs
> to garnish
> ½ cup coconut water

Blend strawberries, cherries, lavender blossoms, and coconut water.
Pour in a glass and add lavender sprigs for garnish.

Yucca Juice

Serves 1

> 2 teaspoons yucca root powder
> ¼ cup noni juice
> 1 teaspoon organic sesame oil
> ½ cup coconut water

Combine all ingredients and stir.

Kiwi Berry Smoothie

Serves 2

2 cups blueberries
1 cup strawberries
1 cup blackberries
2 kiwi fruits, peeled
½ cup brewed and cooled green tea
1 tablespoon acai berry powder
3 tablespoons fresh tarragon leaves

Blend all ingredients until smooth.

Almond Butter Smoothie

Serves 1

1 cup blueberries
2 tablespoons organic almond butter
1 banana
1 tablespoon raw cacao powder
1 tablespoon flaxseed oil
½ cup chocolate-flavored almond milk

Blend all ingredients until smooth.

Triple Chocolate Smoothie

Serves 1 to 2

¼ cup chopped, dark chocolate, plus extra to garnish
1 teaspoon organic cacao powder
1 teaspoon honey
1 teaspoon bee pollen
1 cup unsweetened almond milk

Blend all ingredients until smooth. Garnish with dark chocolate shavings.

Coftea Smoothie

Serves 1

½ cup brewed and cooled organic coffee
3 tablespoons raw cacao powder
1 tablespoon whey protein
½ cup brewed and cooled green tea
15 drops ChlorOxygen (chlorophyll)

Blend all ingredients until smooth.

Avocado Kale Smoothie

Serves 2

1 large ripe avocado, peeled and pitted
8 kale leaves
6 Swiss chard leaves
½ cup canned coconut milk
juice of 1 lime
1 or 2 green apple slices (optional)

Blend all ingredients until smooth. If desired, add honey to taste and garnish with green apple slices.

Peach Orange Smoothie

Serves 1

½ cup sliced peaches
½ cup fresh orange juice
1 tablespoon honey
¼ teaspoon almond or vanilla extract

Blend all ingredients until smooth.

Chunky Coconut Shake
Serves 2

½ cup shredded, dried, unsweetened coconut
2 teaspoons honey
1 cup coconut water
1 teaspoon brewers' yeast
½ cup watercress leaves

Blend all ingredients for about 30 seconds.

Breakfast

Nutty Papaya Yogurt
Serves 1

½ cup low-fat Greek yogurt
1 tablespoon linseed oil
1 cup diced ripe papaya
1 tablespoon almonds, chopped
1 tablespoon walnuts, chopped

Mix Greek yogurt with linseed oil. Top with papaya, almonds, and walnuts.

Blueberry Banana Cottage Cheese with Almonds
Serves 1 to 2

> 1 cup organic cottage cheese
> ½ banana, sliced
> ½ cup blueberries
> 1 tablespoon slivered almonds

Mix fruit and almonds in cottage cheese and serve. For a variation, use yogurt instead of cottage cheese.

Tofu Salad on Whole Grain Pita
Serves 4

> ½ block tofu
> ¼ cup finely chopped scallions
> 2 tablespoons egg-free mayonnaise
> 2 teaspoons Dijon mustard
> ¼ teaspoon turmeric or curry powder
> ¼ teaspoon garlic powder
> ¼ cup broccoli sprouts
> 4 small whole grain pitas
> chopped romaine lettuce
> almond or walnut oil for serving

Mix and mash tofu with scallion, mayonnaise, mustard, spices and broccoli sprouts. Spread on whole grain pita (or fill if pita is pocket-style), garnish with chopped romaine lettuce and drizzle with a little almond or walnut oil.

Steel-Cut Oatmeal with Fresh Berries

Serves 3 to 4

1 cup steel-cut oats
1 tablespoon ghee or butter
3 cups boiling water
½ cup low-fat almond milk
1 tablespoon brown sugar
1 teaspoon honey
¼ teaspoon organic cinnamon
¼ teaspoon nutmeg
½ cup mixed berries (strawberries, raspberries, blackberries)

In a large saucepan over medium heat, melt butter. Add oats and cook, stirring, until the oats look and smell lightly toasted. Carefully add 3 cups of boiling water. Reduce heat to low, cover, and simmer without stirring for 30 minutes. Add milk and stir gently for an additional 10 minutes. Remove oatmeal from heat. Add half of the berries, and brown sugar, honey, cinnamon, and nutmeg to the oatmeal in the pan and mix. Serve the oatmeal and top with remaining fresh berries.

Exotic Banana Pancakes

Serves 4

2 cups whole wheat flour
2 tablespoons brown sugar
¼ teaspoon kosher salt
1 teaspoon baking powder
½ teaspoon baking soda
½ teaspoon organic cinnamon
½ teaspoon curry powder
2 large eggs
2 cups low-fat buttermilk
3 tablespoons ghee or butter, melted and cooled slightly
1 banana, chopped
coconut oil, ghee, or butter for greasing the pan
organic maple syrup for serving

In a large bowl, whisk to combine the flour, sugar, salt, baking powder, baking soda, and spices. In a separate bowl, beat eggs, buttermilk, and ghee. Pour egg mixture into dry ingredients, mix, and let sit for 5 minutes (to allow baking soda and powder to create bubbles). Gently stir in chopped banana. (If banana is extremely ripe, you can mash and stir into the liquid ingredients.)

Heat the griddle and lightly grease. Pour batter and flip pancakes when bubbles form. Remove when golden brown. Serve with organic maple syrup. Makes about 8 pancakes.

Cinnamon Peach Pancakes
Serves 4

2 cups whole wheat flour
2 tablespoons brown sugar
¼ teaspoon sea salt
1 teaspoon baking powder
½ teaspoon baking soda
½ teaspoon organic cinnamon
2 large eggs
2 cups low-fat buttermilk
3 tablespoons ghee butter, melted and cooled slightly
coconut oil, ghee, or butter for greasing pan
1 ½ cups finely chopped peaches
organic maple syrup for serving

In a large bowl, whisk to combine the flour, sugar, salt, baking powder, baking soda, and cinnamon. In a separate bowl, beat eggs, buttermilk, and butter. Pour egg mixture into dry ingredients, mix, and let sit for 5 minutes (to allow baking soda and powder to create bubbles). Stir in 1 cup of the chopped peaches.

Heat the griddle and lightly grease. Pour batter and flip pancakes when bubbles form. Remove when golden brown. Serve topped with remaining peaches and organic maple syrup. Makes about 8 pancakes.

Eggless Cinnamon French Toast
Serves 2

4 slices sprouted whole wheat bread
¾ cup organic low-fat milk
1 teaspoon organic cinnamon
¼ teaspoon salt
½ teaspoon paprika
1 teaspoon almond extract
2 ripe bananas
coconut oil, ghee, or butter for greasing pan
organic maple syrup for serving

Blend milk, cinnamon, salt, paprika, almond extract, and bananas until smooth. Cut 4 slices of bread diagonally. Dip each piece of bread in the mixture.

Heat the griddle and lightly grease. Lay slices in medium-hot pan and fry until golden on both sides. Serve topped with sliced bananas and organic maple syrup if desired.

Almond Butter Waffles
Serves 5 to 6

¼ cup almond butter
¼ cup wheat germ
3 tablespoons butter, softened
2 eggs, lightly beaten
1 ½ cups organic low-fat milk
1 ½ cups whole wheat flour
2 teaspoons baking powder
1 to 2 tablespoons brewers' yeast
¼ teaspoon salt
coconut oil, ghee, or butter for the waffle iron
organic maple syrup for serving

In a large bowl, beat almond butter, wheat germ, and butter until creamy. Add eggs and milk, mixing well. In a separate bowl, whisk together flour, baking powder, brewers' yeast, and salt. Add to the milk mixture and blend thoroughly until smooth. Cook on a preheated and lightly greased waffle iron. Ladle about ½ cup or ¾ cup of batter onto iron and close. Waffle is done cooking when indicator light turns off. Serve with maple syrup if desired. Makes 6 waffles.

Chocolate Super Waffles
Serves 5 to 6

1 ¼ cups whole wheat flour
3 teaspoons baking powder
1 teaspoon salt
1 teaspoon ground ginger
1 teaspoon paprika
1 teaspoon cacao powder
1 cup wheat germ
4 tablespoons butter, melted
2 eggs, lightly beaten
2 tablespoons honey
2 cups organic low-fat milk
coconut oil, ghee, or butter for the waffle iron
organic maple syrup for serving

In a large bowl, whisk together flour, baking powder, salt, and spices. Stir in wheat germ. In a separate bowl, mix together remaining ingredients. Add liquid mixture to flour mixture, and beat or stir until smooth. Cook on a preheated waffle iron lightly greased. Ladle about ½ cup or ¾ cup of batter onto iron and close. Waffle is done cooking when indicator light turns off. Serve with organic maple syrup if desired. Makes 6 waffles.

Breakfast Burrito
Serves 1

2 eggs
½ cup sliced scallions
¼ teaspoon salt
¼ teaspoon pepper
¼ cup cooked pinto beans
2 tablespoons shredded low-fat mozzarella
1 sprouted whole grain tortilla
Chopped onions, bell peppers, salsa, and hot sauce (optional)

Scramble eggs, salt, pepper, and scallions in a lightly greased pan over medium-high heat. Stir in beans and cheese to warm them. Scoop onto tortilla and add onions, bell peppers, salsa, and hot sauce if you like. Fold tortilla and enjoy!

Veggie Frittata
Serves 2

1 tablespoon grapeseed oil
½ cup sliced scallions
3 tablespoons minced parsley
1 small onion, thinly sliced
1 tablespoon fresh rosemary, finely chopped
3 eggs
¼ cup organic low-fat milk
2 tablespoons grated mozzarella cheese
½ teaspoon salt
¼ teaspoon pepper
1 tablespoon extra-virgin olive oil

Preheat oven to 375 degrees. In an ovenproof skillet over medium heat, warm grapeseed oil and cook scallions, parsley, onion, and rosemary until onion is light brown and tender, about 2 to 3 minutes. Remove pan from heat.

In a bowl, beat eggs. Add milk, cheese, salt, and pepper. Pour over vegetables in skillet and cook over medium heat, stirring gently with spatula until eggs begin to set, about 2 minutes. Transfer to the oven for 5 minutes or until the eggs are cooked through. Drizzle with olive oil and serve.

Salads

Very Green Salad with Aloe Dressing
Serves 4

3 cups kale, chopped
2 cups baby arugula
1 small head of romaine lettuce, chopped
½ cup frozen sweet peas, cooked and cooled
½ cup cubed avocado
½ cup broccoli sprouts
½ cup crumbled feta cheese
¼ cup chopped almonds
½ cup Aloe Dressing (see page 285)

Mix ingredients in a bowl. Drizzle with Aloe Dressing. Enjoy!

Mango, Spinach, and Feta Cheese Salad
Serves 2

1 firm red-orange mango
2 cups baby spinach leaves
1 tablespoon lime juice
¼ cup sliced almonds
¼ cup sweetened dried cranberries
¼ cup feta cheese, crumbled
¼ cup Ginger Vinaigrette (see page 284)

Peel mango and grate into a mixing bowl. Combine mango with spinach, lime juice, almonds, and cranberries. Lightly toss with feta cheese and drizzle with vinaigrette.

Arugula and Peach Salad
Serves 2

¼ cup sliced almonds
1 teaspoon coconut oil
½ peach, cut into thin wedges
3 cups arugula
½ cup shredded carrots
¼ cup broccoli sprouts
¼ cup pomegranate seeds
¼ teaspoon salt
¼ teaspoon black pepper
¼ cup Aloe Dressing (see page 285)

In a dry skillet over medium heat, toast almonds, stirring constantly, and remove from pan as soon as they start to color. Add oil to pan and saute peach slices until lightly browned on both sides. Remove from heat. Combine arugula, carrots, sprouts, pomegranate, salt and pepper. Add toasted almonds and peaches to salad. Drizzle with Aloe Dressing and serve.

Sweet Beet Salad
Serves 2

½ pound beets, raw or cooked, cooled, and peeled
2 small avocados, peeled, pitted, and cubed
½ cup walnuts
¼ cup sweetened dried cranberries
¼ cup raisins
1 head of romaine lettuce, chopped
¼ cup Classic Vinaigrette (see page 285)

Grate beets by hand or in a food processor. Gently combine avocado cubes, walnuts, cranberries, and raisins in a bowl. On each
plate, arrange romaine lettuce, then avocado mixture, and top with
grated beets. Drizzle with vinaigrette.

Tofu Spinach Salad with Pomegranate
Serves 4

1 block firm tofu cut into 4 slices and patted dry or packaged tofu
strips
1 tablespoon coconut or grapeseed oil
1 teaspoon cumin
¼ teaspoon black pepper
¼ teaspoon kosher salt
2 9-ounce bags of spinach leaves
1 cup chopped walnuts
½ cup fresh pomegranate seeds
½ cup Ginger Vinaigrette (see page 284)

Preheat a skillet over medium-high heat and add oil. Sprinkle tofu
slices with cumin, salt, and black pepper. Place in the skillet and
cook on both sides until lightly browned. Remove from heat.

In a mixing bowl, combine the spinach, walnuts, and pomegranate seeds and toss with half the dressing until combined. Plate the
tossed salad and top each serving with tofu. Drizzle additional vinaigrette over all if desired.

Cobb Salad

Serves 4

1 pound skinless, boneless chicken breasts
1 tablespoon coconut or grapeseed oil
8 cups romaine lettuce
3 hard-boiled eggs, chopped
2 fresh tomatoes, chopped
6 tablespoons grated pecorino cheese
4 slices cooked turkey bacon, crumbled
1 medium avocado, diced
¼ teaspoon sea salt
¼ teaspoon black pepper
½ cup Creamy Honey Mustard Dressing (see page 283)

Preheat a skillet over medium-high heat and add oil. Season chicken with salt and pepper. Cook, turning once, until cooked through, about 5 to 6 minutes. Cut chicken into bite-size pieces. Combine all remaining salad ingredients in a large bowl and add chicken. Add dressing and toss gently.

Chicken, Apple, and Watercress Salad

Serves 2

2 cups diced or shredded, cooked chicken
1 bunch watercress
½ cucumber, thinly sliced
½ apple, thinly sliced
2 tablespoons walnuts, finely chopped
2 tablespoons golden raisins
1 tablespoon fresh lemon juice
¼ cup Horseradish Vinaigrette (see page 283)

Mix chicken with watercress, cucumbers, apples, walnuts, and raisins. Toss with fresh lemon juice and drizzle with Horseradish Vinaigrette.

Almond Caesar Salad with Grilled Chicken
Serves 4

4 grilled and diced chicken cutlets
10 cups chopped romaine lettuce
3 tablespoons grated Parmesan cheese
¼ cup chopped almonds
¼ cup homemade whole grain croutons (optional)
¼– ½ cup Creamy Honey Mustard Dressing (see page 283)

Mix chicken, lettuce, cheese, nuts, croutons, if desired, and dressing.

Thai Chicken Salad
Serves 4

1 tablespoon coconut or grapeseed oil
1 pound boneless, skinless chicken breast, cut into strips
¼ teaspoon kosher salt
¼ teaspoon black pepper
1 tablespoon red curry paste
¼ cup fresh lime juice
1 tablespoon garlic chili pepper sauce
3 tablespoons minced cilantro
1 medium head of romaine lettuce, chopped or torn
1 cup cherry tomatoes
½ cucumber, peeled and thinly sliced
2 tangerines, peeled and segmented

Preheat a skillet over medium-high heat and add oil. Season chicken with salt and pepper, add to the hot pan and cook, tossing and turning, until cooked through, about 3 to 4 minutes. Remove from heat.

In a large bowl, stir together red curry paste, lime juice, and garlic chili pepper sauce. Add remaining ingredients and the chicken in the bowl. Toss with the sauce, then add tangerines, toss gently again, and serve.

Spicy Tabouleh

Makes about 3 cups

1 cup bulgur wheat
1 ½ cups boiling water
1 ½ teaspoons extra-virgin olive oil
¼ cup extra-virgin olive oil
¼ cup fresh lemon juice
2 bunches parsley, finely chopped
¼ cup chopped fresh mint
½ cup chopped fresh dill
½ cup chopped avocado
½ cup chopped yellow bell pepper
1 firm tomato, chopped
½ onion, chopped
¼ teaspoon salt
¼ teaspoon black pepper
¼ teaspoon chili powder
½ cup crumbled feta cheese

Combine bulgur, boiling water, and 1 ½ teaspoons oil in a large bowl. Cover and let mixture stand for 20 minutes, until wheat is softened and water is absorbed. Whisk olive oil and lemon juice together, then add to bulgur along with remaining ingredients. Toss well. Add additional oil and lemon if desired. Serve at room temperature.

Soups

Cucumber Curry Ginger Soup
Serves 2

1 cup soy milk
1 tablespoon butter
5 raw almonds
1 cup diced cucumber, unpeeled
1 teaspoon curry powder
1 tablespoon fresh lime juice
3 slices fresh ginger
⅛ teaspoon black pepper
1 teaspoon dried holy basil (or tulsi powder)

In a blender, combine milk, butter, and almonds and blend for 30 seconds. Then add the rest of the ingredients and blend for 2 minutes, or until smooth. Pour mixture into medium saucepan and warm over low heat, stirring constantly until just heated through.

Kombu Chicken Soup
Serves 3

Homemade Chicken Stock
1 pound bony chicken pieces
1 celery stalk, cut into chunks
1 carrot, cut into chunks
½ onion, chopped
⅛ teaspoon rosemary
⅛ teaspoon thyme
⅛ teaspoon grated fresh ginger
¼ teaspoon kosher salt
¼ teaspoon freshly ground black pepper

1 6-inch strip dried kombu, cut horizontally into thin strips
2 teaspoons light miso paste

Place chicken and all stock ingredients in a medium pot. Add enough water to cover chicken pieces. Cover pot and bring to a boil. Skim off foam. Lower heat and simmer, partially covered, for an hour. Remove chicken and allow to cool, then remove meat from bones. Discard bones and chop up meat. Strain the broth, setting aside vegetables and chicken.

Gently heat broth along with kombu slices. Mix in miso paste. Add chicken, carrots, and celery from broth back in, but do not allow to boil or simmer. Remove from heat and let steep 3 to 4 minutes. Remove kombu before serving.

Fresh Pea Soup
Serves 4

2 pounds fresh young peas in pods
2 quarts water
1 tablespoon sliced scallions
1 chopped whole potato
2 tablespoons Greek yogurt
salt and pepper to taste

Shell peas, setting aside peas and placing pods in a large saucepan with 8 cups of water. Bring to a boil, reduce heat, cover, and simmer for 15 to 20 minutes. Skim out and discard pods. To the pot, add scallions and chopped potatoes. Return to a boil, reduce heat, cover, and simmer for 10 to 15 minutes, or until potato chunks are fully cooked and starting to fall apart. Add peas and simmer for 3 to 4 minutes, or until just cooked. (Ideally, they'll retain their bright green color.) Using an immersion blender or carefully transferring the mixture to a blender or food processor, purée soup until smooth. Stir in yogurt and salt and pepper to taste. Heat up as needed, but do not allow to boil.

Vegetable Soup
Serves 6

2 tablespoons ghee or butter
½ cup thinly sliced carrots
1 cup diced celery
¼ cup sliced scallions
2 cups diced yam
4 whole tomatoes, coarsely chopped, or 1 can whole or stewed tomatoes
1 or 2 red bell peppers, seeded and cut into small pieces
1 bay leaf
2 quarts vegetable stock
extra virgin olive oil for serving

In a large soup pot, melt butter and sauté carrots, celery, and scallions for 2 to 3 minutes. Add remaining vegetables and stock. Bring to boil, lower heat, and simmer, partially covered, for about 30 minutes. Remove bay leaf before serving. Drizzle each serving with some olive oil.

New England Clam Chowder
Serves 4

1 quart shucked large clams
4 slices organic turkey bacon, chopped
½ cup sliced onions
3 cups diced raw potatoes
2 tablespoons ghee or butter
2 tablespoons whole wheat or unbleached flour
4 cups organic low-fat milk, heated
½ teaspoon salt
½ teaspoon pepper

Wash clams in about 2 cups clean water and save the water, straining if it appears sandy. Grind or chop hard parts of the clams. In a large saucepan or soup pot, brown chopped turkey bacon slowly until crisp, then remove from pan and set aside.

Sauté onions and chopped hard parts of clams in bacon drippings. Stir and cook for 3 to 4 minutes, or until tender. Add potatoes and reserved clam liquid, stir, and simmer until potatoes are fork-tender but not falling apart. Add soft parts of the clams.

In a separate saucepan or double boiler, melt butter. Add flour and cook, stirring, for 1 to 2 minutes, but do not let it brown. Stir in hot milk and cook, stirring, until mixture begins to thicken slightly. Add this into the chowder pot and keep hot until serving. Do not let boil.

Season to taste with salt and pepper. Serve sprinkled with bits of crispy turkey bacon.

Manhattan Shrimp Chowder
Serves 4

4 slices turkey bacon, chopped
½ cup chopped onion
2 cups diced raw red skin, Yukon Gold or other boiling potatoes
1 tablespoon chopped red bell pepper
2 tablespoons chopped celery
½ pound peeled shrimp, chopped
2 cups stewed tomatoes or tomato juice
½ teaspoon salt
½ teaspoon black pepper
½ teaspoon garlic powder
½ teaspoon thyme
½ teaspoon paprika
½ teaspoon pepper
1 bay leaf
2 tablespoons chopped fresh parsley

In a large saucepan or soup pot, brown turkey bacon slowly until crisp, then remove from pan and set aside. Add to drippings the chopped onion and cook, stirring, for 2 minutes or until tender.

Add potatoes, red pepper, celery, and enough water to cover the vegetables. Heat to boiling, lower heat, and simmer until potatoes are fork-tender but not falling apart, about 10 minutes. Add shrimp, to-matoes (or juice), and seasonings. Simmer for 3 to 5 minutes. Remove bay leaf.

Serve sprinkled with bits of crispy turkey bacon and garnish with chopped parsley.

Onion Soup

Serves 8

2 tablespoons ghee or butter
1 pound onions, sliced into very thin crescents
2 tablespoons whole wheat flour
6 to 8 cups organic vegetable broth
salt and pepper to taste
8 slices sprouted whole grain bread
½ cup grated Gruyere cheese

In a large heavy saucepan or Dutch oven over very low heat, melt butter and sauté onions stirring to coat well. Avoid excessive brown-ing. When onions are glazed and lightly golden, sprinkle flour over them, stir, and cook for 1 minute. Add broth slowly, stirring con-stantly. Cover and simmer gently for 20 to 30 minutes.

Sprinkle slices of sprouted whole grain bread with cheese and toast them in the oven until cheese melts and browns. Place bread slices, cut in half if necessary, atop steaming bowls of soup to serve.

Fresh Asparagus Soup

Serves 6

¾ pound fresh asparagus
10 cups organic vegetable broth
1 teaspoon salt
¼ teaspoon black pepper
¼ clove garlic, minced
2 tablespoons plain Greek yogurt

Break tough ends off asparagus and lightly peel the stalks if the outer layer seems tough. Cut into 1-inch pieces. In a large soup pot, bring broth to a simmer, add asparagus, and cook until asparagus is tender, 3 to 5 minutes. Transfer asparagus and 2 cups of the hot broth to a food processor or blender. (Or use an immersion blender.) Purée until smooth, then return purée to the soup pot. Stir in salt, black pepper, and garlic, and bring to a boil. Remove from heat, stir in yogurt, and serve.

Chinese Egg Drop Soup

Serves 4

3 cups organic vegetable broth
3 teaspoons almond flour
2 slices fresh ginger
1 medium egg, beaten
½ teaspoon soy sauce
2 tablespoons minced scallion greens

In a small bowl, combine 3 tablespoons vegetable broth with almond flour. Stir to blend well. Place remaining broth in a medium saucepan, add ginger, and bring to a boil. Stir in almond flour mixture and cook, stirring, until soup thickens slightly, about 1 minute. Gradually add egg and stir to mix egg into the soup well. Add soy sauce and scallion. Discard ginger and serve.

Cilantro Kale Soup

Serves 2

1 cup kale, slivered
4 cups organic vegetable broth
¼ cup chopped cilantro leaves and tender stems
1 6-ounce can sliced water chestnuts, rinsed and drained

Rinse kale leaves. In a medium saucepan, bring vegetable broth to a boil over medium-high heat. Add kale and cilantro. Cook until kale is wilted but still bright green, about 2 minutes. Add water chestnuts and serve immediately.

Winter Squash and Chickpea Soup

Serves 2

4 cups organic vegetable broth
2 medium celery ribs with leaves, diced (1 ⅓ cups)
1 large onion, chopped
1 cup cooked chickpeas
2 cups cubed, peeled butternut or other winter squash
1 garlic clove, minced
½ teaspoon salt
¼ teaspoon pepper
2 tablespoons chopped fresh rosemary
1 tablespoon minced chives
extra virgin olive oil for serving

In a large saucepan, combine vegetable broth, celery, onion, chickpeas, squash, garlic, salt, pepper, and 1 tablespoon rosemary. Bring to a boil, reduce heat to medium-low, and simmer, partially covered, until vegetables are tender, 20 to 25 minutes. Serve sprinkled with remaining rosemary and chives and drizzled with some olive oil.

Sandwiches and Wraps

Salmon Burgers
Serves 4

1 ¼ pounds skinless salmon fillet, cut into 1-inch pieces
4 scallions, thinly sliced
¼ teaspoon kosher salt
¼ teaspoon black pepper
1 tablespoons coconut or grapeseed oil
4 whole wheat rolls
avocado slices
cilantro sprigs

Place salmon pieces in a food processor and pulse 3 to 4 times until coarsely chopped but still chunky. Add scallions, salt, and pepper to the food processor and pulse briefly to combine. Shape the mixture into 4 patties. Preheat a cast iron skillet over medium-high heat, warm oil, and cook patties for 3 to 4 minutes on each side.

Serve salmon burgers on rolls topped with avocado and cilantro sprigs. Goes well with Very Green Salad with Aloe Dressing (see page 241).

Tomato Swiss Melt
Serves 1

2 slices sprouted whole grain bread
¼ teaspoon salt
2 slices organic tomato
2 slices Swiss cheese

Sprinkle each tomato slice with salt. Top each slice of bread with a slice of tomato and cover with cheese. Broil in toaster oven until cheese melts.

Turkey and Cheese Sandwich
Serves 1

2 slices sprouted whole grain bread
4 ounces sliced turkey
1 slice aged pecorino cheese
1 teaspoon spicy mustard
1 leaf romaine lettuce
1 slice organic tomato
3 sprigs of fresh parsley (optional)

Yes, I know you've made a turkey sandwich before. But after watching episodes of some of the nation's most popular TV food shows, I think the number of meat and cheese slices used to make sandwiches is definitely out of sync with the health goals I've discussed. Albeit simple, this sandwich recipe is meant to show you what sensible quantities are.

Turkey Avocado Wrap
Serves 2

2 large sprouted whole grain tortillas
8 ounces sliced turkey
1 avocado, peeled and diced
¼ cup sliced scallions
4 dried figs, chopped
2 tablespoons Balsamic Vinaigrette (see page 284)

Lay tortillas on separate plates. Top each with half the turkey, avocado, scallions, and figs. Drizzle with Balsamic Vinaigrette, roll into a wrap, and serve.

Seitan Veggie Wrap
Serves 4

8 ounces firm seitan, divided into 4 portions
2 to 4 tablespoons tamari (wheat-free soy sauce)
4 sprouted whole grain tortillas
4 tablespoons baba ghanoush
¼ cup sliced red pepper
¼ cup slivered kale
¼ cup diced carrots
¼ cup parsley, chopped fine
¼ cup low-fat Greek yogurt, stirred

Preheat oven to 325 degrees. Place seitan in a small baking dish and drizzle with tamari, saturating the seitan. Bake for 15 minutes or until heated through.

Spread baba ghanoush over each tortilla and add cooked seitan on top. Top tortillas with red pepper, kale, carrots, and parsley.

Drizzle yogurt over vegetables and roll into wraps.

Egg Salad Sandwich
Serves 2

4 eggs
¼ cup diced celery
¼ cup pesto
1 tablespoon low-fat Greek yogurt
1 teaspoon mustard
salt and pepper to taste

For the sandwich
4 pieces sprouted whole grain bread
iceberg lettuce
1 organic tomato, sliced

Place eggs in a small saucepan and cover with water. When water comes to a boil, turn off heat. Cover pan and allow eggs to "cook" for 10 minutes for firm, creamy eggs. Transfer the eggs to an ice water bath for 1 minute, then peel.

In a medium bowl, mash eggs and add celery, pesto, yogurt, mustard, salt, and pepper. Mix together well.

Toast bread before topping with egg salad, lettuce, and tomato slices.

Main Dishes

Basil Salmon and Wild Rice
Serves 4

1 cup wild and long-grain rice blend
2 cups fresh basil leaves
1 cup extra-virgin olive oil, plus 1 tablespoon to cook fish
¾ teaspoon kosher salt, plus ¼ teaspoon to season fish
¼ teaspoon black pepper
4 6-ounce salmon fillets

Cook rice following the package instructions.

Quickly blanch basil leaves by dropping them into a pot of boiling water and scooping them out after 5 seconds. Drain them on paper towel. In a blender, combine basil, 1 cup of olive oil, salt, and black pepper and purée until smooth.

Preheat oven to 400 degrees.

Heat an oven-safe stainless steel pan over medium-high heat and warm 1 tablespoon of olive oil. Season salmon with kosher salt and add to pan. Cook salmon for 3 minutes on each side. Carefully transfer the pan to the oven for 6 minutes or until salmon flakes when tested with a fork. Plate it, drizzle the puréed basil over it, and serve with wild rice.

Cod and Roasted Scallions

Serves 4

10 small red potatoes, sliced ¼ inch thick
2 tablespoons extra-virgin olive oil
½ teaspoon chili powder
kosher salt
black pepper
4 6-ounce pieces of cod, skinless
2 bunches scallions, trimmed
1 lemon

Preheat oven to 425 degrees. In a roasting pan, toss potato slices with 1 tablespoon olive oil, chili powder, salt, and pepper. Roast for 10 to 15 minutes, turning potatoes over halfway through so that both sides appear golden brown.

Arrange cod and scallions on top of potatoes and drizzle with additional oil, salt, and pepper. Squeeze lemon juice over all. Bake cod and scallions for 10 minutes. Serve and enjoy!

Broiled Flounder
with Sautéed Red Pepper and Quinoa

Serves 3 to 4

1 cup quinoa
2 red peppers, seeded and chopped
1 tablespoon extra-virgin olive oil
4 skinless, boneless flounder fillets
2 tablespoons ghee butter
kosher salt and black pepper

Using a fine mesh strainer, rinse quinoa thoroughly. Transfer to a sauce pan with 2 cups of water and cover. Over high heat bring to a boil, lower heat, cover, and simmer for 15 to 20 minutes. Preheat a skillet, gently warm olive oil, and sauté peppers, sprinkling with salt and pepper. Stir into quinoa and set aside.

Preheat broiler at high heat.

Sprinkle salt and pepper over fillets. Heat butter in a saucepan and add over fish. Broil until fillets flake easily with a fork.

Serve the flounder on a bed of quinoa and peppers.

Lemon Dill Halibut with Garlic Cauliflower Purée
Serves 4

4 4-ounce halibut steaks
kosher salt
freshly ground black pepper
2 tablespoons extra-virgin olive oil
1 cup dry white wine
1 teaspoon fresh lemon juice
1 tablespoon ghee butter
4 tablespoons chopped fresh dill

For the cauliflower
1 medium cauliflower, cut into small pieces
½ teaspoon garlic, minced
2 tablespoons lemon juice
1 tablespoon low-fat cream cheese, softened
1 cup organic low-fat milk
¼ cup grated Parmesan cheese
2 tablespoons ghee butter
½ teaspoon dill, chopped

Preheat a sauté pan large enough to hold halibut in one layer with olive oil. Season fish liberally with salt and pepper on both sides. Cook, turning once, until fish flakes easily with fork, about 5 to 7 minutes total, depending on the thickness of the steaks.

In a small saucepan, combine wine and lemon juice and simmer until reduced by half. Remove from heat and stir in butter. Plate halibut, top with wine sauce, and sprinkle with fresh dill.

Over boiling water, steam cauliflower for 6 minutes or until very tender. Transfer to a food processor along with garlic, lemon juice, cream cheese, milk, and Parmesan and purée. Garnish purée with dill and serve with ghee butter alongside fish.

Red Snapper with Red Potatoes and Asparagus
Serves 4

For the vegetables
1 pound small red potatoes
1 bunch fresh asparagus, tough bottoms discarded
2 tablespoons extra-virgin olive oil
½ tablespoon sesame seeds
1 teaspoon finely chopped fresh rosemary
1 teaspoon minced fresh thyme

4 4-ounce snapper fillets
2 tablespoons grapeseed oil
2 tablespoons honey
¼ cup white wine
1 teaspoon ground ginger
kosher salt
freshly ground black pepper

Preheat oven to 350 degrees. In a small roasting pan, toss potatoes and asparagus with olive oil. Sprinkle with sesame seeds, rosemary, and thyme. Bake for 1 hour.

Heat grapeseed oil in a skillet over medium heat. Mix honey, white wine, ginger, salt, and black pepper. Coat fish with mixture, then sauté in oil.

Curried Red Snapper with Asian Pear Cabbage Slaw
Serves 2

For the slaw
2 cups shredded red cabbage
2 cups shredded green cabbage
1 large Asian pear, thinly sliced
1 tablespoon mustard
1 tablespoon honey
¼ cup sour cream
4 tablespoons apple cider vinegar
½ teaspoon minced fresh thyme
1½ tablespoons minced fresh parsley
1 tablespoon minced fresh dill

2 6-ounce red snapper fillets
1 tablespoon coconut oil
kosher salt
freshly ground black pepper
1 medium garlic clove, minced
1 or 2 chili peppers, seeded and chopped
2 scallions, chopped
2 teaspoons fresh parsley, minced
5 fresh mint leaves, chopped
1 to 2 teaspoons curry powder

Combine cabbages and pear in a large bowl. In a separate bowl, whisk together mustard, honey, sour cream, cider vinegar, thyme, parsley, and dill. Pour mixture over cabbage and toss until thoroughly coated. Refrigerate at least 1 hour.

In a lidded sauté pan large enough to hold fish in a single layer, gently heat coconut oil. Season the fillets with salt and pepper, and arrange in pan. Scatter garlic, chili peppers, scallions, parsley, mint, and curry powder over the fish. Cover pan and cook fish just until it flakes easily, 5 to 7 minutes.

Serve red snapper fillets with cabbage slaw, sprinkling chopped dill over slaw.

Ginger Salmon
Serves 4

4 salmon steaks
4 tablespoons grapeseed oil
kosher salt
freshly ground black pepper
¼ cup lemon juice
1 ½ teaspoons ginger
1 tablespoon chopped fresh mint

Coat salmon with oil and season with salt, pepper, lemon juice, and ginger. Bake in oven preheated to 350 degrees until fish flakes with a fork. Sprinkle with chopped mint and serve.

Flounder and Endive Nut Salad
Serves 4

For the salad
½ cup pine nuts, chopped
½ cup walnuts, chopped
1 tablespoon mustard
1 tablespoon red wine vinegar
½ tablespoon lemon juice
3 tablespoons extra-virgin olive oil
4 endives, cored and quartered
1 medium beet, cooked, peeled, and diced
1 tablespoon minced fresh parsley

4 flounder fillets
kosher salt
freshly ground black pepper
½ teaspoon paprika
1 tablespoon coconut oil

In a dry skillet over medium heat, gently toast pine nuts and walnuts until fragrant and starting to change color. Quickly remove from skillet. In a small bowl, whisk mustard, vinegar, and lemon juice, then slowly whisk in olive oil for a creamy consistency.

Separate endive leaves and place them on a plate. Pour dressing and nuts over the salad. Scatter beets over it and garnish with fresh parsley.

Season flounder with salt, pepper, and paprika. In a sauté pan large enough to hold fish in one layer, heat coconut oil and cook flounder over medium-low heat until it flakes easily, 3 to 4 minutes. Plate along with salad and serve.

Olive Baked Salmon
Serves 4

4 salmon fillets (about 3 ounces each)
½ teaspoon salt
½ teaspoon pepper
½ cup chopped brined or oil-cured black olives
½ garlic clove, finely chopped
1 teaspoon fresh dill, finely chopped
½ cup organic vegetable broth
1 teaspoon honey
Juice of 1 lemon

Preheat oven to 450 degrees. Season salmon with salt and pepper. Combine black olives, garlic, dill, broth, honey, and lemon juice in a shallow casserole dish. Arrange salmon fillets in a single layer. Bake 10 minutes, until fish is opaque throughout.

Broiled Snapper with Lime
Serves 4

4 snapper fillets (about 1 pound)
½ teaspoon salt
½ teaspoon pepper
2 tablespoons pumpkin seed oil
1 tablespoon spicy sesame oil
¼ cup fresh lime juice

Season snapper on both sides with salt and pepper. Combine pumpkin seed and sesame oils, mixing to blend well. Spread a generous 2 teaspoons over each fish fillet.

Preheat broiler. Broil fish 4 to 6 inches from heat, about 5 minutes or until fish flakes easily. Remove and drizzle lime juice. Serve with brown rice.

Baked Halibut Fillets with Garlic and Chopped Celery
Serves 4

4 halibut fillets (about 1 pound)
2 tablespoons avocado oil
⅛ teaspoon rosemary
½ teaspoon salt
½ teaspoon pepper
1 tablespoon lime juice
1 onion, thinly sliced
1 celery stalk, coarsely chopped
¼ clove garlic, minced

Preheat oven to 375 degrees. Arrange fish fillets in a casserole dish in a single layer. Coat fish with 1 tablespoon of oil and season with rosemary, salt, and pepper. Pour lime juice over halibut. Toss onion, celery and garlic with remaining avocado oil then scatter on top of fish. Bake for 10 minutes, until cooked throughout.

Barbecue Haddock
Serves 4

1 teaspoon thyme
1 teaspoon paprika
1 teaspoon oregano
1 teaspoon garlic powder
¼ teaspoon salt
½ teaspoon black pepper
¼ teaspoon cayenne pepper
4 haddock fillets
1 tablespoon grapeseed oil

In a small bowl, combine spices, salt, and pepper. Mix well. Pat seasoning mixture into fish fillets using the heel of hand. In a large cast iron skillet, heat oil and tilt pan to coat bottom. Add fish fillets and cook over medium heat, turning once, until browned on both sides, about 6 to 8 minutes.

Spiced Roast Chicken with Watercress Salad
Serves 4

½ teaspoon paprika
½ teaspoon ground black pepper
½ teaspoon kosher salt
3 tablespoons coconut crystals or brown sugar
2 tablespoons chili powder
2 tablespoons saffron
1 chicken, 4 to 5 lbs.
2 bunches watercress, chopped
1 head romaine lettuce, chopped
½ cup broccoli sprouts
2 cucumbers, sliced thinly
½ cup Ginger Vinaigrette (see page 284)

Preheat oven to 325 degrees. Combine black pepper, paprika, salt, brown sugar, chili powder, and saffron to make a dry rub. Season chicken with the rub, arrange it on a rack in a roasting pan, and loosely cover it with aluminum foil. Roast until juices are clear and meat thermometer reads 160 degrees, about 1 hour or 15 minutes per pound.

Arrange watercress, lettuce, sprouts and cucumbers on a serving platter and top which chicken meat removed from the bone. Drizzle with Ginger Vinaigrette.

Orange Fennel Roast Chicken and Baked Garlic Yucca Fries

Serves 4

1 orange
1 chicken, 4 to 5 lbs.
2 tablespoons extra-virgin olive oil
½ teaspoon salt
½ teaspoon freshly ground black pepper
½ teaspoon oregano
1 teaspoon fresh rosemary, chopped
1 teaspoon fennel seeds
1 medium fennel bulb

For the fries
1 yucca
extra-virgin olive oil
kosher salt
freshly ground black pepper
½ teaspoon garlic powder

Arrange oven racks to accommodate roasting pan and baking sheet below. Preheat oven to 325 degrees. Grate orange zest and cut orange into 4 wedges. Rub chicken with an orange wedge, then coat chicken with olive oil and rub with salt, pepper, oregano, rosemary, and fennel seeds. Thinly slice fennel and chop a handful of fennel fronds. Stuff chicken with fennel and remaining orange wedges.

Arrange chicken on a rack in a roasting pan. Roast until juices are clear and meat thermometer reads 160 degrees, about 1 hour or 15 to 20 minutes per pound.

Peel and cut yucca into thin strips. Coat with olive oil and add salt, pepper, and garlic powder. Spray a baking sheet with cooking spray and place yucca strips on it in a single layer. Bake 10 to 15 minutes or until golden brown, and serve alongside the chicken.

Coconut Curry Chicken and Brown Rice
Serves 4

2 cups water
1 cup brown rice
1 teaspoon salt
3 tablespoons coconut oil
2 teaspoons curry powder
1 13 ½ ounce can coconut milk
4 skinless, boneless chicken breasts
1 teaspoon allspice
kosher salt
freshly ground black pepper
½ cup cilantro, chopped (optional)

Bring 2 cups of water to boil in large pot. Add brown rice and salt. Lower heat, cover, and allow rice to simmer for 45 minutes. Fluff rice with fork.

Heat 1 tablespoon of coconut oil in a small saucepan. Add curry powder and stir for 1 minute. Add coconut milk and simmer until liquid is reduced by half.

In a large, heavy skillet heat 2 tablespoons of coconut oil. Then add chicken, allspice, salt, and pepper. Once chicken is cooked, cut into thin strips. Combine coconut curry sauce and chicken and stir. Garnish chicken with cilantro, if desired. Serve with a bed of rice and enjoy!

Chicken and Moroccan Brown Rice Pilaf

Serves 4

4 chicken breasts, cut into bite-size pieces
kosher salt
freshly ground black pepper
½ teaspoon ground coriander (reserve ¼ teaspoon for rice)
2 tablespoons coconut oil
1 clove garlic, minced
½ teaspoon organic cinnammon
¼ teaspoon cumin
1 cup long-grain brown rice
2 cups chicken stock
1 teaspoon honey
¼ cup dried apricots, chopped
¼ cup fresh cilantro, minced
½ cup sliced almonds, chopped pistachios, or a combination

Toss chicken breast chunks with salt, pepper, and coriander to season thoroughly. In a Dutch oven or deep skillet with a tight-fitting lid, heat 1 tablespoon coconut oil over medium heat and sauté chicken until lightly browned on most sides. (It doesn't need to be completely cooked.) Remove chicken from the pan and set aside.

If pan is dry, add remaining coconut oil. Over low heat, gently sauté garlic (don't let it burn) then add cinnamon, cumin, and rice, stirring until rice is coated. Add stock, honey, and apricots and raise the heat. Bring to a boil, then lower the heat, cover, and simmer for 30 minutes. Uncover pot, quickly add chicken along with any juices that have accumulated, and cover the pot again. Simmer for an additional 10 to 15 minutes or until stock has all been absorbed.

Just before serving, fold in chopped cilantro and nuts, saving some of each to sprinkle on top.

Chicken and Vegetable Casserole
Serves 6

4 tablespoons ghee butter
2 cups unsweetened almond milk
1 cup sour cream
3 cups shredded cooked chicken
1 teaspoon rosemary
1 teaspoon thyme
¼ teaspoon kosher salt
¼ teaspoon freshly ground black pepper
2 cups small broccoli florets
1 cup yellow summer squash, cut into quarter-inch slices
1 cup zucchini, cut into quarter-inch slices
1 cup grated carrots
1 tablespoon Parmesan cheese
¼ cup bread crumbs

Preheat oven to 350 degrees. Heat butter in a large saucepan. Whisk in almond milk and sour cream until thickened.

In a large bowl, combine chicken, rosemary, thyme, salt, pepper, and vegetables. Add butter and cream mixture and mix well. Transfer to a baking dish and sprinkle with Parmesan cheese and bread crumbs.

Bake until filling is bubbling and bread crumbs are golden 20 to 25 minutes.

Sesame Chicken with Broccoli and Brown Rice

Serves 4

1 ½ cups brown rice
¼ cup sesame seeds
¼ cup almonds
¼ cup grapeseed oil
3 boneless chicken breasts, cubed
1 tablespoon sesame oil
1 teaspoon ground ginger
½ tablespoon brown sugar
¼ teaspoon kosher salt
¼ teaspoon freshly ground black pepper
⅓ cup light soy sauce
1 teaspoon honey
2 bunches of broccoli

In a medium saucepan, combine rice with 3 ½ cups of water. Bring to a boil, then cover, lower heat, and simmer gently for 45 minutes.

In a large, dry, preheated skillet, toast first seeds and then almonds, stirring constantly and removing from the pan as soon as they start to color. Chop almonds finely, and set seeds and nuts aside.

In the same skillet, heat grapeseed oil over medium heat. Sauté the chicken cubes, turning, until they are lightly browned and cooked through. In a small bowl, combine ground ginger, brown sugar, salt, pepper, soy sauce, and honey. Add to the chicken, stirring to coat and warm through. Remove from the heat, drizzle with sesame oil, and sprinkle with sesame seeds and almonds.

Rinse broccoli and cut into florets. Steam and add over a bed of brown rice.

Saffron Chicken with Sesame Green Beans and Spelt
Serves 4

1 cup spelt
3 tablespoons grapeseed oil
4 boneless chicken breasts
½ teaspoon kosher salt
½ teaspoon freshly ground black pepper
2 teaspoons fresh ginger, grated
4 cloves garlic, minced
¼ cup chopped scallions
¼ cup chopped onions
1 teaspoon saffron
1 pound fresh green beans
1 teaspoon extra-virgin olive oil
1 tablespoon sesame seeds, toasted

In a medium saucepan, combine spelt with 3 cups of water. Bring to a boil, cover, then lower heat and simmer for 90 minutes.

Heat grapeseed oil in a large pan over medium heat. Season chicken with salt and pepper, then brown it in the pan. Once chicken is browned, add ginger, garlic, scallions, onions, and saffron. Cover pan with a lid and let it simmer over low heat for 12 to 15 minutes. Add parsley in the last 5 minutes of cooking.

Steam green beans. Drain beans, drizzle olive oil over them. Top with toasted sesame seeds. Serve saffron chicken next to a bed of spelt topped with sesame green beans.

Chicken Breast in Curry Yogurt

Serves 4

4 skinless, boneless chicken breasts
¼ teaspoon kosher salt
¼ teaspoon freshly ground pepper
1 cup low-fat Greek yogurt
1 teaspoon onion powder
1 teaspoon garlic powder
1 teaspoon yellow mustard
1 tablespoon curry powder
½ cup bread crumbs

Preheat oven to 350 degrees. Season chicken breasts with salt and pepper.

Combine yogurt and seasonings in a bowl and mix. Spread yogurt mixture on both sides of chicken, coat each piece in bread crumbs, and arrange on a lightly greased or parchment-paper-lined baking dish.

Bake for 25 to 30 minutes. Turn on broiler. Broil chicken for 2 minutes, turning once, until bread crumbs are toasted.

Rosemary Baked Chicken with Pineapple Rice and Cauliflower
Serves 4

For the rice
1 cup whole grain brown rice
1½ cups water
1 cup pineapple juice
dash of salt

2 boneless, skinless chicken breasts
½ cup Balsamic Vinaigrette (see page 284)
dried rosemary

For the cauliflower
3 to 4 cups cauliflower florets
¼ teaspoon nutmeg

Preheat oven to 350 degrees. In a medium saucepan, combine 1 cup of rice, water, pineapple juice, and salt. Bring to a boil, cover, lower heat and simmer about 40 to 45 minutes.

Place chicken breasts in an oven-safe baking dish and pour vinaigrette over chicken. Sprinkle with a generous amount of rosemary, then bake 25 to 30 minutes or until chicken is cooked through.

Sprinkle cauliflower with nutmeg and steam for 8 to 10 minutes or until cauliflower is soft.

Slice chicken. Fold cauliflower into rice. Arrange slices of chicken on a bed of rice and serve.

Tangy Barbecue Chicken
Serves 2 (Serves 4 with sides)

1 2½-pound chicken, quartered
1 tablespoon sesame oil
4 tablespoons tomato paste
2 garlic cloves, minced
2 tablespoons Worcestershire sauce
2 tablespoons rice wine vinegar
2 tablespoons Dijon or yellow mustard
1 teaspoon honey
dash of cayenne

Rinse chicken pieces and pat dry. In a medium bowl, combine oil, tomato paste, garlic, Worcestershire, vinegar, mustard, honey, and cayenne. Stir to mix well. Add chicken pieces and turn to coat. Marinate at room temperature, turning once or twice, for 30 to 60 minutes.

Prepare a medium-hot fire in a grill, or preheat boiler. Set chicken about 6 inches from heat. Grill or broil and turn, basting with marinade every 10 minutes, until browned outside and light to the bone but still moist, about 25 minutes.

Stir-Fried Chicken with Eggplant and Onion
Serves 4

3 skinless, boneless chicken breasts
1 medium eggplant
1 medium onion
3 scallions
1 teaspoon arrowroot starch
¼ cup organic vegetable broth
¼ cup rice vinegar
1 tablespoon mustard
¼ cup coconut oil
1 teaspoon grated fresh ginger
1 teaspoon salt

Cut chicken crosswise on the diagonal into very thin slices. Cut eggplant lengthwise in half, then crosswise into thin slices. Cut onion into thin 1 ½-inch strips. Slice 2 scallions (chop one scallion and set aside).

In a small bowl, dissolve arrowroot starch in vegetable broth and rice vinegar, then stir in mustard. Set sauce aside.

Heat a wok or large skillet until hot. Add oil and heat until shimmering. Add chicken and stir-fry 2 minutes, separating slices. Add eggplant, onion, scallions, ginger, and salt. Cook over high heat, tossing constantly, until chicken is white throughout and vegetables are crisp-tender, 2 to 3 minutes.

Stir sauce and add to pan. Cook, stirring, until sauce thickens and coats chicken and vegetables, 1 to 2 minutes. Plate and garnish with chopped scallions. Serve and enjoy!

Herb Roasted Turkey Breast with Mustard Caper Sauce
Serves 4

1 whole bone-in turkey breast (6 to 7 pounds)
1 tablespoon fresh rosemary leaves, chopped
2 to 3 fresh basil leaves, finely chopped
1 tablespoon minced garlic
2 tablespoons extra-virgin olive oil
2 tablespoons freshly squeezed lemon juice
1 teaspoon kosher salt
1 teaspoon freshly ground black pepper
1 ½ pounds fresh broccoli, cut into small pieces
1 pound baby carrots

For the sauce
½ cup dry white wine
½ cup sour cream
2 teaspoons Dijon mustard
2 tablespoons ghee butter
¼ tablespoon capers, drained

Preheat oven to 325 degrees. Arrange turkey breast in a roasting pan. Combine herbs, garlic, olive oil, and lemon juice and rub all over turkey breast, then sprinkle with salt and pepper. Roast skin side up and roast 1 ½ to 2 hours until the skin is golden brown and a meat thermometer reads 160 degrees. Remove from oven and let rest.

Steam broccoli and carrots.

In a small saucepan, bring wine to boil until reduced by half. Whisk in sour cream, mustard, ghee butter, and capers, and simmer until slightly thickened.

Carve turkey breast and serve, drizzling mustard caper sauce over turkey and vegetables.

Wine-Braised Lamb and Vegetables
Serves 4

2 tablespoons extra-virgin olive oil
5 garlic cloves, peeled
3 to 4 pounds lamb breast with bone
kosher salt
black pepper
3 cups dry white wine
1 tablespoon chopped fresh sage

½ cup fresh or frozen corn kernels
½ cup fresh or frozen green peas
1 cup baby carrots
1 cup cauliflower florets

In a Dutch oven, heat olive oil and sauté garlic cloves until just barely golden. Increase heat to high, season lamb with salt and pepper, then brown each side. Add white wine and fresh sage. Reduce heat to low and cover. Cook lamb until tender, 2 ½ to 3 hours. Transfer the lamb to a cutting board with rib bones facing up and carve around the bone to remove meat. Skim fat from cooking juices. Add vegetables and lamb to pot and return to heat for 5 to 6 minutes.

Sesame Pork Tenderloin and Pine Nut Salad

Serves 4

1 pound pork tenderloin, trimmed
¼ cup extra-virgin olive oil
½ teaspoon kosher salt
½ teaspoon freshly ground black pepper
1 teaspoon ground ginger
1 teaspoon ground cumin
¼ cup sesame seeds

For the salad
1 pound brussels sprouts
½ small red cabbage
4 cups organic chicken broth
½ cup pine nuts
½ red onion, chopped
1 cup shredded carrots
¼ cup sweetened dried cranberries

Preheat oven to 425 degrees. Set pork in a shallow roasting pan or ovenproof skillet. Coat pork with olive oil. Combine salt, pepper, ginger, cumin, and sesame seeds and rub into the pork tenderloin all over. Roast in oven until a meat thermometer reads 145 degrees, about 20 minutes.

Boil brussels sprouts and cabbage in chicken broth until tender, then drain, and set aside. Toast pine nuts in a small pan. Combine cabbage, brussels sprouts, nuts, onions, carrots, and cranberries. Drizzle with Classic Vinaigrette (see page 285) or Aloe Dressing (see page 285). Serve sliced tenderloin on a bed of dressed vegetables.

Eggplant and Lentil Stew

Serves 4

1 large eggplant
½ cup green lentils
1 small Spanish onion, finely diced
4 garlic cloves, minced
2 tomatoes, chopped
2 green chili peppers, seeded and chopped
2 tablespoons mint leaves, chopped
1 tablespoon tomato paste
¼ teaspoon crushed red pepper flakes
2 teaspoons salt
¾ cup extra-virgin olive oil
4 tablespoons of pomegranate molasses

Preheat oven to 350 degrees. Peel and cut eggplant into ½-inch rounds and sprinkle with salt.

In a mixing bowl, combine lentils, onions, garlic, tomatoes, chilies, mint, tomato paste, crushed red pepper flakes, and salt.

Rinse salt from eggplant and pat dry. Add to vegetable mixture and mix well.

Coat a large gratin dish with olive oil and transfer eggplant mixture along with 1 ½ cups of water. Drizzle olive oil over mixture and pour pomegranate molasses over eggplant mix. Cover with foil and bake for 1 ½ hours. Remove foil and bake for an additional 30 minutes uncovered.

Ziti with Zucchini

Serves 3

1 large yellow onion, cut into thin wedges
1 cup fresh celery, sliced thin diagonally
3 cloves garlic, coarsely chopped
1 tablespoon extra-virgin olive oil
1 teaspoon dried thyme
freshly ground black pepper and salt to taste
½ pound whole grain or vegetable ziti
1 sliced zucchini
¾ cup ricotta cheese, at room temperature
1 14.5-ounce can tomatoes, coarsely chopped and drained
⅓ cup roasted pickled okra, rinsed, drained, and diced (optional)
2 tablespoons grated Parmesan cheese

Preheat oven to 350 degrees. In a large, shallow baking dish (about 2-quart size), combine onion, celery, garlic, and oil. Sprinkle with thyme, salt, and pepper, and stir to blend. Bake, stirring occasionally, until vegetables are tender and begin to brown, about 25 minutes.

Cook ziti until just al dente. Reserving ½ cup of cooking liquid, drain pasta and set aside.

In a large bowl, combine zucchini, ricotta, tomatoes, okra, ziti, and cooking liquid. Pour into baking dish with onion and celery. Stir gently to blend and sprinkle with Parmesan. Cover with foil and bake until ingredients are just warmed through, about 15 minutes. Remove foil and bake until top is lightly browned, about 10 minutes more.

Fettuccine Alfredo
Serves 2

½ pound whole grain or vegetable fettuccine
1 tablespoon unsalted butter or ghee, melted
¼ cup low-fat Greek yogurt
2 tablespoons light cream
3 tablespoons grated Parmesan cheese
2 tablespoons grated mozzarella cheese
¼ teaspoon salt
crushed red pepper flakes to taste

Bring a large pot filled with salted water to a boil. Add fettuccine and cook until tender but still firm, 3 to 4 minutes. Reserve ¼ cup cooking liquid, then drain fettuccine. In a mixing bowl, stir together butter, reserved cooking liquid, yogurt, and cream. Add fettucine, Parmesan cheese, mozzarella cheese, salt, and red pepper flakes, and toss.

Rigatoni with Pesto Tomato Sauce
Serves 2

1 tablespoon extra-virgin olive oil
½ cup chopped onion
1 tablespoon tomato paste
1 tablespoon anchovy paste or 2 flat anchovy fillets, rinsed, dried, and chopped
1 cup canned chopped tomatoes with purée
¼ cup bottled or homemade Pesto Sauce (see page 282)
½ pound whole grain or vegetable rigatoni
½ cup grated Parmesan cheese (reserve 2 teaspoons)
2 tablespoons basil, chopped
pinch crushed red pepper flakes

Heat oil in a skillet and cook onions on low until clear and increase heat to slightly caramelize. Add tomato paste and anchovy paste. Stir to coat the onions for 2 minutes. Add canned chopped tomatoes with purée and as much of the pesto as desired. Simmer for 10 minutes.

Add water and salt to a large pot and bring to a boil. While sauce simmers, cook the pasta. Drain cooked pasta and mix in with sauce. Top with grated parmesan and chopped fresh basil. Sprinkle with red pepper flakes.

Easy Salmon Pesto Pasta
Serves 2

½ pound whole grain or vegetable conchiglie or other shell pasta
1 6.5-ounce can water-packed organic salmon
3 teaspoons chopped almonds
¼ cup Pesto Sauce (see below)

Bring a large pot filled with salted water to a boil. Cook pasta until tender but still firm. Reserve ¼ cup cooking liquid, then drain pasta. In a large serving bowl, toss together salmon and almonds. Add pesto sauce and reserved cooking liquid and mix well. Add pasta and toss to coat.

Halibut and Broccoli over Pasta
Serves 3

½ pound whole grain or vegetable penne pasta
1 cup broccoli florets
grapeseed oil
2 to 3 halibut fillets
1 cup low-fat Greek yogurt
¼ cup chopped scallions
½ cup grated mozzarella cheese
dash of salt

In a large pot, boil water with salt. Cook pasta according to the package directions, adding broccoli florets to pasta cooking water about 3 minutes before pasta is done. Drain and return it to the pot.

Lightly coat stainless steel pan with grapeseed oil. Cook halibut fillets in pan for 3 minutes on each side.

Stir pan-seared halibut into pot of drained pasta and broccoli. Toss over low heat, breaking up fish. In a medium bowl, mix yogurt and scallions together. Add to pasta, halibut, and broccoli, stirring well. Top with mozzarella cheese and serve warm.

Pesto Sauce

2 cups fresh basil leaves
4 garlic cloves
½ cup Italian parsley leaves
½ cup extra-virgin olive oil
¼ cup grated Parmesan cheese
¼ teaspoon salt
¼ teaspoon pepper

In a food processor or blender, combine basil, garlic, and parsley and whirl to chop. Add olive oil, Parmesan cheese, salt, and pepper. Process until fairly smooth. Use pesto at once, refrigerate for up to two days, or pack into clean 4- or 8-ounce jars, cover tightly with lids, and freeze to use as needed.

Dressings, Dips, and Spreads

Creamy Honey Mustard Dressing
Makes about ½ to ¾ cup

½ cup low-fat Greek yogurt
¼ teaspoon dry mustard
1 tablespoon honey
dash of garlic powder
¼ teaspoon salt
⅛ teaspoon black pepper

Whisk together. Thin with water if desired.

Horseradish Dressing
Makes about a cup

4 tablespoons wheat germ oil
½ cup extra-virgin olive oil
4 tablespoons fresh lime juice
2 teaspoons coconut crystals
½ teaspoon grated nutmeg
2 tablespoons horseradish
½ teaspoon salt
1 clove garlic, minced

Combine all ingredients except garlic in a bowl or electric blender. Mix vigorously. Pour into a container and add garlic. Refrigerate and shake before each use. Discard dressing mix after one week.

Balsamic Vinaigrette

Makes about a cup

¼ cup balsamic vinegar
½ cup extra-virgin olive oil
1 clove garlic, sliced or minced
½ teaspoon salt
1 tablespoon chopped fresh thyme
1 tablespoon scallions

Combine all ingredients in a bottle. Shake and chill. Discard dressing mix after 1 week.

Ginger Vinaigrette

Makes about ¾ cup

¼ cup fresh lime juice
¼ teaspoon brown sugar
½ teaspoon kosher salt
2 teaspoons finely grated ginger
¼ teaspoon freshly ground black pepper
½ cup extra-virgin olive oil

In a bowl, whisk together lime juice, brown sugar, and salt in a small bowl until completely blended. Add ginger, black pepper, and olive oil.

Classic Vinaigrette

Makes about ¾ cup

1 teaspoon Dijon mustard
¼ cup red wine vinegar
½ cup extra-virgin olive oil
2 tablespoons minced tarragon or cilantro (optional)
¼ teaspoon freshly ground black pepper
½ teaspoon kosher salt

Mix all ingredients well.

Aloe Dressing

Makes about a quarter cup

2 tablespoons extra-virgin olive oil
2 tablespoons balsamic vinegar
2 tablespoons aloe vera gel (Lily of the Desert)
1 teaspoon lecithin granules

Combine olive oil, balsamic vinegar, aloe gel, and lecithin granules.

Avocado and Cheese Spread

Makes about 2 cups (depends on size of avocado)

1 large ripe avocado, peeled and pitted
1 cup low-fat Greek yogurt
1 tablespoon wheat germ or brewer's yeast
1 tablespoon fresh lime juice
1 teaspoon chopped scallions
2 tablespoons cottage cheese
¼ teaspoon salt

In a food processor or by hand, mash avocado then combine with the other ingredients and mix well.

Garlic Cheese Spread

Makes about 1⅓ cups

½ cup cottage cheese
2 tablespoons low-fat Greek yogurt
1 clove garlic
¼ cup chopped pimento
½ cup pitted green olives, chopped
½ teaspoon Worcestershire sauce
¼ teaspoon nutmeg
¼ teaspoon salt

Mash cottage cheese and yogurt together to create a smooth paste. Put garlic through garlic press and stir into mixture. Add remaining ingredients and blend thoroughly.

Mediterranean Vegetarian Spread

Makes about 3 cups

1 cup chopped zucchini
1 cup chopped eggplant
2 tablespoons extra-virgin olive oil
⅓ cup cooked chickpeas
1 tomato, peeled, seeded, and diced
¼ cup scallions
⅓ cup low-fat sour cream
1 cup feta cheese, crumbled
2 tablespoons fresh basil
½ teaspoon dried oregano

Preheat oven to 375 degrees. Toss zucchini and eggplant with 1 tablespoon olive oil. Place zucchini and eggplant on pan and bake for 30 minutes. Let cool slightly. Transfer to a food processor along with remaining 1 tablespoon olive oil and all other ingredients and process until smooth and spreadable.

Vegetarian Spread

Makes 2 cups

1 cup organic cottage cheese
¼ cup low-fat Greek yogurt
¼ cup onions or scallions, chopped
¼ cup chopped apple
¼ cup chopped celery
¼ cup chopped red bell pepper
1 tablespoon chopped pimento
salt and pepper to taste

Mix all ingredients well. Let spread sit for 10 minutes to allow flavors to come out.

Three Cs Dip

Makes 1 ⅔ cups

1 cup low-fat Greek yogurt
4 tablespoons ghee butter
½ teaspoon curry powder
½ teaspoon caraway seeds, toasted
2 teaspoons finely chopped fresh cilantro
1 tablespoon ground nutmeg
1 teaspoon salt

Blend yogurt and butter together until soft and creamy. Mix remaining ingredients together. Refrigerate at least 1 hour to allow flavors to blend. Bring to room temperature before serving.

Summary of Gene Therapy Foods and Health Benefits

Weight Management	Heart Disease	Cancer	Diabetes	Aging
Aloe vera	Almonds	Beets	Aloe	Bok choy
Asparagus	Apples	Blueberries	Bay leaves	Carrots
Celery	Blueberries	Carrots	Black beans	Collard
Curry powder	Brazil nuts	Cooked	Blueberry and	greens
Flounder	Brown rice	tomatoes	grape juice	Corn
Grapefruit	Chicken	Cruciferous	Broccoli	Cruciferous
Miso soup	Coldwater fish	vegetables	Cashew nuts	vegetables
Romaine lettuce	Cranberries	Curry powder	Coldwater fish	Green tea
Wheatgrass	Cruciferous	Garlic	Cruciferous	Kale
Yogurt	vegetables	Ginger	vegetables	Lettuce
	Flaxseeds	Olive oil	Curry powder	Mangoes
	Kale	Rosemary	Olive oil	Olive oil
	Lentils	Walnuts	Omega-3 fatty	Romaine
	Oats		acids walnuts	Spinach
	Olive oil		Onions	Squash
	Pecans		Sesame seeds	Sweet
			Soybeans	potatoes

Weight Management	Heart Disease	Cancer	Diabetes	Aging
	Pumpkin seeds		Spinach	Tomatoes
	Purple plums		Steel-cut oats	Whole grains
	Quinoa		Tomatoes	Yucca
	Red cabbage		Whole grains	Zucchini
	Scallions		Yucca	
	Sesame seeds			
	Sunflower seeds			
	Tomatoes			
	Walnuts			
	Watercress			
	Yellow or red onions			

Sleep	Healthy Hair	Healthy Skin	Prostate	Urinary Tract	Liver Support
Aloe vera	Chicken	Apricots	Basil leaves	Black raspberries	Blueberries
Asparagus	Eggs	Brazil nuts	Blueberries	Celery	Brazil nuts
Celery	Greek yogurt	Green tea	Brussels sprouts	Cranberries	Grapes
Curry powder	Kale	Peas	Cilantro	Garlic	Kale
Flounder	Lentils	Plums	Dandelion leaves	Greek yogurt with kefir cultures	Lentils
Grapefruit	Pumpkins and squash	Salmon	Linseed oil	Oregano	Olive oil
Miso soup	Salmon	Spinach	Miso	Parsley	Pumpkin seeds
Romaine lettuce	Shrimp	Walnuts	Rosemary	Peaches	Salmon
Wheatgrass	Strawberries	Water—eight glasses per day	Thyme	Thyme	Turmeric
Yogurt	Walnuts		Tofu	Wheatgrass	Wheatgrass
			Watercress		

Calcium	Omega-3	URI & Fighting Infection	Preventing Food and Chemical Sensitivities	Combating Fatigue
Almonds	Arugula	Almonds	Apples	Cashews
Dried figs	Basil	Edible camphor	Bananas	Dark
Greek yogurt	Cod	Garlic	Brown rice	chocolate
Kale	Flaxseed oil	Ginger	Garlic	Ginger
Oatmeal	Haddock	Turmeric	Greek yogurt with	Greek yogurt
Salmon	Oregano	powder	kefir cultures	with kefir
Sardines	Salmon		Leeks	cultures
Sesame seeds	Walnuts		Raw asparagus	Green tea
Soybeans	Watercress		Sprouted whole	Pumpkin
Tofu	Wheat germ		grain bread	seeds
	oil		Sweet potatoes	Red bell
			Winter squash	peppers
				Steel-cut
				oatmeal
				Watermelon
				Wheatgrass
				juice

Gene Therapy Foods and Corresponding Recipes

Ingredients	Disease focus	Recipes
Almonds	Heart disease	Recipes include raw almonds, almond milk and almond butter: Almond Butter Smoothie Almond Butter Waffles Almond Caesar Salad with Grilled Chicken Aloe juice Arugula and Peach Salad Berrylicious Smoothie Blueberry Banana Cottage Cheese with Almonds Coconut Cream and Almond Smoothie Coconut milk Cucumber Curry Ginger Soup Easy Salmon Pesto Pasta Mango, Spinach, and Feta Cheese Salad Nutty Papaya Yogurt Sesame Chicken with Broccoli and Brown Rice Steel-Cut Oatmeal and Fresh Berries Triple Chocolate Smoothie

Ingredients	Disease focus	Recipes
Aloe	Weight management Diabetes	Aloe Juice Coconut Cream and Almond Smoothie Aloe Dressing
Apples	All areas	ABC Smoothie Apple Ginger Juice Avocado Kale Smoothie Carrot Kale Wheatgrass Juice Chicken, Apple, and Watercress Salad Fruit Smoothie Go Green Smoothie Spiced Apple Smoothie Vegetarian Spread
Asparagus	Weight management	Fresh Asparagus Soup Red Snapper with Red Potatoes and Asparagus
Bay leaves	Diabetes	Manhattan Shrimp Chowder Vegetable Soup
Beets	Cancer	ABC Smoothie Acai Berry Juice Flounder and Endive Nut Salad Spiced Apple Smoothie Sweet Beet Salad
Blueberries	Heart disease Cancer Diabetes	Almond Butter Smoothie Berrylicious Smoothie Blueberry Banana Cottage Cheese with Almonds Blueberry Coconut Juice Kiwi Berry Smoothie Orange Berry Slushie
Brown rice	Heart disease	Broiled Snapper with Lime Chicken and Moroccan Brown Rice Pilaf Coconut Curry Chicken and Brown Rice Rosemary Baked Chicken with Pineapple Rice and Cauliflower Sesame Chicken with Broccoli and Brown Rice
Carrots	Cancer Aging	ABC Smoothie Acai Berry Juice Arugula and Peach Salad Carrot Kale Wheatgrass Juice

Ingredients	Disease focus	Recipes
Carrots	Cancer Aging	Chicken and Vegetable Casserole
		Herb Roasted Turkey Breast with Mustard Caper Sauce
		Kombu Chicken Soup
		Seitan Veggie Wrap
		Sesame Pork Tenderloin and Pine Nut Salad
		Vegetable Soup
		Wine-Braised Lamb and Vegetables
Celery	Weight management	Baked Halibut Fillets with Garlic and Chopped Celery
		Egg Salad Sandwich
		Go Green Smoothie
		Manhattan Shrimp Chowder
		Spiced Apple Smoothie
		Tomato Juice
		Vegetable Soup
		Winter Squash and Chickpea Soup
		Ziti with Zucchini
Chicken	Heart disease	Almond Caesar Salad with Grilled Chicken
		Chicken and Moroccan Brown Rice Pilaf
		Chicken and Vegetable Casserole
		Chicken Breast in Curry Yogurt
		Chicken, Apple and Watercress Salad
		Cobb Salad
		Coconut Curry Chicken and Brown Rice
		Kombu Chicken Soup
		Orange Fennel Roast Chicken and Baked Garlic Yucca Fries
		Rosemary Baked Chicken with Pineapple Rice and Cauliflower
		Saffron Chicken with Sesame Green Beans and Spelt
		Sesame Chicken with Broccoli and Brown Rice
		Spiced Roast Chicken with Watercress Salad
		Stir–Fried Chicken with Eggplant and Onion
		Tangy Barbecue Chicken Stir-Fried
		Thai Chicken Salad

Ingredients	Disease focus	Recipes
Coldwater fish	Heart disease	Baked Halibut Fillets with Garlic and Chopped Celery
		Barbecue Haddock
		Basil Salmon and Wild Rice
		Broiled Flounder with Sauteed Red Pepper and Quinoa
		Broiled Snapper with Lime
		Curried Red Snapper with Asian Pear Cabbage Slaw
		Flounder and Endive Nut Salad
		Ginger Salmon
		Olive Baked Salmon
Corn	Aging	Wine-Braised Lamb and Vegetables
Cranberries	Heart disease	Berrylicious Smoothie
		Mango, Spinach, and Feta Cheese Salad
		Sesame Pork Tenderloin and Pine Nut Salad
		Sweet Beet Salad
Cruciferous vegetables	All areas	**Arugula:**
		Go Green Salad with Aloe Dressing
		Arugula and Peach Salad
		Broccoli:
		Chicken and Vegetable Casserole
		Halibut and Broccoli over Pasta
		Herb Roasted Turkey Breast with Mustard Caper Sauce
		Sesame Chicken with Broccoli and Brown Rice
		Broccoli spouts:
		Arugula and Peach Salad
		Very Green Salad with Aloe Dressing
		Brussels sprouts:
		Sesame Pork Tenderloin and Pine Nut Salad

Ingredients	Disease focus	Recipes
Cruciferous vegetables	All areas	**Cabbage:** Curried Red Snapper with Asian Pear Cabbage Slaw Sesame Pork Tenderloin and Pine Nut Salad **Cauliflower:** Lemon Dill Halibut with Garlic Cauliflower Purée Rosemary Baked Chicken with Pineapple Rice and Cauliflower Wine-Braised Lamb and Vegetables **Horseradish:** Horseradish Dressing **Kale:** Avocado Kale Smoothie Carrot Kale Wheatgrass Juice Cilantro Kale Soup Very Green Salad with Aloe Dressing Go Green Smoothie Seitan Veggie Wrap **Watercress:** Chicken, Apple, and Watercress Salad Chunky Coconut Shake Spiced Apple Smoothie
Curry powder	Weight management Cancer Diabetes	Chicken Breast in Curry Yogurt Coconut Curry Chicken and Brown Rice Cucumber Curry Ginger Soup Curried Red Snapper with Asian Pear Cabbage Slaw Exotic Banana Pancakes
Flaxseeds	Heart disease	Aloe Juice
Flounder	Weight management	Broiled Flounder with Sauteed Red Pepper and Quinoa Flounder and Endive Nut Salad
Garlic	Cancer	Baked Halibut Fillets with Garlic and Chopped Celery Balsamic Vinaigrette

Ingredients	Disease focus	Recipes
Garlic	Cancer	Chicken and Moroccan Brown Rice
		Chicken Breast in Curry Yogurt
		Creamy Honey Mustard Dressing
		Curried Red Snapper with Asian Pear Cabbage Slaw
		Eggplant and Lentil Stew
		Fresh Asparagus Soup
		Garlic Cheese Spread
		Herb Roasted Turkey Breast with Mustard Caper Sauce
		Horseradish Dressing
		Lemon Dill Halibut with Garlic Cauliflower Purée
		Manhattan Shrimp Chowder
		Olive Baked Salmon
		Orange Fennel Roast Chicken and Baked Garlic Yucca Fries
		Pesto Sauce
		Rigatoni with Pesto Tomato Sauce
		Rosemary Baked Chicken with Pineapple Rice and Cauliflower
		Saffron Chicken with Sesame Green Beans and Spelt
		Tangy Barbecue Chicken
		Thai Chicken Salad
		Wine-Braised Lamb and Vegetables
		Winter Squash and Chickpea Soup
		Ziti with Zucchini
Ginger	Cancer	ABC Smoothie
		Apple Ginger Juice
		Basil Tomato Juice
		Carrot Kale Wheatgrass Juice
		Chinese Egg Drop Soup
		Chocolate Super Waffles
		Citrus Juice
		Cucumber Curry Ginger Soup
		Ginger Vinaigrette
		Go Green Smoothie
		Red Snapper with Red Potatoes and Asparagus
		Saffron Chicken with Sesame Green Beans and Spelt
		Sesame Chicken with Broccoli and Brown Rice

Ingredients	Disease focus	Recipes
Ginger	Cancer	Sesame Pork Tenderloin and Pine Nut Salad
		Stir-Fried Chicken with Eggplant and Onion
Grape juice (or blueberry juice)	Diabetes	Acai Grape Juice
Grapefruit	Weight management	Acai Grape Juice
Green tea	Aging	Acai Berry Juice
		Coftea Smoothie
		Kiwi Berry Smoothie
Kale	Heart disease	Avocado Kale Smoothie
	Aging	Carrot Kale Wheatgrass Juice
		Cilantro Kale Soup
		Go Green Smoothie
		Very Green Salad with Aloe Dressing
Lentils	Heart disease	Eggplant and Lentil Stew
Lettuce	Weight management	Almond Caesar Salad with Grilled Chicken
		Cobb Salad
	Aging	Egg Salad Sandwich
		Go Green Smoothie
		Sweet Beet Salad
		Thai Chicken Salad
		Turkey and Cheese Sandwich
		Very Green Salad with Aloe Dressing
Mangoes	Aging	Mango, Spinach, and Feta Cheese Salad
Miso paste	Weight management	Kombu Chicken Soup
Oats	Heart disease	Steel-Cut Oatmeal with Fresh Berries
Olive oil	All areas	Aloe Dressing
		Basil Salmon and Wild Rice
		Broiled Flounder with Sauteed Red Pepper and Quinoa
		Classic Vinagrette
		Cod and Roasted Scallions
		Eggplant and Lentil Stew
		Flounder and Endive Nut Salad
		Ginger Vinaigrette

Ingredients	Disease focus	Recipes
Olive oil	All areas	Herb Roasted Turkey Breast with Mustard Caper Sauce
		Horseradish Dressing
		Lemon Dill Halibut with Garlic Cauliflower Purée
		Mediterranean Vegetarian Spread
		Orange Fennel Roast Chicken and Baked Garlic Yucca Fries
		Pesto Sauce
		Rigatoni with Pesto Tomato Sauce
		Sesame Pork Tenderloin and Pine Nut Salad
		Spicy Tabouleh
		Veggie Frittata
		Very Green Salad with Aloe Dressing
		Wine-BraisedLamb and Vegetables
		Ziti with Zucchini
Onions	Heart disease Diabetes	Baked Halibut Fillets with Garlic and Chopped Celery
		Breakfast Burrito
		Chicken Breast in Curry Yogurt
		Eggplant and Lentil Stew
		Manhattan Shrimp Chowder
		New England Clam Chowder
		Onion Soup
		Rigatoni with Pesto Tomato Sauce
		Saffron Chicken with Sesame Green Beans and Spelt
		Sesame Pork Tenderloin and Pine Nut Salad
		Spicy Tabouleh
		Stir-Fried Chicken with Eggplant and Onion
		Vegetarian Spread
		Veggie Frittata
		Winter Squash and Chickpea Soup
		Ziti with Zucchini
Pumpkin seeds	Heart disease	Broiled Snapper with Lime
Red cabbage	Heart disease	Curried Red Snapper with Asian Pear Cabbage Slaw
		Sesame Pork Tenderloin and Pine Nut Salad

Ingredients	Disease focus	Recipes
Romaine lettuce	Weight management	Cobb Salad
		Go Green Smoothie
		Sweet Beet Salad
		Thai Chicken Salad
		Turkey and Cheese Sandwich
		Very Green Salad with Aloe Dressing
Rosemary	Cancer	Baked Halibut Fillets with Garlic and Chopped Celery
		Chicken and Vegetable Casserole
		Herb Roasted Turkey Breast with Mustard Caper Sauce
		Red Snapper with Red Potatoes and Asparagus
		Roast Orange Chicken and Baked Garlic Yucca Fries
		Rosemary Baked Chicken with Pineapple Rice and Cauliflower
		Veggie Frittata
		Winter Squash and Chickpea Soup
Scallions	Heart disease	Avocado and Cheese Spread
		Balsamic Vinaigrette
		Breakfast Burrito
		Cod and Roasted Scallions
		Curried Red Snapper with Asian Pear Cabbage Slaw
		Fresh Pea Soup
		Halibut and Broccoli over Pasta
		Mediterranean Vegetarian Spread
		Saffron Chicken with Sesame Green Beans and Spelt
		Salmon Burgers
		Stir-Fried Chicken with Eggplant and Onion
		Turkey Avocado Wrap
		Vegetable Soup
		Vegetarian Spread
		Veggie Frittata

Ingredients	Disease focus	Recipes
Sesame seeds	Heart disease Diabetes	Broiled Snapper with Lime Red Snapper with Red Potatoes and Asparagus Saffron Chicken with Sesame Green Beans and Spelt Sesame Chicken with Broccoli and Brown Rice Sesame Pork Tenderloin and Pine Nut Salad Tangy Barbecue Chicken Yucca Juice
Spinach	Diabetes Aging	Mango, Spinach, and Feta Cheese Salad Tofu Spinach Salad with Pomegranate
Squash	Aging	Chicken and Vegetable Casserole
Steel-cut oats	Diabetes	Steel-Cut Oatmeal and Fresh Berries
Sunflower seeds	Heart disease	Acai Berry Juice
Tomatoes	Heart disease Cancer	Acai Berry Juice Basil Tomato Juice Cobb Salad Egg Salad Sandwich Eggplant and Lentil Stew Manhattan Shrimp Chowder Mediterranean Vegetarian Spread Rigatoni with Pesto Tomato Sauce Spicy Tabouleh Tangy Barbecue Chicken Thai Chicken Salad Tomato Juice Tomato Swiss Melt Vegetable Soup Ziti with Zucchini
Walnuts	Heart disease Cancer Diabetes	Chicken, Apple, and Watercress Salad Flounder and Endive Nut Salad Nutty Papaya Yogurt Sweet Beet Salad Tofu Spinach Salad with Pomegranate

Ingredients	Disease focus	Recipes
Watercress	Heart disease	Chicken, Apple and Watercress Salad Chunky Coconut Shake Spiced Apple Smoothie Spiced Roast Chicken with Watercress Salad
Wheatgrass	Weight management	Carrot Kale Wheatgrass Juice
Whole grains	All areas	**Bulgur:** Spicy Tabouleh **Oats:** Steel-Cut Oatmeal and Fresh Berries **Spelt:** Saffron Chicken with Sesame Green Beans and Spelt
Yogurt, Greek	All areas	Avocado and Cheese Spread Chicken Breast in Curry Yogurt Creamy Honey Mustard Dressing Egg Salad Sandwich Fettuccine Alfredo Fresh Asparagus Soup Fresh Pea Soup Garlic Cheese Spread Halibut and Broccoli over Pasta Nutty Papaya Yogurt Seitan Veggie Wrap Three Cs Dip Vegetarian Spread
Yucca	Diabetes Aging	Orange Fennel Chicken and Baked Garlic Yucca Fries Yucca Juice
Zucchini	Aging	Chicken and Vegetable Casserole Mediterranean Vegetarian Spread Ziti with Zucchini

Juicers and Other Resources

Juicers

Juicing is an important way to prevent and treat diseases. It extracts bioactive compounds in food and helps the body fight harmful environmental toxins. But juicing should also be a fun, exciting process that you look forward to. Here's some advice to help guide you.

I've been juicing for over twenty years, and in that time I've gone through many machines in my kitchen. The appliance section of a store can be overwhelming if you don't know what you want ahead of time, so I recommend first doing some research online. Should you buy a blender? Juicer? Food processor? Mixer?

I think the first step in your decision process should be to realize that there is no one best juicer—only the juicer that works best for your lifestyle. Here are a few factors to help you narrow down your choices:

Cost: What's your budget? Are you looking to keep the cost down or are you willing to spend hundreds of dollars on a juicer? Starting with a budget will help you narrow down your choices. But no matter what you end up with—a cost-effective or an expensive juicer—know that high-quality juicers exist at various price points, so everyone can afford to make natural, healthy juices at home.

Kitchen real estate: How much countertop or storage space do you have available? Do you want an upright or horizontal juicer? If you want juicing to become a daily part of your life, then consider buying a juicer you can store in plain view. Because if you can see your juicer, you're more likely to put it to good use.

Earplugs, anyone? A noisy juicer can be a deal breaker, so you may want to test for volume, especially if you plan on making your juice in the morning.

Versatility: Will you just be juicing? If not, you may want to look into a juicer that allows you the freedom to make other foods, like smoothies, sorbets, and nut butters.

There are five basic types of machines to choose from:

The Basic Blender

Blenders can be found in a price range that is easy on your budget. Unfortunately, blenders don't work best for juicing because a blender cannot separate the fiber and pulp from the juice. It may seem obvious, but it's important to stress that a blender chops and blends fruits and vegetables, which yields very different quantities and calories than a juicer. A blender uses everything you add in it. A juicer, in contrast, yields less because it removes all the fiber and pulp, leaving only the juice.

If you plan on using your blender for smoothies, pour the liquid ingredients in the blender first, which acts as a lubricant for the blades and helps make chopping the fruit and vegetables easier. Be sure to start at the lowest speed. Increase the speed slowly as you notice the chunks of fruit breaking up.

The Vitamix, a high-performing blender, gives juicers a run for their money. This kind of blender can offer you the versatility that a basic blender cannot. It mixes the juice with the pulp and fiber so you can reap the health benefits of the whole fruit or vegetable. It can be pricey, but it will last you a long time.

Manual Juicers

Hand-operated juicers are inexpensive, but they work best when juicing with either wheatgrass or citrus fruit. Otherwise, your juicing choices will be limited.

Centrifugal Juicers

These machines spin at high speeds to release the juice and extract the nutrients from fresh produce. Although they are inexpensive and the most commonly purchased type of juicer, they are less versatile than gear juicers. You may have to replace your centrifugal juicer often, because they don't have a long life span.

Single-Gear Juicers

These machines are affordable, highly functional juicers that shred and crush to ensure the optimal release of nutrients. This type of juicer is also versatile—you can make natural ice cream, nut butters, and fresh pasta.

Twin-Gear Juicers

These juicers pulverize produce and are considered to be top of the line. With two gears, they crush and grind fruits and vegetables at low speeds to yield the best nutrient content possible. Their high performance and versatility make them expensive, but they will last you a very long time.

Once you've made your choice, read the instructions carefully to ensure that you're handling your new machine with care. Get familiar enough with it that setup and cleanup become second nature.

Here are some additional tips for successful juicing.

Thoroughly wash your fruits and vegetables. Some may need to be peeled, while others need to have their peel intact for optimal nutrition. Most often you'll be chopping the produce into pieces so that it can fit into the juicer's chute. Depending on your machine, you may also have to remove apple cores.

Prepare the night before. Things can be rushed in the morning, so do your washing and chopping ahead of time. Store your ingredients in a ziplock bag or container in your refrigerator. That way, in the morning all you have to do is run your ingredients through the juicer. Or juice the night before and keep it in an airtight bottle so you can just grab it and go in the morning.

Keep it simple. Those processed juices and smoothies have a smorgasbord of ingredients. And while you may be excited to replicate a fresher version of your favorite store-bought juice, put on the brakes. Mixing too many ingredients together is a recipe for a natural juice disaster. The taste can be awful for the overzealous newbie juicer who mixes a variety of produce. Keep it to three types of produce for ease and an enjoyable flavor!

Clean your juicer ASAP! The longer pulp remnants and juices stay sitting in your juicer, the harder it'll be to clean things up.

Store leftover juice in an airtight container to keep it fresh. An airtight Tupperware or Mason jar will work just fine. Juicing creates a nutrient-rich product that is preservative-free, so it doesn't have a long time in your refrigerator. Drink it within forty-eight hours.

Don't pitch the pulp. Pulp is loaded with nutrients, so don't let it go to waste. Use it in smoothies, make popsicles for the kids, or dehydrate it and mix it in with your favorite raw nuts and seeds as a trail mix. Or add it to stews, soups, or broths as a nutritious thickener. You can also add pulp to soil as compost.

Brands and Models

Breville Juice Fountain Elite
www.brevilleusa.com

NutriBullet (vegetable extractor)
www.nutribullet.com

Hurom Slow Juicer
www.hurom.com

Omega J8003 (masticating juicer)
www.omegajuicers.com

Juiceman Pro
www.juiceman.com

Other Resources

The following is a list of recommended supplement, nutritional resource, and nontoxic home product companies. Contact them directly for information about products and where to find them.

Beauty and Skincare Products

Aveda
www.aveda.com

Aubrey Organics
www.aubrey-organics.com

Burt's Bees
www.burtsbees.com

Tom's of Maine
www.tomsofmaine.com

June Jacobs
www.junejacobs.com

Children's Health

Agency for Healthcare Research and Quality
www.ahrq.gov

Children's Defense Fund
www.childrensdefense.org

Children's Environmental Health Network
www.cehn.org

Partnership for Children's Health and the Environment
www.partnersforchildren.org

Home

Green America's National Green Pages
www.greenpages.org

The Green Guide
www.greenguide.com

Furniture

Furnature (chemical-free upholstered furniture and mattresses)
www.furnature.com

Green Design Furniture
(wood furnishings)
www.greendesigns.com

Garden

Burpee Seeds
www.burpee.com

Organic Garden
www.organicgardening.com

Gardens Alive
www.gardensalive.com

Planet Natural
www.planetnatural.com

Household Cleaners

Bon Ami
www.faultless.com

Sun and Earth
www.sunandearth.com

Seventh Generation
www.seventhgeneration.com

Supplements and Foods

Allergy Research Group
www.allergyresearchgroup.com

Alvarado Street Bakery Organic and
Sprouted Grain Breads
www.alvaradostreetbakery.com

Avemar
www.avemar.com

Barlean's Organic Oils
www.barleans.com

Biotics Research
www.bioticsresearch.com

Chi's Enterprises
www.chi-health.com

Designs for Health
www.designsforhealth.com

Eat Wild (information about
pasture-based farming)
www.eatwild.com

Enerhealth Botanicals
www.enerhealthbotanicals.com

Environmental Working Group
(includes food news)
www.ewg.org/foodnews

Enzymatic Therapy
www.enzymatictherapy.com

Euro Pharma
www.europharmausa.com

Gaia Herbs
www.gaiaherbs.com

Gaynor Integrative Oncology
215 East 72nd Street
New York, NY 11021
www.drgaynor.com

Gaynor Wellness
215 East 72nd Street
New York, NY 11021
www.gaynorwellness.com

Gene Response, Inc.
www.genechanger.com
www.drgaynorsgenechangerblog.com

Harney and Sons Fine Teas
www.harney.com

Herbs, Etc.
www.herbsetc.com

Host Defense
www.hostdefense.com

Integrative Therapeutics
www.integrativepro.com

Jarrow Formulas
www.jarrow.com

JHS Natural Products
www.jhsnp.com

Metagenics
www.metagenics.com

Montana Naturals
http://mtnaturals.com

Mushroom Science
www.mushroomscience.com

Mushroom Wisdom
www.mushroomwisdom.com

Nature's Way
www.naturesway.com

Nordic Naturals
www.nordicnaturals.com

NOW Foods
www.nowfoods.com

NutriCology
www.nutricology.com

Nutri-Fruit (all-natural dried
fruit powders)
www.nutrifruit.com

Oregon's Wild Harvest
www.oregonswildharvest.com

Pure Bar (organic snacks)
www.thepurebar.com

Pure Encapsulations
www.puréencapsulations.com

Quercegen
www.quercegen.com

Savesta Life Sciences
www.savestalife.com

Scenic Fruit
www.scenicfruit.com

Seanol (a patented extract of
marine polyphenols)
www.jprenew.com

Solaray
www.solaray.com

Source Naturals
www.sourcenaturals.com

Sun Chlorella
www.sunchlorellausa.com

Thorne Research
www.thorne.com

Vital Nutrients
www.vitalnutrients.net

Wakunaga (Kyolic Aged Garlic Extract)
www.kyolic.com

Well Wisdom
www.wellwisdom.com

Whole Foods Market
www.wholefoods.com

Xymogen
www.xymogen.com

Toxins Information

Agency for Toxic Substances and Disease
Registry
www.atsdr.cdc.gov

EnviroLink
www.envirolink.org

Trade and Quality Assurance Organizations

ConsumerLab
www.consumerlab.com

NSF International
www.nsf.org

Organic Trade Organization
www.ota.com

United States Pharmacopeia (USP)
www.usp.org

Acknowledgments

This book describes a new paradigm that forms the basis of both health and disease: we are born with genes from each parent, but our genetic destiny can be changed throughout our lives through diet and lifestyle.

I am indebted to the physicians and scientists who supported and influenced my medical and scientific career: Dr. Mehmet Oz, Dr. Jeff Milsom, Dr. Andrew Dannenberg, Dr. Joseph Nevins, Dr. James Darnell, Dr. Devra Davis, Dr. Connie Mariano, Dr. Michael Osborne, Dr. Sheldon Feldman, Dr. Anne Moore, Dr. Orli Ettingen, Dr. Robert Zieve, Dr. Michael Roizen, and Dr. Alex Swistel.

I would like to thank the editorial team at Viking whose tireless input and support greatly assisted in the creation of this work: Carole Desanti, Christopher Russell, and Clare Ferraro. I would also like to thank the creative work of the Viking marketing team: Carolyn Coleburn, Lindsay Prevette, Nancy Sheppard, Sarah Janet, and Emma Mohney.

I would additionally like to thank Richard Prudhomme, Priscilla Gilman, Leslie Perkins, William Patrick, Emily Kessler, and Jaimie Lazare whose input and editorial suggestions contributed so much to this book.

I am most indebted to my agent, Lynn Nesbit, for believing in the book and guiding me the whole way.

Introduction

1. P. Anand, A. B. Kunnumakara, C. Sundaram, et al., "Cancer Is a Preventable Disease That Requires Major Lifestyle Changes," *Pharmaceutical Research* 25, no. 9 (2008): 2097–116.
2. M. Gaynor et al., "Complete Remission of Widely Metastatic Melanoma," *Cancer Strategies Journal* 2, no. 2 (2014): 10–13.

Chapter 1: The Basic Plan

1. C. D. Gardner, A. Kiazand, S. Alhassan, et al., "Comparison of the Atkins, Zone, Ornish, and LEARN Diets for Change in Weight and Related Risk Factors among Overweight Premenopausal Women. *JAMA: The Journal of the American Medical Association* 297, no. 9 (2007): 969.
2. F. M. Sacks, G. A. Bray, V. J. Carey, et al., "Comparison of Weight-Loss Diets with Different Compositions of Fat, Protein, and Carbohydrates," *New England Journal of Medicine* 360, no. 9 (2009): 859–73.
3. V. Chajès, ACM Thiébaut, M. Rotival, et al., "Association between Serum Trans-Monounsaturated Fatty Acids and Breast Cancer Risk in the E3N-EPIC Study," *American Journal of Epidemiology*, 167, no. 11 (2008): 1312–20.
4. J. E. Chavarro, M. J. Stampfer, H. Campos, T. Kurth, W. C. Willett, and J. Ma, "A Prospective Study of Trans-Fatty Acid Levels in Blood and Risk of Prostate Cancer," *Cancer Epidemiology Biomarkers & Prevention* 17, no. 1 (January 1, 2008): 95–101.

5. J. D. Furtado, H. Campos, A. E. Sumner, L. J. Appel, V. J. Carey, and F. M. Sacks, "Dietary Interventions That Lower Lipoproteins Containing Apolipoprotein C-III Are More Effective in Whites Than in Blacks: Results of the Omniheart Trial," *The American Journal of Clinical Nutrition* 92, no. 4 (October 1, 2010): 714–22.

6. M. M. Mamerow, J. A. Mettler, K. L. English, et al., "Dietary Protein Distribution Positively Influences 24-h Muscle Protein Synthesis in Healthy Adults," *Journal of Nutrition* (2014).

7. S. Li, A. Flint, J. K. Pai, et al., "Dietary Fiber Intake and Mortality Among Survivors of Myocardial Infarction: Prospective Cohort Study," *British Medical Journal* (2014): 348.

8. S. H. Lee, T. Oe, and I. A. Blair, "Vitamin C-Induced Decomposition of Lipid Hydroperoxides to Endogenous Genotoxins," *Science* 5524, no. 292 (2001): 2083–86.

9. E. R. Miller, R. Pastor-Barriuso, D. Dalal, R. A. Riemersma, L. J. Appel, E. Guallar, "Meta-Analysis: High-Dosage Vitamin E Supplementation May Increase All-Cause Mortality," *Annals of Internal Medicine* 142, no. 1 (2005): 37–46.

Chapter 2: Obesity

1. M. Hatori, C. Vollmers, A. Zarrinpar, et al., "Time-Restricted Feeding Without Reducing Caloric Intake Prevents Metabolic Diseases in Mice Fed a High-Fat Diet," *Cell Metabolism* 15, no. 6 (2012): 848–60.

2. J. A. Vinson, B. R. Burnham, and M. V. Nagendran, "Randomized, Double-Blind, Placebo-Controlled, Linear Dose, Crossover Study to Evaluate the Efficacy and Safety of a Green Coffee Bean Extract in Overweight Subjects," *Diabetes, Metabolic Syndrome and Obesity: Targets and Therapy* 5, no. 21 (2012).

3. S. J. Song et al., "Decaffeinated Green Coffee Bean Extract Attenuates Diet-Induced Obesity and Insulin Resistance in Mice," *Evidence-Based Complementary and Alternative Medicine*, 2014.

4. H. Shimoda et al., "Inhibitory Effect of Green Coffeebean Extract on Fat Accumulation and Body Weight Gain in Mice," *BMC Complement Altern Med.* 6, no. 9 (2006).

5. I. Onakpoya et al., "The Use of Green Coffee Extract as a Weight Loss Supplement: A Systematic Review and Meta-Analysis of Randomised Clinical Trials," *Gastroenterology research and practice*, 2011.

6. K. L. Teff, S. S. Elliott, M. Tschöp, et al., "Dietary Fructose Reduces Circulating Insulin and Leptin, Attenuates Postprandial Suppression of Ghrelin, and Increases Triglycerides in Women," *Journal of Clinical Endocrinology & Metabolism* 89, no. 6 (2004): 2963–72.

7. K. L. Stanhope, J. M. Schwarz, N. L. Keim, et al., "Consuming Fructose-Sweetened, Not Glucose-Sweetened, Beverages Increases Visceral Adiposity and Lipids and Decreases Insulin Sensitivity in Overweight/Obese Humans," *Journal of Clinical Investigation* 119, no. 5 (2009): 1322.

8. Y. Nagai, S. Yonemitsu, D. M. Erion, et al., "The Role of Peroxisome Proliferator-Activated Receptor [gamma] Coactivator-1 [beta] in the Pathogenesis of Fructose-Induced Insulin Resistance," *Cell Metabolism* 9, no. 3 (2009): 252–64.

9. K. Spiegel, E. Tasali, P. Penev, and E. Van Cauter, "Brief Communication: Sleep Curtailment in Healthy Young Men Is Associated with Decreased Leptin Levels, Elevated Ghrelin Levels, and Increased Hunger and Appetite," *Annals of Internal Medicine* 141, no. 11 (2004): 846–50.

10. A. K. Gosby, A. D. Conigrave, N. S. Lau, et al., "Testing Protein Leverage in Lean Humans: A Randomised Controlled Experimental Study," *PLOS ONE* 6, no. 10 (2011): e25929.

11. T. M. Larsen, S. M. Dalskov, M. Van Baak, et al., "Diets with High or Low Protein Content and Glycemic Index for Weight-Loss Maintenance," *New England Journal of Medicine* 363, no. 22 (2010): 2102–13.

12. S. Tulipani, R. Llorach, O. Jauregui, et al., "Metabolomics Unveils Urinary Changes in Subjects with Metabolic Syndrome Following 12-Week Nuts Consumption," *Journal of Proteome Research* 10, no. 11 (2011): 5047–58.

13. H. K. Sung, K. O. Doh, J. E. Son, et al., "Adipose Vascular Endothelial Growth Factor Regulates Metabolic Homeostasis Through Angiogenesis," *Cell Metabolism* 17, no. 1 (2013): 61–72.

14. J. G. Neels, T. Thinnes, and D. J. Loskutoff, "Angiogenesis in an In Vivo Model of Adipose Tissue Development," *FASEB Journal* 18, no. 9 (2004): 983–85.

15. E. Bråkenhielm, R. Cao, B. Gao, et al., "Angiogenesis Inhibitor, TNP-470, Prevents Diet-Induced and Genetic Obesity in Mice," *Circulation Research* 94, no. 12 (2004): 1579–88.

16. A. Ejaz, D. Wu, P. Kwan, and M. Meydani, "Curcumin Inhibits Adipogenesis in 3T3-L1 Adipocytes and Angiogenesis and Obesity in C57/BL Mice," *Journal of Nutrition* 139, no. 5 (2009): 919–25.

17. J. Y. Yang, M. A. Della-Fera, C. Nelson-Dooley, and C. A. Baile, "Molecular Mechanisms of Apoptosis Induced by Ajoene in 3T3-L1 Adipocytes," *Obesity* 14, no. 3 (2006): 388–97.

18. J. Y. Yang, M. A. Della-Fera, and C. A. Baile, "Guggulsterone Inhibits Adipocyte Differentiation and Induces Apoptosis in 3T3-L1 Cells," *Obesity* 16, no. 1 (2007): 16–22.

19. U. H. Park, H. S. Jeong, E. Y. Jo, et al., "Piperine, a Component of Black Pepper, Inhibits Adipogenesis by Antagonizing PPARγ Activity in 3T3-L1 Cells," *Journal of Agricultural and Food Chemistry* 60, no. 15 (2012): 3853–60.

20. S. Rayalam, M. A. Della-Fera, and C. A. Baile, "Phytochemicals and Regulation of the Adipocyte Life Cycle," *Journal of Nutritional Biochemistry* 19, no. 11 (2008): 717–26.

21. S. S. Tworoger, Y. Yasui, M. V. Vitiello, et al., "Effects of a Yearlong Moderate-Intensity Exercise and a Stretching Intervention on Sleep Quality In Postmenopausal Women," *Sleep* 26, no. 7 (2003): 830–36.

Chapter 3: Heart Disease

1. H. C. Stary, A. B. Chandler, S. Glagov, et al., "A Definition of Initial, Fatty Streak, and Intermediate Lesions of Atherosclerosis. A Report from the Committee on Vascular Lesions of the Council on Arteriosclerosis, American Heart Association," *Arteriosclerosis, Thrombosis, and Vascular Biology* 14, no. 5 (1994): 840–56.

2. J. L. Carwile, X. Ye, X. Zhou, A. M. Calafat, and K. B. Michels, "Canned Soup Consumption and Urinary Bisphenol A: A Randomized Crossover Trial," *JAMA* 306, no. 20 (2011): 2218–20.

3. E. Chavakis et al., "Oxidized LDL Inhibits Vascular Endothelial Growth Factor–Induced Endothelial Cell Migration by an Inhibitory Effect on the Akt/Endothelial Nitric Oxide Synthase Pathway," *Circulation* 103, no. 16 (2001): 2102–7.

4. P. Basu et al., "Chronic Hyperhomocysteinemia Causes Vascular Remodelling by Instigating Vein Phenotype in Artery," *Archives of Physiology and Biochemistry* 117, no. 5 (2011): 270–82.

5. R. Hambrecht, E. Fiehn, C. Weigl, et al., "Regular Physical Exercise Corrects Endothelial Dysfunction and Improves Exercise Capacity in Patients with Chronic Heart Failure," *Circulation* 98, no. 24 (1998): 2709–15.

6. This is actually ironic, since it was in the context of heart disease that these personality types were first developed. Back then, in the 1950s, the As were supposedly overstressing themselves to an early grave.

7. M. A. Austin, M. C. King, K. M. Vranizan, and R. M. Krauss, "Atherogenic Lipoprotein Phenotype: A Proposed Genetic Marker for Coronary Heart Disease Risk," *Circulation* 82, no. 2 (1990): 495–506.

8. K. El Harchaoui, W. A. Van der Steeg, E. S. Stroes, et al., "Value of Low-Density Lipoprotein Particle Number and Size as Predictors of Coronary Artery Disease in Apparently Healthy Men and Women: The EPIC-Norfolk Prospective Population Study," *Journal of the American College of Cardiology* 49, no. 5 (2007): 547–53.

9. M. Miller, N. J. Stone, C. Ballantyne, et al., "Triglycerides and Cardiovascular Disease: A Scientific Statement from the American Heart Association," *Circulation* 123, no. 20 (2011): 2292–333.

10. W. C. Willett, M. J. Stampfer, J. Manson, et al., "Intake of Trans Fatty Acids and Risk of Coronary Heart Disease Among Women," *Lancet* 341, no. 8845 (1993): 581–85.

11. T. M. Brasky, A. K. Darke, X. Song, et al., "Plasma Phospholipid Fatty Acids and Prostate Cancer Risk in the SELECT Trial," *Journal of the National Cancer Institute* 105, no. 15 (2013): 1132–41.

12. M. Zakkar, K. Van der Heiden, L. A. Luong, et al., "Activation of Nrf2 in Endothelial Cells Protects Arteries from Exhibiting a Proinflammatory State," *Arteriosclerosis, Thrombosis, and Vascular Biology* 29, no. 11 (2009): 1851–57.

13. M. L. Assunção et al., "Effects Of Dietary Coconut Oil on the Biochemical and Anthropometric Profiles of Women Presenting Abdominal Obesity," *Lipids* 44, no. 7 (2009): 593–601.

14. R. A. Koeth et al., "Intestinal Microbiota Metabolism of L-Carnitine, a Nutrient in Red Meat, Promotes Atherosclerosis," *Nature Medicine* 19, no. 5 (2013): 576–85.

15. R. Ferrari et al., "Therapeutic Effects of L-Carnitine And Propionyl-L-Carnitine on Cardiovascular Diseases: A Review," *Annals of the New York Academy of Sciences* 1033, no. 1 (2004): 79–91.

16. P. J. Turnbaugh et al., "The Effect of Diet on the Human Gut Microbiome: A Metagenomic Analysis in Humanized Gnotobiotic Mice," *Science Translational Medicine* 1, no. 6 (2009): 6ra14-16ra14.

17. P. W. Siri-Tarino et al., "Saturated Fat, Carbohydrate, and Cardiovascular Disease," *The American Journal of Clinical Nutrition* 91, no. 3 (2010): 502–9.

18. L. Cordain et al., "Origins and Evolution of the Western Diet: Health Implications for the 21st Century," *The American Journal of Clinical Nutrition* 81, no. 2 (2005): 341–54.

19. A. P. Liou et al., "Conserved Shifts in the Gut Microbiota Due to Gastric Bypass Reduce Host Weight and Adiposity," *Science Translational Medicine* 5, no. 178 (2013): 178ra141–178ra141.

20. S. Liu et al., "Whole-Grain Consumption and Risk of Coronary Heart Disease: Results from the Nurses' Health Study," *The American Journal of Clinical Nutrition* 70, no. 3 (1999): 412–19.

21. J. F. Wang-Polagruto, A. C. Villablanca, J. A. Polagruto, et al., "Chronic Consumption of Flavanol-Rich Cocoa Improves Endothelial Function and Decreases Vascular Cell Adhesion Molecule in Hypercholesterolemic Postmenopausal Women," *Journal of Cardiovascular Pharmacology* 47 (2006): S177–S186.
22. K. Courage, "Why Is Dark Chocolate Good for You? Thank Your Microbes," 2014; http://www.scientificamerican.com/article/why-is-dark-chocolate-good-for-you-thank-your-microbes/. Accessed August 22, 2014.
23. M. G. Hertog et al., "Dietary Antioxidant Flavonoids and Risk of Coronary Heart Disease: The Zutphen Elderly Study," *The Lancet* 342, no. 8878 (1993): 1007–1011.
24. A. Lynn, H. Hamadeh, W. C. Leung, J. M. Russell, and M. E. Barker, "Effects of Pomegranate Juice Supplementation on Pulse Wave Velocity and Blood Pressure in Healthy Young and Middle-Aged Men and Women," *Plant Foods for Human Nutrition* 67, no. 3 (2012): 309–14.
25. A. Rao, "Lycopene, Tomatoes, and the Prevention of Coronary Heart Disease," *Experimental Biology and Medicine* 227, no. 10 (2002): 908–13.
26. M. H. Carlsen, B. L. Halvorsen, K. Holte, et al., "The Total Antioxidant Content of More Than 3,100 Foods, Beverages, Spices, Herbs and Supplements Used Worldwide," *Nutrition Journal* 9, no. 3 (2010): 1–11.
27. E. Susalit et al., "Olive (*Olea Europaea*) Leaf Extract Effective In Patients With Stage-1 Hypertension: Comparison With Captopril," *Phytomedicine* 18, no. 4 (2011): 251–58.
28. P. M. Kris-Etherton, F. B. Hu, E. Ros, and J. Sabaté, "The Role of Tree Nuts and Peanuts in the Prevention of Coronary Heart Disease: Multiple Potential Mechanisms," *Journal of Nutrition* 138, no. 9 (2008): 1746S–51S.
29. D. J. Jenkins, P. J. Jones, B. Lamarche, et al., "Effect of a Dietary Portfolio of Cholesterol-Lowering Foods Given at 2 Levels of Intensity of Dietary Advice on Serum Lipids in Hyperlipidemia: A Randomized Controlled Trial," *JAMA* 306, no. 8 (2011): 831–39.
30. Kris-Etherton et al., "Role of Tree Nuts."
31. D. J. A. Jenkins, C. W. C. Kendall, A. Marchie, et al., "Effects of a Dietary Portfolio of Cholesterol-Lowering Foods vs. Lovastatin on Serum Lipids and C-Reactive Protein," *JAMA* 290, no. 4 (2003): 502–10; D. J. A. Jenkins, C. W. C. Kendall, A. Marchie, et al., "Dose Response of Almonds on Coronary Heart Disease Risk Factors: Blood Lipids, Oxidized Low-Density Lipoproteins, Lipoprotein (a), Homocysteine, and Pulmonary Nitric Oxide," *Circulation* 106, no. 11 (2002): 1327–32.
32. C. Dalgård, F. Nielsen, J. D. Morrow, et al., "Supplementation with Orange and Blackcurrant Juice, but Not Vitamin E, Improves Inflammatory Markers in Patients with Peripheral Arterial Disease," *British Journal of Nutrition* 101 (2009): 263–69.
33. Y. Jin, X. Cui, U. P. Singh, et al., "Systemic Inflammatory Load in Humans Is Suppressed by Consumption of Two Formulations of Dried, Encapsulated Juice Concentrate," *Molecular Nutrition & Food Research* 54, no. 10 (2010): 1506–14.
34. K. Jacob, M. J. Periago, V. Bohm, and G. R. Berruezo, "Influence of Lycopene and Vitamin C from Tomato Juice on Biomarkers of Oxidative Stress and Inflammation," *British Journal of Nutrition* 99, no. 1 (2008):137.
35. Q. Sun, L. Shi, E. B. Rimm, et al., "Vitamin D Intake and Risk of Cardiovascular Disease in US Men and Women," *American Journal of Clinical Nutrition* 94, no. 2 (2011): 534–42.
36. S. C. Larsson, N. Orsini, and A. Wolk, "Dietary Magnesium Intake and Risk of Stroke: A Meta-Analysis of Prospective Studies," *American Journal of Clinical Nutrition* 95, no. 2 (2012): 362–66.

37. F. L. Rosenfeldt, S. J. Haas, H. Krum, et al., "Coenzyme Q10 in the Treatment of Hypertension: A Meta-Analysis of the Clinical Trials," *Journal of Human Hypertension* 21, no. 4 (2007): 297–306.
38. A. Shakeri, H. Tabibi, and M. Hedayati, "Effects of L-Carnitine Supplement on Serum Inflammatory Cytokines, C-Reactive Protein, Lipoprotein (a), and Oxidative Stress in Hemodialysis Patients with Lp(a) Hyperlipoproteinemia," *Hemodialysis International* 14, no. 4 (2010): 498–504.
39. T. L. Zern, R. J. Wood, C. Greene, et al., "Grape Polyphenols Exert a Cardioprotective Effect in Pre- and Postmenopausal Women by Lowering Plasma Lipids and Reducing Oxidative Stress," *Journal of Nutrition* 135, no. 8 (2005): 1911.

Chapter 4: Cancer

1. F. L. Chan, H. L. Choi, Z. Y. Chen, P. S. F. Chan, and Y. Huang, "Induction of Apoptosis in Prostate Cancer Cell Lines by a Flavonoid, Baicalin," *Cancer Letters* 160, no. 2 (2000): 219–28.
2. C. Lee, L. Raffaghello, S. Brandhorst, et al., "Fasting Cycles Retard Growth of Tumors and Sensitize a Range of Cancer Cell Types to Chemotherapy," *Science Translational Medicine* 4, no. 24 (2012): 124–27.
3. F. M. Safdie, T. Dorff, D. Quinn, et al., "Fasting and Cancer Treatment in Humans: A Case Series Report," *Aging* 1, no. 12 (2009):988.
4. F. Jonsson, L. Yin, C. Lundholm, K. Smedby, K. Czene, and Y. Pawitan, "Low-Dose Aspirin Use and Cancer Characteristics: A Population-Based Cohort Study," *British Journal of Cancer* 109, no. 7 (2013): 1921–25.
5. A. M. Algra and P. M. Rothwell, "Effects of Regular Aspirin on Long-Term Cancer Incidence and Metastasis: A Systematic Comparison of Evidence from Observational Studies versus Randomised Trials," *Lancet Oncology* 13, no. 5 (2012): 518–27.
6. X. Ye, J. Fu, Y. Yang, and S. Chen, "Dose-Risk and Duration-Risk Relationships Between Aspirin and Colorectal Cancer: A Meta-Analysis of Published Cohort Studies," *PLOS ONE* 8, no. 2 (2013): e57578.
7. *Report on Carcinogens* available at http://ntp.niehs.nih.gov/pubhealth/roc/roc12/index.html.
8. A. C. Just, R. M. Whyatt, R. L. Miller, et al., "Children's Urinary Phthalate Metabolites and Fractional Exhaled Nitric Oxide in an Urban Cohort," *American Journal of Respiratory and Critical Care Medicine* 186, no. 9 (2012): 830–37.
9. R. Prentice, D. Thompson, C. Clifford, S. Gorbach, B. Goldwin, and D. Byar, "Dietary Fat Reduction and Plasma Estradiol Concentration in Healthy Postmenopausal Women," *Journal of the National Cancer Institute* 82, no.2 (1990): 129–34.
10. E. Cho, D. Spiegelman, D. J. Hunter, et al., "Premenopausal Fat Intake and Risk of Breast Cancer," *Journal of the National Cancer Institute* 95, no. 14 (2003): 1079–85.
11. A. B. Miller et al., "Twenty-Five-Year Follow-Up for Breast Cancer Incidence and Mortality of the Canadian National Breast Screening Study: Randomised Screening Trial," *BMJ: British Medical Journal* (2014): 348.
12. S. B. Mohr et al., "Meta-Analysis of Vitamin D Sufficiency for Improving Survival of Patients with Breast Cancer," *Anticancer Research* 34, no. 3 (2014): 1163–66.
13. P. J. Goodwin et al., "Prognostic Effects of 25-Hydroxyvitamin D Levels in Early Breast Cancer," *Journal of Clinical Oncology* 27, no. 23 (2009): 3757–63.

14. M. S. Pearce, J. A. Salotti, M. P. Little, et al., "Radiation Exposure from CT Scans in Childhood and Subsequent Risk of Leukaemia and Brain Tumours: A Retrospective Cohort Study," *Lancet* 380, no. 9840 (2012): 499–505.

15. P. C. Norris and E. A. Dennis, "Omega-3 Fatty Acids Cause Dramatic Changes in TLR4 and Purinergic Eicosanoid Signaling," *Proceedings of the National Academy of Sciences* 109, no. 22 (2012): 8517–22.

16. P. Bougnoux, S. Koscielny, V. Chajes, P. Descamps, C. Couet, and G. Calais, "α-Linolenic Acid Content of Adipose Breast Tissue: A Host Determinant of the Risk of Early Metastasis in Breast Cancer," *British Journal of Cancer* 70, no. 2 (1994): 330–34.

17. Z. R. Zhu, J. Ågren, S. Männistö, et al., "Fatty Acid Composition of Breast Adipose Tissue in Breast Cancer Patients and in Patients with Benign Breast Disease," *Nutrition and Cancer* 24, no. 2 (1995): 151–60.

18. S. P. Mehta, A. P. Boddy, J. Cook, et al., "Effect of N-3 Polyunsaturated Fatty Acids on Barrett's Epithelium in the Human Lower Esophagus," *American Journal of Clinical Nutrition* 87, no. 4 (2008): 949–56.

19. M. Anti et al., "Effect of 3 Fatty Acids on Rectal Mucosal Cell Proliferation in Subjects at Risk for Colon Cancer," *Gastroenterology* 103, no. 3 (1992): 883–91.

20. A. Aro, S. Männistö, I. Salminen, M. L. Ovaskainen, V. Kataja, and M. Uusitupa, "Inverse Association Between Dietary and Serum Conjugated Linoleic Acid and Risk of Breast Cancer in Postmenopausal Women," *Nutrition and Cancer* 38, no. 2 (2000): 151–57.

21. N. E. Hubbard et al., "Reduction of Murine Mammary Tumor Metastasis by Conjugated Linoleic Acid," *Cancer Letters* 150, no. 1 (2000): 93-100.

22. C. J. Lopez-Bote et al., "Effect of Free-Range Feeding on Omega-3 Fatty Acids and Alpha-Tocopherol Content and Oxidative Stability of Eggs," *Animal Feed Science and Technology* 72: 33–40.

23. F. Song et al., "Increased Caffeine Intake Is Associated with Reduced Risk of Basal Cell Carcinoma of the Skin," *Cancer Research* 72, no. 13 (2012): 3282–89.

24. R. Sinha, A. J. Cross, C. R. Daniel, et al., "Caffeinated and Decaffeinated Coffee and Tea Intakes and Risk of Colorectal Cancer in a Large Prospective Study," *American Journal of Clinical Nutrition* 96, no. 2 (2012): 374–81.

25. Norman H. Edelman and Mark Rosen, scientific abstracts, *Chest* 2011, Annual Meeting of the American College of Chest Physicians, Honolulu, October 22–26, 2011.

26. S. Cimino, G. Sortino, V. Favilla, et al., "Polyphenols: Key Issues Involved in Chemoprevention of Prostate Cancer," *Oxidative Medicine and Cellular Longevity* 2012 (2012): 632959.

27. S. Haratifar and M. Corredig, "Interactions Between Tea Catechins and Casein Micelles and Their Impact on Renneting Functionality," *Food Chemistry* 143 (2014): 27-32; S. Tewari, et al., "Comparative Study of Antioxidant Potential of Tea with and Without Additives," *Indian Journal of Physiology and Pharmacology* 44, no. 2 (2000): 215–19.

28. Y. Fang, V. G. DeMarco, and M. B. Nicholl, "Resveratrol Enhances Radiation Sensitivity in Prostate Cancer by Inhibiting Cell Proliferation and Promoting Cell Senescence and Apoptosis," *Cancer Science* 103, no. 6 (2012): 1090–98.

29. W. M. Schoonen et al., "Alcohol Consumption and Risk of Prostate Cancer in Middle-Aged Men," *International Journal of Cancer* 113, no. 1 (2005): 133–40.

30. S. Shabbeer, M. Sobolewski, S. Kachhap, N. Davidson, M. A. Carducci, and S. Khan, "Fenugreek: A Naturally Occurring Edible Spice as an Anticancer Agent," *Cancer Biology & Therapy* 8, no. 3 (2009): 272.

31. M. Kakarala, D. E. Brenner, H. Korkaya, et al., "Targeting Breast Stem Cells with the Cancer Preventive Compounds Curcumin and Piperine," *Breast Cancer Research and Treatment* 122, no. 3 (2010): 777–85.

32. M. A. Azuine and S. V. Bhide, "Adjuvant Chemoprevention of Experimental Cancer: Catechin and Dietary Turmeric in Forestomach and Oral Cancer Models," *Journal of Ethnopharmacology* 44, no. 3 (1994): 211–17.

33. B. E. Bachmeier, P. Killian, U. Pfeffer, and A. G. Nerlich, "Novel Aspects for the Application of Curcumin in Chemoprevention of Various Cancers," *Frontiers in Bioscience (Scholar Edition)* 2 (2010): 697–717; E. Sikora, A. Bielak-Zmijewska, G. Mosieniak, and K. Piwocka, "The Promise of Slow Down Ageing May Come from Curcumin," *Current Pharmaceutical Design* 16, no. 7 (2010): 884–92.

34. G. B. Sajithlal, P. Chithra, and G. Chandrakasan, "Effect of Curcumin on the Advanced Glycation and Cross-Linking of Collagen in Diabetic Rats," *Biochemical Pharmacology* 56, no. 12 (1998): 1607–14.

35. J. Ravindran, S. Prasad, and B. B. Aggarwal, "Curcumin and Cancer Cells: How Many Ways Can Curry Kill Tumor Cells Selectively?," *AAPS Journal* 11, no. 3 (2009): 495–510.

36. C. A. Clark, M. D. McEachern, S. H. Shah, et al., "Curcumin Inhibits Carcinogen and Nicotine-Induced Mammalian Target of Rapamycin Pathway Activation in Head and Neck Squamous Cell Carcinoma," *Cancer Prevention Research* 3, no. 12 (2010): 1586–95.

37. Ibid.

38. B. E. Bachmeier, P. Killian, U. Pfeffer, and A. G. Nerlich, "Novel Aspects for the Application of Curcumin in Chemoprevention of Various Cancers," *Frontiers in Bioscience (Scholar Edition)* 2 (2010): 697–717; G. Bar-Sela, R. Epelbaum, and M. Schaffer, "Curcumin as an Anti-Cancer Agent: Review of the Gap Between Basic and Clinical Applications," *Current Medicinal Chemistry* 17, no. 3 (2010): 190–97; L. Wang, Y. Shen, R. Song, Y. Sun, J. Xu, and Q. Xu, "An Anticancer Effect of Curcumin Mediated by Down-Regulating Phosphatase of Regenerating Liver-3 Expression on Highly Metastatic Melanoma Cells," *Molecular Pharmacology* 76, no. 6 (2009): 1238–45.

39. M. Schmidt, G. Betti, and A. Hensel, "Saffron in Phytotherapy: Pharmacology and Clinical Uses," *Wiener Medizinische Wochenschrift* 157, no. 13 (2007): 315–19.

40. A. Amin, A. A. Hamza, K. Bajbouj, S. S. Ashraf, and S. Daoud, "Saffron: A Potential Candidate for a Novel Anticancer Drug Against Hepatocellular Carcinoma," *Hepatology* 54, no. 3 (2011): 857–67.

41. W. G. Gutheil, G. Reed, A. Ray, and A. Dhar, "Crocetin: An Agent Derived from Saffron for Prevention and Therapy for Cancer," *Current Pharmaceutical Biotechnology* 13, no. 1 (2011): 173–79.

42. K. Singletary, C. MacDonald, and M. Wallig, "Inhibition by Rosemary and Carnosol of 7,12-Dimethylbenz[a]anthracene (DMBA)-Induced Rat Mammary Tumorigenesis and In Vivo DMBA-DNA Adduct Formation," *Cancer Letters* 104, no. 1 (1996): 43–48.

43. K. A. Scheckel, S. C. Degner, and D. V. Romagnolo, "Rosmarinic Acid Antagonizes Activator Protein-1-Dependent Activation of Cyclooxygenase-2 Expression in Human Cancer and Nonmalignant Cell Lines," *Journal of Nutrition* 138, no. 11 (2008): 2098–105.

44. S. A. Bingham, N. E. Day, R. Luben, et al., "Dietary Fibre in Food and Protection Against Colorectal Cancer in the European Prospective Investigation into Cancer and Nutrition (EPIC): An Observational Study," *Lancet* 361, no. 9368 (2003): 1496–501.

45. C. Miglio, E. Chiavaro, A. Visconti, V. Fogliano, and N. Pellegrini, "Effects of Different Cooking Methods on Nutritional and Physicochemical Characteristics of Selected Vegetables," *Journal of Agricultural and Food Chemistry* 56, no. 1 (2007): 139–47.

46. L. Song and P. J. Thornalley, "Effect of Storage, Processing and Cooking on Gluco-sinolate Content of Brassica vegetables," *Food and Chemical Toxicology* 45, no. 2 (2007): 216–24.

47. T. K. Lee, R. T. P. Poon, J. Y. Wo, et al., "Lupeol Suppresses Cisplatin-Induced Nuclear Factor-κB Activation in Head and Neck Squamous Cell Carcinoma and Inhibits Local Invasion and Nodal Metastasis in an Orthotopic Nude Mouse Model," *Cancer Research* 67, no. 18 (2007): 8800–8809.

48. M. Saleem, "Lupeol, a Novel Anti-Inflammatory and Anti-Cancer Dietary Triter-pene," *Cancer Letters* 285, no. 2 (2009): 109–15.

49. C. Tilli, A. J. W. Stavast-Kooy, J. D. D. Vuerstaek, et al., "The Garlic-Derived Organo-sulfur Component Ajoene Decreases Basal Cell Carcinoma Tumor Size by Inducing Apoptosis," *Archives of Dermatological Research* 295, no. 3 (2003): 117–23.

50. O. Kucuk et al., "Phase II Randomized Clinical Trial of Lycopene Supplementation Before Radical Prostatectomy," *Cancer Epidemiology Biomarkers & Prevention* 10, no. 8 (2001): 861–68; O. Kucuk et al., "Effects of Lycopene Supplementation In Patients with Localized Prostate Cancer. *Experimental Biology and Medicine* 227, no. 10 (2002): 881–85.

51. A. J. Pantuck et al., "Phase II Study of Pomegranate Juice for Men With Rising Prostate-Specific Antigen Following Surgery or Radiation for Prostate Cancer," *Clinical Cancer Research* 12, no. 13 (2006): 4018–26.

52. J. H. Fowke, F. L. Chung, F. Jin, et al., "Urinary Isothiocyanate Levels, Brassica, and Human Breast Cancer," *Cancer Research* 63, no. 14 (2003): 3980–86; M. S. Donaldson, "Nutrition and Cancer: A Review of the Evidence for an Anti-Cancer Diet," *Nutrition Journal* 3 (2004): 19; J. D. Hayes, M. O. Kelleher, and I. M. Eggleston, "The Cancer Chemopreventive Actions of Phytochemicals Derived from Glucosinolates," *European Journal of Nutrition* 47, no. 2 (2008): 73–88.

53. S. A. Ritz, J. Wan, and D. Diaz-Sanchez, "Sulforaphane-Stimulated Phase II Enzyme Induction Inhibits Cytokine Production by Airway Epithelial Cells Stimulated with Diesel Extract," *American Journal of Physiology–Lung Cellular and Molecular Physiology* 292, no. 1 (2007): L33–L39; D. James, S. Devaraj, P. Bellur, S. Lakkanna, J. Vicini, and S. Boddupalli, "Novel Concepts of Broccoli Sulforaphanes and Disease: Induction of Phase II Antioxidant and Detoxification Enzymes by Enhanced-Glucoraphanin Broccoli," *Nutrition Reviews* 70, no. 11 (2012): 654–65.

54. D. Cervi, B. Pak, N. Venier, et al., "Micronutrients Attenuate Progression of Prostate Cancer by Elevating the Endogenous Inhibitor of Angiogenesis, Platelet Factor–4," *BMC Cancer* 10, no. 1 (2010):258.

55. M. Vijayababu et al., "Quercetin-Induced Growth Inhibition and Cell Death in Prostatic Carcinoma Cells (PC-3) Are Associated with Increase in P21 and Hypo-phosphorylated Retinoblastoma Proteins Expression," Journal of Cancer Research and Clinical Oncology 131, no. 11 (2005): 765–71; M. Russo et al., "The Flavonoid Quercetin in Disease Prevention and Therapy: Facts and Fancies," *Biochemical Pharmacology* 83, no. 1 (2012): 6-15.

56. A. J. Butt, C. G. Roberts, A. A. Seawright, et al., "A Novel Plant Toxin, Persin, with In Vivo Activity in the Mammary Gland, Induces Bim-Dependent Apoptosis in Human Breast Cancer Cells," *Molecular Cancer Therapeutics* 5, no. 9 (2006): 2300–2309.

57. Ibid.

58. C. G. Roberts et al., "Synergistic Cytotoxicity Between Tamoxifen and the Plant Toxin Persin in Human Breast Cancer Cells Is Dependent on Bim Expression and Mediated by Modulation of Ceramide Metabolism," *Molecular Cancer Therapeutics* 6, no. 10 (2007): 2777–85.

59. V. A. Kirsh, U. Peters, S. T. Mayne, et al., "Prospective Study of Fruit and Vegetable Intake and Risk of Prostate Cancer," Journal of the National Cancer Institute 99, no. 15 (2007): 1200–1209.

60. J. W. Fahey et al., "Sulforaphane Inhibits Extracellular, Intracellular, and Antibiotic-Resistant Strains of Helicobacter Pylori and Prevents Benzo [A] Pyrene-Induced Stomach Tumors," *Proceedings of the National Academy of Sciences* 99, no. 11 (2002): 7610–15.

61. J. D. Clarke, R. H. Dashwood, and E. Ho, "Multi-Targeted Prevention of Cancer by Sulforaphane," *Cancer Letters* 269, no. 2 (2008): 291–304.

62. M. Traka, A. V. Gasper, A. Melchini, et al., "Broccoli Consumption Interacts with GSTM1 to Perturb Oncogenic Signalling Pathways in the Prostate," *PLOS ONE* 3, no. 7 (2008): e2568.

63. W. S. Yang, P. Va, M. Y. Wong, H. L. Zhang, and Y. B. Xiang, "Soy Intake Is Associated with Lower Lung Cancer Risk: Results from a Meta-Analysis of Epidemiologic Studies," *American Journal of Clinical Nutrition* 94, no. 6 (2011): 1575–83.

64. B. Lazarevic et al., "Efficacy and Safety of Short-Term Genistein Intervention in Patients with Localized Prostate Cancer Prior to Radical Prostatectomy: A Randomized, Placebo-Controlled, Double-Blind Phase 2 Clinical Trial," *Nutrition and Cancer* 63, no. 6 (2011): 889–98.

65. J. Sforcin, "Propolis and the Immune System: A Review," *Journal of Ethnopharmacology* 113, no. 1 (2007): 1–14; H. Li et al., "Antiproliferation of Human Prostate Cancer Cells by Ethanolic Extracts of Brazilian Propolis and Its Botanical Origin," *International Journal of Oncology* 31, no. 3 (2007): 601–6; N. Samet et al., "The Effect of Bee Propolis on Recurrent Aphthous Stomatitis: A Pilot Study," *Clinical Oral Investigations* 11, no. 2 (2007): 143–47; K. Shimizu et al., "Artepillin C In Brazilian Propolis Induces G0/G1 Arrest Via Stimulation of Cip1/P21 Expression in Human Colon Cancer Cells," *Molecular Carcinogenesis* 44, no. 4 (2005): 293–99; M. J. Valente et al., "Biological Activities of Portuguese Propolis: Protection Against Free Radical-Induced Erythrocyte Damage and Inhibition of Human Renal Cancer Cell Growth In Vitro," *Food and Chemical Toxicology* 49, no. 1 (2011): 86-92.

66. D. C. Plais, J. Gardner-Thorpe, H. Ito, S. W. Ashley, and E. E. Whang, "Vitamin B6 Inhibits the Growth of Human Pancreatic Carcinoma," *Nutrition Research* 23, no. 5 (2003): 673–79.

67. S. C. Larsson, N. Orsini, and A. Wolk, "Vitamin B6 and Risk of Colorectal Cancer," *JAMA* 303, no. 11 (2010): 1077–83.

68. B. Frei, I. Birlouez-Aragon, and J. Lykkesfeldt, "Authors' Perspective: What Is the Optimum Intake of Vitamin C in Humans?," *Critical Reviews in Food Science and Nutrition* 52, no. 9 (2012): 815–29.

69. J. Y. Tang, T. Fu, E. LeBlanc, et al., "Calcium Plus Vitamin D Supplementation and the Risk of Nonmelanoma and Melanoma Skin Cancer: Post Hoc Analyses of the Women's Health Initiative Randomized Controlled Trial," *Journal of Clinical Oncology* 29, no. 22 (2011): 3078–84.

70. M. T. Brinkman, M. R. Karagas, M. S. Zens, A. Schned, R. C. Reulen, and M. P. Zeegers, "Minerals and Vitamins and the Risk of Bladder Cancer: Results from the New Hampshire Study," *Cancer Causes and Control* 21, no. 4 (2010): 609–19.

71. A. Barve, T. O. Khor, K. Reuhl, B. Reddy, H. Newmark, and A. N. Kong, "Mixed Tocotrienols Inhibit Prostate Carcinogenesis in TRAMP Mice," *Nutrition and Cancer* 62, no. 6 (2010): 789–94.

72. K. Nimptsch, S. Rohrmann, R. Kaaks, and J. Linseisen, "Dietary Vitamin K Intake in Relation to Cancer Incidence and Mortality: Results from the Heidelberg Cohort of the European Prospective Investigation into Cancer and Nutrition (EPIC-Heidelberg)," *American Journal of Clinical Nutrition* 91, no. 5 (2010): 1348–58.

Chapter 5: Diabetes

1. "National Diabetes Fact Sheet: National Estimates and General Information on Diabetes and Prediabetes in the United States, 2011," U.S. Department of Health and Human Services, Centers for Disease Control and Prevention, Atlanta, Georgia (2011): 201.

2. A. R. Saltiel and C. R. Kahn, "Insulin Signalling and the Regulation of Glucose and Lipid Metabolism," *Nature* 414, no. 6865 (2001): 799–806.

3. S. Jiralerspong et al., "Metformin and Pathologic Complete Responses to Neoadjuvant Chemotherapy in Diabetic Patients with Breast Cancer," *Journal of Clinical Oncology* 27, no. 20 (2009): 3297–302.

4. E. Giovannucci, D. M. Harlan, M. C. Archer, et al., "Diabetes and Cancer: A Consensus Report," *Diabetes Care* 33, no. 7 (2010): 1674–85.

5. G. Blandino, M. Valerio, M. Cioce, et al., "Metformin Elicits Anticancer Effects Through the Sequential Modulation of DICER and c-MYC," *Nature Communications* 3 (2012): 865; I. B. Sahra, Y. Le Marchand–Brustel, J. F. Tanti, and F. Bost, "Metformin in Cancer Therapy: A New Perspective for an Old Antidiabetic Drug?," *Molecular Cancer Therapeutics* 9, no. 5 (2010): 1092–99.

6. D. Margel, D. R. Urbach, L. L. Lipscombe, et al., "Metformin Use and All-Cause and Prostate Cancer–Specific Mortality Among Men with Diabetes," *Journal of Clinical Oncology* 31, no. 25 (2013): 3069–75.

7. A. González-Périz and J. Clària, "Resolution of Adipose Tissue Inflammation," *Scientific World Journal* 10 (2010): 832–56.

8. M. P. St. Onge and P. J. Jones, "Physiological Effects of Medium-Chain Triglycerides: Potential Agents in the Prevention of Obesity," *Journal of Nutrition* 132, no. 3 (2002): 329–32.

9. P. J. White, M. Arita, R. Taguchi, J. X. Kang, and A. Marette, "Transgenic Restoration of Long-Chain n-3 Fatty Acids in Insulin Target Tissues Improves Resolution Capacity and Alleviates Obesity-Linked Inflammation and Insulin Resistance in High-Fat-Fed Mice," *Diabetes* 59, no. 12 (2010): 3066–73.

10. A. González-Périz, R. Horrillo, N. Ferré, et al., "Obesity-Induced Insulin Resistance and Hepatic Steatosis Are Alleviated by ω-3 Fatty Acids: A Role for Resolvins and Protectins," *FASEB Journal* 23, no. 6 (2009):194657.

11. M. Jastroch, A. S. Divakaruni, S. Mookerjee, J. R. Treberg, and M. D. Brand, "Mitochondrial Proton and Electron Leaks," *Essays in Biochemistry* 47 (2010): 53–67.

12. G. A. Nichols, T. A. Hillier, and J. B. Brown, "Normal Fasting Plasma Glucose and Risk of Type 2 Diabetes Diagnosis," *American Journal of Medicine* 121, no. 6 (2008): 519–24.

13. T. Nakagami and DECODA Study Group, "Hyperglycaemia and Mortality from All Causes and from Cardiovascular Disease in Five Populations of Asian Origin," *Diabetologia* 47, no. 3 (2004): 385–94.

14. A. M. W. Petersen and B. K. Pedersen, "The Anti-Inflammatory Effect of Exercise," *Journal of Applied Physiology* 98, no. 4 (2005): 1154–62.

15. J. Neustadt, and S. Pieczenik, *A Revolution in Health Through Nutritional Biochemistry,* iUniverse, 2007.

16. Y. Son et al., "Dietary Magnesium Intake in Relation to Plasma Insulin Levels and Risk of Type 2 Diabetes in Women," *Diabetes Care* 27, no. 1 (2004): 59-65; M. Barbagallo et al., "Effects of Vitamin E and Glutathione on Glucose Metabolism Role of Magnesium *Hypertension* 34, no. 4 (1999): 1002–6.

17. A. C. B. López et al.," Flour Mixture of Rice Flour, Corn and Cassava Starch in the Production of Gluten-Free White Bread," *Brazilian Archives of Biology and Technology* 47, no. 1 (2004): 63–70.

18. M. Kim, and H. K. Shin, "The Water-Soluble Extract of Chicory Reduces Glucose Uptake from the Perfused Jejunum in Rats, *The Journal of Nutrition* 126, no. 9 (1996): 2236–42.

19. R. C. Noland, T. R. Koves, S. E. Seiler, et al., "Carnitine Insufficiency Caused by Aging and Overnutrition Compromises Mitochondrial Performance and Metabolic Control," *Journal of Biological Chemistry* 284, no. 34 (2009): 22840–52.

20. S. D. R. Galloway, T. P. Craig, and S. J. Cleland, "Effects of Oral L-Carnitine Supplementation on Insulin Sensitivity Indices in Response to Glucose Feeding in Lean and Overweight/Obese Males," *Journal of Amino Acids* 41, no. 2 (2011): 507–15.

21. P. Ruggenenti et al., "Ameliorating Hypertension and Insulin Resistance in Subjects at Increased Cardiovascular Risk Effects of Acetyl-l-Carnitine Therapy," *Hypertension* 54, no. 3 (2009): 567–74.

22. A. Al-Romaiyan, B. Liu, H. Asare-Anane, et al., "A Novel *Gymnema sylvestre* Extract Stimulates Insulin Secretion from Human Islets In Vivo and In Vitro," *Phytotherapy Research* 24, no. 9 (2010): 1370–76.

23. K. Srinivasan, "Fenugreek (*Trigonella foenum-graecum*): A Review of Health Beneficial Physiological Effects," *Food Reviews International* 22, no. 2 (2006): 203–24; P. Khosla, D. Gupta, and R. Nagpal, "Effect of *Trigonella foenum-graecum* (Fenugreek) on Blood Glucose in Normal and Diabetic Rats," *Indian Journal of Physiology and Pharmacology* 39, no. 2 (1995): 173–4; D. Puri, K. Prabhu, and P. Murthy, "Mechanism of Action of a Hypoglycemic Principle Isolated from Fenugreek Seeds," *Indian Journal of Physiology and Pharmacology* 46, no. 4 (2002): 457–62; A. Gupta, R. Gupta, and B. Lal, "Effect of *Trigonella foenum-graecum* (Fenugreek) Seeds on Glycaemic Control and Insulin Resistance in Type 2 Diabetes Mellitus: A Double Blind Placebo Controlled Study," *Journal of the Association of Physicians of India* 49 (2001): 1057–61.

24. G. Preethi, C. Jayanthi, and D. Sonal, "Effect of *Trigonella foenum-graecum* Seeds on the Glycemic Index of Food: A Clinical Evaluation," *International Journal of Diabetes in Developing Countries* 27 (2007).

25. S. Chanda, S. Kushwaha, and R. Kumar Tiwari, "Garlic as Food, Spice and Medicine: A Perspective," *Journal of Pharmacy Research* 4, no. 6 (2011):1857.

26. M. Thomson, K. K. Al-Qattan, T. Bordia, and M. Ali, "Including Garlic in the Diet May Help Lower Blood Glucose, Cholesterol, and Triglycerides," *Journal of Nutrition* 136, no. 3 (2006): 800S–802S.

27. M. A. Bang, H. A. Kim, and Y. J. Cho, "Alterations in the Blood Glucose, Serum Lipids and Renal Oxidative Stress in Diabetic Rats by Supplementation of Onion (*Allium cepa.*

Linn)," *Nutrition Research and Practice* 3, no. 3 (2009): 242–46; S. Kelkar, G. Kaklij, and V. Bapat, "Determination of Antidiabetic Activity in *Allium cepa* (Onion) Tissue Cultures," *Indian Journal of Biochemistry and Biophysics* 38, no. 4 (2001): 277–79.

28. A. F. Fidan and Y. Dündar, "The Effects of *Yucca Schidigera* and *Quillaja Saponaria* on DNA Damage, Protein Oxidation, Lipid Peroxidation, and Some Biochemical Parameters in Streptozotocin-Induced Diabetic Rats," *Journal of Diabetes and Its Complications* 22, no. 5 (2008): 348–56.

29. E. Sukandar, H. Permana, I. Adnyana, et al., "Clinical Study of Turmeric (*Curcuma longa* L.) and Garlic (*Allium sativum* L.) Extracts as Antihyperglycemic and Antihyperlipidemic Agent in Type-2 Diabetes-Dyslipidemia Patients," *International Journal of Pharmacology* 4 (2010): 456–63.

30. M. Kuroda, Y. Mimaki, T. Nishiyama, et al., "Hypoglycemic Effects of Turmeric (*Curcuma longa* L. Rhizomes) on Genetically Diabetic KK-Ay Mice," *Biological and Pharmaceutical Bulletin* 28, no. 5 (2005): 937–39.

31. P. Lekshmi, R. Arimboor, K. Raghu, and A. N. Menon, "Turmerin, the Antioxidant Protein from Turmeric (*Curcuma longa*) Exhibits Antihyperglycaemic Effects," *Natural Product Research* 26, no. 17 (2012): 1654–58.

32. S. Chuengsamarn, S. Rattanamongkolgul, R. Luechapudiporn, C. Phisalaphong, and S. Jirawatnotai, "Curcumin Extract for Prevention of Type 2 Diabetes," *Diabetes Care* 35, no. 11 (2012): 2121–27.

33. M. Tanaka, E. Misawa, Y. Ito, et al., "Identification of Five Phytosterols from Aloe Vera Gel as Anti-Diabetic Compounds," *Biological & Pharmaceutical Bulletin* 29, no. 7 (2006): 1418–22.

34. K. Biswas, I. Chattopadhyay, R. K. Banerjee, and U. Bandyopadhyay, "Biological Activities and Medicinal Properties of Neem (*Azadirachta indica*)," *Current Science* 82, no. 11 (2002): 1336–45.

35. A. Saxena and N. K. Vikram, "Role of Selected Indian Plants in Management of Type 2 Diabetes: A Review," *Journal of Alternative and Complementary Medicine* 10, no. 2 (2004): 369–78.

36. P. Khosla, S. Bhanwra, J. Singh, S. Seth, and R. K. Srivastava, "A Study of Hypoglycaemic Effects of *Azadirachta indica* (Neem) in Normal and Alloxan Diabetic Rabbits," *Indian Journal of Physiology and Pharmacology* 44, no. 1 (2000): 69–74.

37. R. T. Narendhirakannan, S. Subramanian, and M. Kandaswamy, "Biochemical Evaluation of Antidiabetogenic Properties of Some Commonly Used Indian Plants on Streptozotocin-Induced Diabetes in Experimental Rats," *Clinical and Experimental Pharmacology and Physiology* 33, no. 12 (2006): 1150–57.

38. S. Gholap and A. Kar, "Hypoglycaemic Effects of Some Plant Extracts Are Possibly Mediated Through Inhibition in Corticosteroid Concentration," *Die Pharmazie* 59, no. 11 (2004): 876–78.

39. A. Khan, G. Zaman, and R. A. Anderson, "Bay Leaves Improve Glucose and Lipid Profile of People with Type 2 Diabetes," *Journal of Clinical Biochemistry and Nutrition* 44, no. 1 (2009): 52–56.

40. C. Ulbricht, T. Rae Abrams, S. Brent, et al., "Reishi Mushroom (*Ganoderma lucidum*): Systematic Review by the Natural Standard Research Collaboration," *Journal of the Society for Integrative Oncology* 8, no. 4 (2010): 148–59.

41. A. Thyagarajan-Sahu, B. Lane, and D. Sliva, "ReishiMax, Mushroom Based Dietary Supplement, Inhibits Adipocyte Differentiation, Stimulates Glucose Uptake and Activates AMPK," *BMC Complementary and Alternative Medicine* 11, no. 1 (2011): 74–88.

42. S. Fatmawati, K. Shimizu, and R. Kondo, "Ganoderol B: A Potent α-Glucosidase Inhibitor Isolated from the Fruiting Body of *Ganoderma lucidum*," *Phytomedicine* 18, no. 12 (2011): 1053–55.

43. Y. Chen, J. Qiao, J. Luo, et al., "Effects of *Ganoderma lucidum* Polysaccharides on Advanced Glycation End Products and Receptor of Aorta Pectoralis in T2DM rats" [In Chinese], *Zhongguo Zhong yao za zhi* [China Journal of Chinese Materia Medica] 36, no. 5 (2011):624.

44. M. V. Nagendran, "Effect of Green Coffee Bean Extract (GCE), High in Chlorogenic Acids, on Glucose Metabolism," Poster presentation number 45-LB-P, *Obesity* (2011).

45. T. Murase, K. Misawa, Y. Minegishi, et al., "Coffee Polyphenols Suppress Diet-Induced Body Fat Accumulation by Downregulating SREBP-1c and Related Molecules in C57BL/6J Mice," *American Journal of Physiology–Endocrinology and Metabolism* 300, no. 1 (2011): E122–E133.

46. E. Salazar-Martinez, W. C. Willett, A. Ascherio, et al., "Coffee Consumption and Risk for Type 2 Diabetes Mellitus," *Annals of Internal Medicine* 140, no. 1 (2004): 1–8; M. A. Pereira, E. D. Parker, and A. R. Folsom, "Coffee Consumption and Risk of Type 2 Diabetes Mellitus: An 11-Year Prospective Study of 28,812 Postmenopausal Women," *Archives of Internal Medicine* 166, no. 12 (2006): 1311–16; K. L. Johnston, M. N. Clifford, and L. M. Morgan, "Coffee Acutely Modifies Gastrointestinal Hormone Secretion and Glucose Tolerance in Humans: Glycemic Effects of Chlorogenic Acid and Caffeine," *American Journal of Clinical Nutrition* 78, no. 4 (2003): 728–33; S. Bidel, G. Hu, J. Sundvall, J. Kaprio, and J. Tuomilehto, "Effects of Coffee Consumption on Glucose Tolerance, Serum Glucose and Insulin Levels: A Cross-Sectional Analysis," *Hormone and Metabolic Research* 38, no. 1 (2006): 38–43; R. M. Van Dam and E. J. M. Feskens, "Coffee Consumption and Risk of Type 2 Diabetes Mellitus," *Lancet* 360, no. 9344 (2002): 1477–78.

47. B. K. Bassoli, P. Cassolla, G. R. Borba-Murad, et al., "Chlorogenic Acid Reduces the Plasma Glucose Peak in the Oral Glucose Tolerance Test: Effects on Hepatic Glucose Release and Glycaemia," *Cell Biochemistry and Function* 26, no. 3 (2008): 320–28; C. Henry-Vitrac, A. Ibarra, M. Roller, J. M. Mérillon, and X. Vitrac, "Contribution of Chlorogenic Acids to the Inhibition of Human Hepatic Glucose-6-Phosphatase Activity in Vitro by Svetol, a Standardized Decaffeinated Green Coffee Extract," *Journal of Agricultural and Food Chemistry* 58, no. 7 (2010): 4141–44.

48. T. Matsui, T. Tanaka, S. Tamura, et al., "α-Glucosidase Inhibitory Profile of Catechins and Theaflavins," *Journal of Agricultural and Food Chemistry* 55, no. 1 (2006): 99–105.

49. Y. Shoji and H. Nakashima, "Glucose-Lowering Effect of Powder Formulation of African Black Tea Extract in KK-Ay/Tajcl Diabetic Mouse," *Archives of Pharmacal Research* 29, no. 9 (2006): 786–94.

50. Y. H. Kao et al., "Tea, Obesity, and Diabetes," *Molecular Nutrition & Food Research* 50, no. 2 (2006): 188-210; S. Rudelle et al., "Effect of a Thermogenic Beverage on 24-Hour Energy Metabolism in Humans," *Obesity* 15, no. 2 (2007): 349–55.

51. R. A. Anderson and M. M. Polansky, "Tea Enhances Insulin Activity," *Journal of Agricultural and Food Chemistry* 50, no. 24 (2002): 7182–86.

52. J. K. Lin and S. Y. Lin-Shiau, "Mechanisms of Hypolipidemic and Anti-Obesity Effects of Tea and Tea Polyphenols," *Molecular Nutrition & Food Research* 50, no. 2 (2006): 211–17.

53. M. E. Waltner-Law et al., "Epigallocatechin Gallate, a Constituent of Green Tea, Represses Hepatic Glucose Production," *The Journal of Biological Chemistry* 277, no. 38 (Sept. 20, 2002): 34933–40.

54. Y. Kobayashi et al., "Green Tea Polyphenols Inhibit the Sodium-Dependent Glucose Transporter of Intestinal Epithelial Cells by a Competitive Mechanism," *Journal of Agricultural and Food Chemistry* 48, no. 11 (2000): 5618–23.

55. A. T. H. Glow, "Magnesium Supplements May Reduce Diabetes Risk," *Diabetes, Obesity and Metabolism* 13, no. 3 (2011): 281–84.

56. S. Larsson and A. Wolk, "Magnesium Intake and Risk of Type 2 Diabetes: A Meta-Analysis," *Journal of Internal Medicine* 262, no. 2 (2007): 208–14.

57. R. Villegas, Y. T. Gao, Q. Dai, et al., "Dietary Calcium and Magnesium Intakes and the Risk of Type 2 Diabetes: The Shanghai Women's Health Study," *American Journal of Clinical Nutrition* 89, no. 4 (2009): 1059–67.

58. R. Chatterjee, H. C. Yeh, T. Shafi, et al., "Serum and Dietary Potassium and Risk of Incident Type 2 Diabetes Mellitus: The Atherosclerosis Risk in Communities (ARIC) Study," *Archives of Internal Medicine* 170, no. 19 (2010): 1745–51.

59. T. N. Akbaraly, J. Arnaud, M. P. Rayman, et al., "Plasma Selenium and Risk of Dysglycemia in an Elderly French Population: Results from the Prospective Epidemiology of Vascular Ageing Study," *Nutrition and Metabolism* 7, no. 1 (2010):21.

60. A. Mancini, M. Magini, R. Festa, et al., "Effects of Natural Dietary Antioxidants on Insulin and IGF1 in Obese Patients with Insulin Resistance," *Endocrine Abstracts* 26 (2011).

61. J. W. J. Beulens, "Dietary Phylloquinone and Menaquinones Intakes and Risk of Type 2 Diabetes," *Diabetes Care* 33, no. 8 (2010): 1699–705.

62. E. Hitt, "Higher Vitamin D Levels Linked to Lower Diabetes Risk," *Medscape Medical News*, June 25, 2011, www.medscape.com/viewarticle/745335.

63. J. Mitri, M. D. Muraru, and A. G. Pittas, "Vitamin D and Type 2 Diabetes: A Systematic Review," *European Journal of Clinical Nutrition* 65, no. 9 (2011): 1005–15.

64. J. Kositsawat, V. L. Freeman, B. S. Gerber, and S. Geraci, "Association of A1c Levels with Vitamin D Status in US Adults," *Diabetes Care* 33, no. 6 (2010): 1236–38.

65. P. Gervois et al., "Regulation of Lipid and Lipoprotein Metabolism by PPAR Activators," *Clinical Chemistry and Laboratory Medicine* 38, no. 1 (2000): 3-11; A. M. Rimando, et al., "Pterostilbene, a New Agonist for the Peroxisome Proliferator-Activated Receptor Alpha-Isoform, Lowers Plasma Lipoproteins and Cholesterol in Hypercholesterolemic Hamster," *Journal of Agricultural Food Chemistry* 53, no. 9 (May 4, 2005): 3403–7.

66. E. M. Seymour, M. R. Bennink, S. W. Watts, and S. F. Bolling, "Whole Grape Intake Impacts Cardiac Peroxisome Proliferator-Activated Receptor and Nuclear Factor κB Activity and Cytokine Expression in Rats with Diastolic Dysfunction," *Hypertension* 55, no. 5 (2010): 1179–85.

67. J. C. Milne, P. D. Lambert, S. Schenk, et al., "Small Molecule Activators of SIRT1 as Therapeutics for the Treatment of Type 2 Diabetes," *Nature* 450, no. 7170 (2007): 712–16.

68. P. Brasnyó, G. A. Molnár, M. Mohás, et al., "Resveratrol Improves Insulin Sensitivity, Reduces Oxidative Stress and Activates the Akt Pathway in Type 2 Diabetic Patients," *British Journal of Nutrition* 106, no. 3 (2011): 383–89.

69. R. Gupta et al., "An Overview of Indian Novel Traditional Medicinal Plants with Anti-Diabetic Potentials," *African Journal of Traditional, Complementary, and Alternative Medicines* 5, no. 1 (2008): 1; P. Patel et al., "Antidiabetic Herbal Drugs, a Review," *Pharmacophore* 3, no. 1 (2012): 18–29.

70. J. A. Joseph et al., "Reversals of Age-Related Declines in Neuronal Signal Transduction, Cognitive, and Motor Behavioral Deficits with Blueberry, Spinach, or Strawberry Dietary Supplementation," *The Journal of Neuroscience* 19, no. 18 (1999): 8114–21.

71. J. Urban, C. J. Dahlberg, B. J. Carroll, and W. Kaminsky, "Absolute Configuration of Beer's Bitter Compounds," *Angewandte Chemie* 125, no. 5 (2013): 1593–95.

72. C. S. Johnston et al., "Examination of the Antiglycemic Properties of Vinegar in Healthy Adults," *Annals of Nutrition and Metabolism* 56, no. 1 (2010): 74–79.

73. C. S. Johnston et al., "Preliminary Evidence That Regular Vinegar Ingestion Favorably Influences Hemoglobin A1c Values in Individuals with Type 2 Diabetes Mellitus," *Diabetes Research and Clinical Practice* 84, no. 2 (2009): e15–e17.

Chapter 6: Aging

1. J. G. Hogervorst, L. J. Schouten, E. J. Konings, R. A. Goldbohm, and P. A. Van den Brandt, "A Prospective Study of Dietary Acrylamide Intake and the Risk of Endometrial, Ovarian, and Breast Cancer," *Cancer Epidemiology, Biomarkers & Prevention* 16, no. 11 (2007): 2304–13.

2. P. T. Olesen, A. Olsen, H. Frandsen, K. Frederiksen, K. Overvad, and A. Tjønneland, "Acrylamide Exposure and Incidence of Breast Cancer Among Postmenopausal Women in the Danish Diet, Cancer and Health Study," *International Journal of Cancer* 122, no. 9 (2008): 2094–2100.

3. R. Krikorian, T. A. Nash, M. D. Shidler, B. Shukitt-Hale, and J. A. Joseph, "Concord Grape Juice Supplementation Improves Memory Function in Older Adults with Mild Cognitive Impairment," *British Journal of Nutrition* 103, no. 5 (2010): 730–34.

4. R. Krikorian and C. Boespflag, "Concord Grape Juice Supplementation and Neurocognitive Function in Human Aging," *Journal of Agricultural and Food Chemistry* 60, no. 23 (2012): 5736–42.

5. J. Uribarri et al., "Advanced Glycation End Products in Foods and a Practical Guide to Their Reduction in the Diet," *Journal of the American Dietetic Association* 110, no. 6 (2010): 911–16; T. Goldberg et al., "Advanced Glycoxidation End Products in Commonly Consumed Foods," *Journal of the American Dietetic Association* 104, no. 8 (2004): 1287–91.

6. A. O. Odegaard, W. P. Koh, J. M. Yuan, M. D. Gross, and M. A. Pereira, "Western-Style Fast Food Intake and Cardiometabolic Risk in an Eastern Country," *Circulation* 126, no. 2 (2012): 182–88.

7. J. A. Lemon et al., "A Complex Dietary Supplement Extends Longevity of Mice," *Journal of Gerontology and Biological Science Medicine* 60, no. 3 (2005): 275–79; V. Aksenov et al., "A Complex Dietary Supplement Augments Spatial Learning, Brain Mass, and Mitochondrial Electron Transport Chain Activity in Aging Mice," *Age,* Nov. 27, 2011; V. Aksenov, et al. Dietary Amelioration of Locomotor, Neurotransmitter and Mitochondrial Aging," *Experimental Biology and Medicine* 235, no. 1 (2010): 66–76.

8. A. M. Sanchez-Sanchez et al., "Intracellular Redox State As Determinant for Melatonin Antiproliferative Vs Cytotoxic Effects in Cancer Cells," *Free Radical Research* 45, no. 11-12 (2011): 1333–41; O. Weinreb et al., "Neurological Mechanisms of Green Tea Polyphenols in Alzheimer's and Parkinson's Diseases," *Journal of Nutritional*

Biochemistry 15, no. 9 (2004): 506–16; B. Catalgol and N. K. Ozer, "Protective Effects of Vitamin E Against Hypercholesterolemia-Induced Age-Related Diseases," *Genes and Nutrition* 7, no. 1 (2012): 91–98; S. Inami et al., "Tea Catechin Consumption Reduces Circulating Oxidized Low-Density Lipoprotein," *International Heart Journal* 48, no. 6 (2007): 725–32; A. Sahebkar, "Potential Efficacy of Ginger As a Natural Supplement for Nonalcoholic Fatty Liver Disease," *World Journal of Gastroenterology* 17, no. 2 (2011): 271-72; H. Y. Ahn and C. H. Kim, "Epigallocatechin-3-Gallate Regulates Inducible Nitric Oxide Synthase Expression in Human Umbilical Vein Endothelial Cells," *Laboratory Animal Research* 27, no. 2 (2011): 85–90; P. V. Babu and D. Liu, "Green Tea Catechins and Cardiovascular Health: An Update," *Current Medicinal Chemistry* 15, no. 18 (2008): 1840-50; K. C. Chiang et al., "Hepatocellular Carcinoma and Vitamin D: A Review," *Journal of Gastroenterology and Hepatology* 26, no. 11 (2011): 1597-603; K. Prasad, "Flaxseed and Cardiovascular Health," *Journal of Cardiovascular Pharmacology* 54, no. 5 (2009): 369-77; D. Moertl et al., "Dose-Dependent Effects of Omega-3-Polyunsaturated Fatty Acids on Systolic Left Ventricular Function, Endothelial Function, and Markers of Inflammation in Chronic Heart Failure of Nonischemic Origin: A Double-Blind, Placebo-Controlled, 3-Arm Study," *American Heart Journal* 161, no. 5 (2011): 915 e1-9.

9. C. Middelmann-Whitney, *Zest for Life: The Mediterranean Anti-Cancer Diet* (Leicester, UK: Matador, 2010).

10. G. Buckland, A. L. Mayén, A. Agudo, et al., "Olive Oil Intake and Mortality Within the Spanish Population (EPIC-Spain)," *American Journal of Clinical Nutrition* 96, no. 1 (2012): 142–49.

11. A. Camargo, J. Ruano, J. Fernandez, et al., "Gene Expression Changes in Mononuclear Cells in Patients with Metabolic Syndrome After Acute Intake of Phenol-Rich Virgin Olive Oil," *BMC Genomics* 11 (2010): 253.

12. P. R. Cheeke, S. Piacente, and W. Oleszek, "Anti-Inflammatory and Anti-Arthritic Effects of *Yucca schidigera*: A Review," *Journal of Inflammation* 3 (2006): 6.

13. S. Sontakke et al., "Open, Randomized, Controlled Clinical Trial of Boswellia Serrata Extract As Compared to Valdecoxib in Osteoarthritis of Knee," *Indian Journal of Pharmacology* 39, no. 1 (2007): 27; R. Kulkarni et al., "Treatment of Osteoarthritis with a Herbomineral Formulation: A Double-Blind, Placebo-Controlled, Cross-Over Study," *Journal of Ethnopharmacology* 33, no. 1 (1991): 91–95.

14. I. Gupta et al., "Effects of Boswellia Serrata Gum Resin in Patients with Bronchial Asthma: Results of a Double-Blind, Placebo-Controlled, 6-Week Clinical Study," *European Journal of Medical Research* 3, no. 11 (1998): 511–14.

15. C. F. Krieglstein et al. "Acetyl-11-Keto-B-Boswellic Acid, a Constituent of a Herbal Medicine From Boswellia Serrata Resin, Attenuates Experimental Ileitis," *International Journal of Colorectal Disease* 16, no. 2 (2001): 88–95.

16. J. L. Quiles, J. J. Ochoa, J. R. Huertas, and J. Mataix, "Coenzyme Q Supplementation Protects from Age-Related DNA Double-Strand Breaks and Increases Lifespan in Rats Fed on a PUFA-Rich Diet," *Experimental Gerontology* 39, no. 2 (2004): 189–94.

17. H. Masaki, "Role of Antioxidants in the Skin: Anti-Aging Effects," *Journal of Dermatological Science* 58, no. 2 (2010): 85–90.

18. H. Sogabe and T. Terado, "Open Clinical Study of Effects of Pumpkin Seed Extract/Soybean Germ Extract Mixture Containing Processed Foods on Nocturia," *Jpn J Med Pharm Sci* 46, no. 5 (2001): 727–37.

19. T. Terado, "Clinical Study of Mixed Processed Food Containing Pumpkin Seed Extract and Soybean Germ Extract on Pollakiuria in Night in Elderly Men," *Jpn J Med Pharm Sci* 52, no. 4 (2004): 551–61.

20. H. Hong et al., "Effects of Pumpkin Seed Oil and Saw Palmetto Oil in Korean Men with Symptomatic Benign Prostatic Hyperplasia," *Nutrition Research and Practice* 3, no. 4 (2009): 323–27.

21. J. H. Dwyer et al., "Progression of Carotid Intima-Media Thickness and Plasma Antioxidants: The Los Angeles Atherosclerosis Study," *Arteriosclerosis, Thrombosis, and Vascular Biology* 24, no. 2 (2004): 313–19.

22. J. A. Joseph, B. Shukitt-Hale, N. A. Denisova, et al., "Reversals of Age-Related Declines in Neuronal Signal Transduction, Cognitive, and Motor Behavioral Deficits with Blueberry, Spinach, or Strawberry Dietary Supplementation," *Journal of Neuroscience* 19, no. 18 (1999): 8114–21.

23. H. Sies and W. Stahl, "Nutritional Protection Against Skin Damage from Sunlight," *Annual Review of Nutrition* 24 (2004): 173-200.

24. M. Schäffer et al., "Vitamin A, Vitamin E, Lutein and β-Carotene in Lung Tissues from Subjects with Chronic Obstructive Pulmonary Disease and Emphysema," *Open Journal of Respiratory Diseases* 3, no. 2 (2013): 44–51.

25. R. M. Van Vugt et al., "Antioxidant Intervention in Rheumatoid Arthritis: Results of An Open Pilot Study," *Clinical Rheumatology* 27, no. 6 (2008): 771–75.

26. B. B. Aggarwal and S. Shishodia, "Molecular Targets of Dietary Agents for Prevention and Therapy of Cancer," *Biochemical Pharmacology* 71, no. 10 (2006): 1397–1421.

27. L. Thal et al., "A 1-Year Multicenter Placebo-Controlled Study of Acetyl-L-Carnitine in Patients with Alzheimer's Disease," *Neurology* 47, no. 3 (1996): 705–11.

28. R. Chan, J. Woo, E. Suen, J. Leung, and N. Tang, "Chinese Tea Consumption Is Associated with Longer Telomere Length in Elderly Chinese Men," *British Journal of Nutrition* 103 (2010): 107–13.

29. S. Kuriyama et al., "Green Tea Consumption And Cognitive Function: A Cross-Sectional Study From The Tsurugaya Project," *The American Journal of Clinical Nutrition* 83, no. 2 (2006): 355–61.

30. C. J. Maxwell, M. S. Hicks, D. B. Hogan, J. Basran, and E. M. Ebly, "Supplemental Use of Antioxidant Vitamins and Subsequent Risk of Cognitive Decline and Dementia," *Dementia and Geriatric Cognitive Disorders* 20, no. 1 (2005): 45–51.

31. P. P. Zandi, J. C. Anthony, A. S. Khachaturian, et al., "Reduced Risk of Alzheimer Disease in Users of Antioxidant Vitamin Supplements: The Cache County Study," *Archives of Neurology* 61, no. 1 (2004): 82–88.

32. F. Mangialasche, M. Kivipelto, P. Mecocci, et al., "High Plasma Levels of Vitamin E Forms and Reduced Alzheimer's Disease Risk in Advanced Age," *Journal of Alzheimer's Disease* 20, no. 4 (2010): 1029–37.

33. P. Knekt et al., "Serum Vitamin D and the Risk of Parkinson Disease," *Archives of Neurology* 67, no. 7 (2010): 808–11.

34. P. Liu, L. J. Kemper, J. Wang, K. R. Zahs, K. H. Ashe, and G. M. Pasinetti, "Grapeseed Polyphenolic Extract Specifically Decreases aβ*56 in the Brains of Tg2576 Mice," *Journal of Alzheimer's Disease* 26, no. 4 (2011): 257–66.

35. T. Kakuda, "Neuroprotective Effects of Theanine and Its Preventive Effects on Cognitive Dysfunction," *Pharmacological Research* 64, no. 2 (2011): 162–68.

36. K. Murakami, Y. Miyake, S. Sasaki, et al., "Dietary Intake of Folate, Vitamin B6, Vitamin B12 and Riboflavin and Risk of Parkinson's Disease: A Case-Control Study in Japan," *British Journal of Nutrition* 104 (2010): 757–64.

37. P. Scheltens, P. J. G. H. Kamphuis, F. R. J. Verhey, et al., "Efficacy of a Medical Food in Mild Alzheimer's Disease: A Randomized, Controlled Trial," *Alzheimer's and Dementia* 6, no. 1 (2010): 1–10.

38. L. De Lau, P. Koudstaal, J. Witteman, A. Hofman, and M. Breteler, "Dietary Folate, Vitamin B12, and Vitamin B6 and the Risk of Parkinson Disease," *Neurology* 67, no. 2 (2006): 315–18.

39. K. Yurko-Mauro, D. McCarthy, D. Rom, et al., "Beneficial Effects of Docosahexaenoic Acid on Cognition in Age-Related Cognitive Decline," *Alzheimer's and Dementia* 6, no. 6 (2010): 456–64.

40. "Higher Levels of Active Form of Vitamin B3 Could Help Prevent Paralysis Following Injury," Life Extension, 2009, www.lef.org/whatshot/2009_11.htm.

41. M.-N. Horcajada et al., "Hesperidin Inhibits Ovariectomized-Induced Osteopenia and Shows Differential Effects on Bone Mass and Strength in Young and Adult Intact Rats," *Journal of Applied Physiology* 104, no. 3 (2008): 648–54.

42. Y. Miwa et al., "Effects of Glucosyl Hesperidin on Serum Lipids In Hyperlipidemic Subjects: Preferential Reduction in Elevated Serum Triglyceride Level," *Journal of Nutritional Science and Vitaminology* 50, no. 3 (2004): 211–18.

43. H. Chiba, M. Uehara, J. Wu, et al., "Hesperidin, a Citrus Flavonoid, Inhibits Bone Loss and Decreases Serum and Hepatic Lipids in Ovariectomized Mice," *Journal of Nutrition* 133, no. 6 (2003): 1892–97.

44. G. Belcaro, M. R. Cesarone, M. Dugall, et al., "Product-Evaluation Registry of Meriva, a Curcumin-Phosphatidylcholine Complex, for the Complementary Management of Osteoarthritis." *Panminerva Medica*. 2010; 52: 55–62.

45. C. L. Shen, M. C. Chyu, J. K. Yeh, et al., "Effect of Green Tea and Tai Chi on Bone Health in Postmenopausal Osteopenic Women: A 6-Month Randomized Placebo-Controlled Trial," *Osteoporosis International* 2011: 1–12.

46. S. Sahni, M. T. Hannan, D. Gagnon, et al., "Protective Effect of Total and Supplemental Vitamin C Intake on the Risk of Hip Fracture: A 17-Year Follow-up from the Framingham Osteoporosis Study," *Osteoporosis International* 20, no. 11 (2009): 1853–61.

47. M. Chung, J. Lee, T. Terasawa, J. Lau, and T. A. Trikalinos, "Vitamin D With or Without Calcium Supplementation for Prevention of Cancer and Fractures: An Updated Meta-Analysis for the U.S. Preventive Services Task Force," *Annals of Internal Medicine* 155, no. 12 (2011): 827–38.

48. L. Rejnmark, A. Avenell, T. Masud, et al., "Vitamin D with Calcium Reduces Mortality: Patient Level Pooled Analysis of 70,528 Patients from Eight Major Vitamin D Trials," *Journal of Clinical Endocrinology & Metabolism* 97, no. 8 (2012): 2670–80.

49. J. Lappe et al., "Calcium and Vitamin D Supplementation Decreases Incidence of Stress Fractures in Female Navy Recruits," *Journal of Bone and Mineral Research* 23, no. 5 (2008): 741–49.

50. P. Bucheli, K. Vidal, L. Shen, et al., "Goji Berry Effects on Macular Characteristics and Plasma Antioxidant Level," *Optometry & Vision Science* 88, no. 2 (2011): 257–62.

51. S. J. Wu, L. T Ng, and C. C. Lin, "Antioxidant Activities of Some Common Ingredients of Traditional Chinese Medicine, *Angelica sinensis*, *Lycium barbarum* and *Poria cocos*," *Phytotherapy Research* 18, no. 12 (2004): 1008–12.

52. H. Zhao, A. Alexeev, E. Chang, G. Greenburg, and K. Bojanowski, "*Lycium barbarum* Glycoconjugates: Effect on Human Skin and Cultured Dermal Fibroblasts," *Phytomedicine* 12, no. 1 (2005): 131–37.

53. S. Mirunalini and M. Krishnaveni, "Therapeutic Potential of *Phyllanthus emblica* (Amla): The Ayurvedic Wonder," *Journal of Basic and Clinical Physiology and Pharmacology* 21, no. 1 (2010): 93–105.

54. M. D. Adil, P. Kaiser, N. K. Satti, A. M. Zargar, R. A. Vishwakarma, and S. A. Tasduq, "Effect of *Emblica officinalis* (Fruit) Against UVB-Induced Photo-Aging in Human Skin Fibroblasts," *Journal of Ethnopharmacology* 132, no. 1 (2010): 109–14.

55. P. Chanvorachote, V. Pongrakhananon, S. Luanpitpong, B. Chanvorachote, S. Wannachaiyasit, and U. Nimmannit, "Type I Pro-Collagen Promoting and Anti-Collagenase Activities of *Phyllanthus emblica* Extract in Mouse Fibroblasts," *Journal of Cosmetic Science* 60, no. 4 (2009): 395–403.

56. W. J. Chen and G. Abatangelo, "Functions of Hyaluronan in Wound Repair," *Wound Repair and Regeneration* 7, no. 2 (1999): 79–89.

57. M. Sumitra, P. Manikandan, V. S. Gayathri, P. Mahendran, and L. Suguna, "*Emblica officinalis* Exerts Wound Healing Action Through Upregulation of Collagen and Extracellular Signal-Regulated Kinases (ERK½)," *Wound Repair and Regeneration* 17, no. 1 (2009): 99–107.

58. C. Saliou et al., "Solar Ultraviolet-Induced Erythema in Human Skin and Nuclear Factor-Kappa-B–Dependent Gene Expression In Keratinocytes Are Modulated by a French Maritime Pine Bark Extract," *Free Radical Biology and Medicine* 30, no. 2 (2001): 154–60; D. Segger and F. Schonlau, "Supplementation with Evelle Improves Skin Smoothness and Elasticity in a Double-Blind, Placebo-Controlled Study with 62 Women," *Journal of Dermatological Treatment* 15, no. 4 (2004): 222–26.

Chapter 7: The Gene Therapy Questionnaire

1. "What Is Osteoporosis? Fast Facts: An Easy-to-Read Series of Publications for the Public," http://www.niams.nih.gov/Health_Info/Bone/Osteoporosis/osteoporosis_ff.asp. Accessed August 24, 2014; M. J. Bolland et al., "Effect of Calcium Supplements on Risk of Myocardial Infarction and Cardiovascular Events: Meta-Analysis," *BMJ* (2010): 341; J. J. Anderson et al., "Calcium Intakes and Femoral and Lumbar Bone Density of Elderly U.S. Men and Women: National Health and Nutrition Examination Survey 2005–2006 Analysis," *The Journal of Clinical Endocrinology & Metabolism* 97, no. 12 (2012): 4531–39; H. A. Bischoff et al., "Calcium Intake and Hip Fracture Risk in Men and Women: A Meta-Analysis of Prospective Cohort Studies and Randomized Controlled Trials," *The American Journal of Clinical Nutrition* 86, no. 6 (2007): 1780–90; K. Li et al., "Associations Of Dietary Calcium Intake And Calcium Supplementation With Myocardial Infarction And Stroke Risk And Overall Cardiovascular Mortality In The Heidelberg Cohort Of The European Prospective Investigation Into Cancer And Nutrition Study," *Heart* 98, no. 12 (2012): 920–25; Q. Xiao et al., "Dietary and Supplemental Calcium Intake and Cardiovascular Disease Mortality: The National Institutes of Health–Aarp Diet and Health Study," *JAMA Internal Medicine* 173, no. 8 (2013): 639–46; I. R. Reid and M. J. Bolland, "Calcium Supplements: Bad for the Heart?" *Heart* 98, no. 12 (2012): 895–96; M. J. Favus, "The Risk of Kidney Stone Formation: The Form of Calcium Matters," *The American Journal of Clinical Nutrition* 94,

no. 1 (2011): 5-6; K. Michaëlsson et al., "Long Term Calcium Intake and Rates of All Cause and Cardiovascular Mortality: Community Based Prospective Longitudinal Cohort Study." *British Medical Journal* (2013): 346.

2. J. L. Frestedt et al., "A Natural Seaweed Derived Mineral Supplement (Aquamin F) for Knee Osteoarthritis: A Randomised, Placebo Controlled Pilot Study," *Nutrition Journal* 8, no. 1 (2009): 7; J. L. Frestedt et al., "A Natural Mineral Supplement Provides Relief from Knee Osteoarthritis Symptoms: A Randomized Controlled Pilot Trial," *Nutrition Journal* 7, no. 9 (2008); D. M. O'Gorman et al., "The Marine-Derived, Multi-Mineral Formula, Aquamin, Enhances Mineralisation of Osteoblast Cells in Vitro," *Phytotherapy Research* 26, no. 3 (2012): 375–80; M. N. Aslam et al., "A Mineral-Rich Extract from the Red Marine Algae Lithothamnion Calcareum Preserves Bone Structure and Function in Female Mice on a Western-Style Diet," *Calcified Tissue International* 86, no. 4 (2010): 313–24; B. D. Nielsen et al., "A Marine Mineral Supplement Alters Markers of Bone Metabolism in Yearling Arabians," *Journal of Equine Veterinary Science* 30, no. 8 (2010): 419–24; H. G. Lee et al., "The Effects of a Mineral Supplement (Aquamin F®) and Its Combination with Multi-Species Lactic Acid Bacteria (LAB) on Bone Accretion in an Ovariectomized Rat Model," *J. Exp. Biomed. Sci.* 16, no. 4 (2010): 213–20.

dietary fats. *See* fats and oils
dips. *See* dressings, dips, spreads
DNA
   chromosomes and telomeres, 155–56
   damage from superoxide, 160
   methylation, 53, 59–60, 83
   transcription errors, 80–81, 82–83,
     155–56
dressings, dips, spreads
   Aloe Dressing, 285
   Avocado and Cheese Spread, 285
   Balsamic Vinaigrette, 284
   Classic Vinaigrette, 285
   Creamy Honey Mustard Dressing, 283
   Garlic Cheese Spread, 286
   Ginger Vinaigrette, 284
   Horseradish Dressing, 283
   Mediterranean Vegetarian Spread, 286
   Pesto Sauce, 282
   Three Cs Dip, 287
   Vegetarian Spread, 287
drinks. *See* alcoholic drinks; coffee and
   green coffee bean extract; juices and
   smoothies; tea
drug-induced nutritional deficiencies,
   185–88

Easy Salmon Pesto Pasta, 281
Eggless Cinnamon French Toast, 238
Eggplant and Lentil Stew, 278
Eggplant and Onion, Stir-Fried Chicken
   with, 274–75
eggs
   Chinese Egg Drop Soup, 252
   Cobb Salad, 244
   Egg Salad Sandwich, 256–57
   free-range chicken eggs, 104
   Veggie Frittata, 240–41
Endive Nut Salad, Flounder and, 262–63
estrogens, 90–91, 103
exercise
   amount and types, 26, 199
   anti-inflammatory benefit, 135, 162
   to build muscle mass, 37, 39, 135, 199
   foods and supplements to maximize
     benefits, 199–201
   in healthy living, 41–42, 136
   increase in rate of blood flow, 54–55

   lack of, as carcinogen, 82
   morning routine, 42
   weight management, 41–43
Exotic Banana Pancakes, 236

fads and faux foods, 12–14
fat. *See* obesity and weight management
fatigue, 206–7, 291
fats and oils
   for cooking, 61, 127, 195, 215
   olive oil, 56, 97, 167, 212
   omega-3 fatty acids, 57–58, 97, 98–99,
     195, 196, 197, 291
   in Rule of One-Thirds, 6–8
   shopping guidelines, 212
   trans fats, 7, 57
   types, sources, and effects, 6–7, 57
fenugreek, 106, 144
fermented foods, 64, 151–52
Fettuccine Alfredo, 280
fish. *See also list of recipes on page 296*
   omega-3 and omega-6 fats, 196–97
   toxins, 99
fish oil supplements, 57, 97, 99
flavonoids, 67–69
Flounder, Broiled, with Sautéed Red
   Pepper and Quinoa, 258–59
Flounder and Endive Nut Salad, 262–63
food and chemical sensitivities, 203–5, 291
free radicals, 16, 130–32, 156–58, 162
French Toast, Eggless Cinnamon, 238
Fresh Asparagus Soup, 252
Fresh Pea Soup, 248
Frittata, Veggie, 240–41
fruits and vegetables. *See also* juices and
   smoothies; *specific types*
   anticancer choices, 109–14
   daily servings, 191
   grocery staples, 212–13
   juicing, 74, 307
   organically grown, 110, 212
   top ten ecogenetic, 192
   total antioxidant capacity, 70
Fruit Smoothie, 228

garlic, 41, 111, 144 (*See also list of recipes
   on pages 297–98*)
Garlic Cheese Spread, 286